DIFFERENTIAL DIAGNOSIS OF COMMON COMPLAINTS

ROBERT H. SELLER, M.D.

Professor of Medicine and Professor of Family Medicine
Medical School of the State University of New York
Buffalo, New York

1986

W. B. SAUNDERS COMPANY

Philadelphia   London   Toronto   Mexico City   Rio de Janeiro   Sydney   Tokyo   Hong Kong

W. B. Saunders Company: West Washington Square
Philadelphia, PA 19105

Library of Congress Cataloging in Publication Data

Seller, Robert H., 1931–

Differential diagnosis of common complaints.

1. Diagnosis, Differential.   I. Title.
   [DNLM: 1. Diagnosis, Differential. WB 141.5 S467d]

RC71.5.S45 1986   616.07′5   85–8377

ISBN 0–7216–1648–8

Differential Diagnosis of Common Complaints   ISBN   0-7216-1648-8

Last digit is the print number: 9   8   7   6   5   4   3   2   1

This book is dedicated to

My father, David S. Seller, M.D., a superb family physician who showed me the joy of practicing medicine;

My professor, Peter Kuo, M.D., who introduced me to the fun of research and teaching;

My chief, Samuel Bellet, M.D., who encouraged me to do research; and

My friend and former chairman John H. Moyer III, M.D., who gave me the opportunity to develop as a clinician and academician.

ACKNOWLEDGMENTS

My special thanks go to Mrs. Joyce Vana, who assisted me extensively in assembling the material for this book, and to Donnica Moore, who assisted in the final editing of the manuscript. Martha E. Manning, Senior Reference Librarian, provided invaluable assistance in the literature reviews. Patti Villepigue typed, and to accommodate my revisions, retyped each chapter more times than either of us wish to remember. Finally, I wish to thank my faculty colleagues of the Medical School of the State University of New York at Buffalo who reviewed each of the chapters.

PREFACE

The purpose of this text is to help physicians accurately diagnose the most common complaints. Most medical school curricula, texts, and continuing education courses deal with diseases. Patients, however, usually come to their physicians complaining of headache, backache, or fatigue—not migraine, spinal stenosis or depression. To address this reality this book is organized around common presenting complaints, the patients' symptoms rather than their diseases. The 31 symptoms reviewed account for more than 70 per cent of the chief complaints with which physicians are confronted. The physician who has mastered the differential diagnosis of these symptoms will be able to accurately diagnose nearly all the problems seen in a typical medical practice.

Each chapter deals with a different common complaint. The chapters are organized to approximate the problem solving process that most physicians use to make a diagnosis. Initially, the presenting symptom suggests several diagnostic possibilities. Then this diagnostic list is further defined and reduced by additional, more specific, historical findings; by the patient's physical findings; and then by the results of diagnostic studies. The index lists all complaints, symptoms, and diagnoses mentioned in the text.

Each chapter is divided into the following sections:

Introduction. Includes relevant definitions as well as a list of the most common causes of the symptom.

Nature of the patient. Identifies those conditions which are most prevalent within a particular patient subgroup (children, elderly, premenopausal, diabetic, hypertensive, immunocompromised, etc.).

Nature of symptom. Further identifies conditions by amplifying additional characteristics of the symptoms (how, when, where, radiation, acute/chronic, etc.).

Associated symptoms

Precipitating and aggravating factors

Ameliorating factors

Physical findings

Diagnostic studies

Less common diagnostic considerations

Selected references. Most articles represent an approach to differential diagnosis of problems rather than a review of a specific disease.

A concise summary table is located at the end of each chapter. These tables summarize the salient differential diagnostic features of each of the most common clinical entities that cause a particular complaint.

The text does not deal extensively with pathophysiology or therapy except in situations where this information is particularly useful in the diagnostic process. The most useful diagnostic studies for differential diagnosis are reviewed. The text concentrates on the most likely diagnoses and common illnesses which include many serious illnesses. It also notes when there is a need to rule out grave diagnostic possibilities.

Clinicians and students may use this book for general information about the many causes of common chief complaints. They can also use it as a reference text when presented with a patient who has a specific symptom (such as facial pain, shortness of breath or fever) when the diagnosis is not apparent.

"Differential Diagnosis of Common Complaints" was written to be useful. I hope you find it so . . . Remember the adage "If you don't think about it—you will never diagnose it."

CONTENTS

1

ABDOMINAL PAIN IN ADULTS

The most common causes of abdominal pain are discussed here, with special attention given to the acute abdomen and recurrent abdominal pain. The term *acute abdomen* is medical jargon that refers to any acute condition within the abdomen that requires immediate surgical attention. It must be noted that acute abdominal pain may be of non-abdominal origin and does not always need surgery. The majority of patients who consult a physician for abdominal pain do not have an acute abdomen, although their chief complaint may be a sudden or acute onset of abdominal pain. In studies involving analysis of large series of patients presenting to emergency rooms with acute abdominal pain, NSAP (nonspecific abdominal pain) was the most common diagnosis. Most patients with this symptom probably have gastroenteritis.

The common causes of abdominal pain include *gastroenteritis, gastritis, peptic ulcer disease, reflux esophagitis, irritable bowel syndrome, dysmenorrhea, salpingitis, appendicitis, cholecystitis, cholelithiasis, intestinal obstruction, mesenteric adenitis, diverticulitis, pancreatitis, ureterolithiasis, incarcerated hernias, gas entrapment syndromes,* and *ischemic bowel disease* (particularly in the elderly). All the aforementioned conditions can present with an acute or sudden onset of abdominal pain, many can cause recurrent abdominal pain, and a few require surgical intervention. Any acute abdominal condition requires the physician to make an early, precise diagnosis, since in many instances prognosis depends on prompt initiation of therapy (particularly surgical therapy).

The more serious the problem, the more urgent the need for an accurate diagnosis.

The examiner can best establish a complete and accurate diagnosis by noting carefully age and sex, past medical history, precipitating factors, location of the pain itself and of radiated discomfort, associated vomiting, altered bowel habits, chills and fever, and findings yielded on physical examination, particularly of the abdomen. **Abdominal pain without other symptoms or signs is rarely a serious problem.**

The physician must be particularly aware of the conditions that cause abdominal pain and that usually require surgical intervention. According to one large study, the most common conditions requiring surgical intervention are *appendicitis, cholecystitis,* and *perforated peptic ulcer.* Others include *acute intestinal obstruction, torsion of a viscus or ovary, perforation of a viscus, tumors, ectopic pregnancy, dissecting* and *ruptured aneurysms, mesenteric occlusion,* and *embolizations* and *infarctions of the bowel.*

Several authors warn against the practice of "pattern matching" in the diagnosis of acute abdominal surgical conditions; they have found that typical findings occur in only 60 to 70 per cent of patients. This means that if physicians attempt to match acute problems with patterns or stereotypes of the disease, they will fail to make the correct diagnosis in 30 to 40 per cent of cases. Therefore, to improve diagnostic accuracy, physicians must know the standard and typical presentations and must also be aware of the subtleties involved in the differential diagnosis. The "best test" method is more accurate than "pattern matching" in establishing the diagnosis.

The "best test" method involves elicitation of specific information that correlates well with the correct diagnosis. This method suggests that when a specific symptom or physical sign is noted, its presence is highly useful in establishing the correct diagnosis. For instance, the finding of pain in the right upper quadrant most frequently suggests *cholecystitis.* Likewise, if pain is aggravated by movement it most frequently indicates *appendicitis* but also suggests *perforated peptic ulcer* to a lesser degree. A "best test" question used to differentiate the most common causes of abdominal pain—nonspecific abdominal pain (NSAP) and appendicitis—is whether the pain is aggravated by coughing or movement. The pain of appendicitis is aggravated by movement or coughing, whereas the pain of NSAP is not. Abdominal pain that is aggravated by movement or coughing is probably due to peritoneal inflammation. "Best test" signs that are helpful in differential diagnosis include the presence of a *palpable mass* in diverticular disease, *hyperactive bowel sounds* in small bowel obstruction, *reduced bowel sounds* in perforation, and *involuntary guarding* in the right lower quadrant with appendicitis. The validity of "best test" findings has been supported by retrospective studies in which the diagnosis is known.

NATURE OF PATIENT

In elderly patients, it is often difficult for the physician to elicit an accurate description of the nature of the pain. These patients may be unable to distinguish new symptoms from pre-existing complaints. They often present late in their illnesses, often after treating themselves for indigestion or constipation. In contrast to the high frequency of appendicitis, cholecystitis, and perforated ulcers in most general surgical series, the most frequent causes of acute surgical abdomen in patients over 70 years of age are *strangulated hernias* (45 per cent) and other forms of *intestinal obstruction* (25 per cent).

It must be remembered that cancer is a common cause of abdominal pain in the elderly. In a study of patients over the age of 50 years presenting with nonspecific abdominal pain, 10 per cent had cancer. The majority of these patients with cancer had large bowel cancer. *Colonic cancer* is almost as common as perforated peptic ulcer, pancreatitis, and renal colic in patients over the age of 50 years. Cancer should be strongly suspected if the patient is older than 50 years and has had previous bouts of unexplained abdominal pain, if the present abdominal pain has lasted at least 4 days, and if constipation is present.

Elderly patients also have a higher frequency of uncommon causes of surgical abdomen, including *ruptured aortic aneurysm, acute mesenteric infarction,* and *inflammatory diverticular disease.*

The age of the individual also offers clues to diagnosis in other groups of patients. *Appendicitis* has its peak incidence in the second decade, although it can occur in patients older than 60 years as well as in infants. The incidence of *cholecystitis* increases with age.

Cholecystitis is more common in whites than in blacks, more prevalent in females than in males, and more common in women taking birth control pills or estrogens than in those who are not. Drugs that increase cholesterol saturation also increase the incidence of *cholelithiasis.* They include clofibrate (Atromid), conjugated estrogens, and estrogen-progesterone combinations.

Nonspecific abdominal pain (NSAP) is an imprecise diagnosis, yet it is the most common diagnosis given to patients presenting to an emergency room with abdominal pain as their chief complaint. This diagnosis is most common in patients under the age of 40 years.

Irritable colon seems to be most common in young women, particularly those who have young children. This frequency has been attributed to the life pressures to which these women are subjected. Symptoms of irritable colon are also more frequent in others under stress, including children. The abdominal pain from an irritable colon may be a vague discomfort or pain in the left lower quadrant, right lower quadrant, or midabdomen. It occasionally radiates to the back. This pain may be relieved by defecation and may be associated with other well-recognized symptoms of irritable colon—mucus in the stool, constipation alternating with diarrhea, and small marble-like stools.

Peptic ulcer pain is most common between ages 30 and 50 years but may occur in teenagers and, rarely, in young children. It is considerably more common in men than in women. This diagnosis should not be entirely disregarded in women, however, because there is a significant incidence of perforated peptic ulcer among them that may be a result of the physician's failure to consider peptic ulcer in the diagnosis. Although only 15 per cent of patients with ulcer symptoms are older than 60 years, 80 per cent of deaths due to ulcers occur in this group since ulcer disease in the elderly is more likely to run a virulent course.

Acute intestinal obstruction occurs in all age groups. In the elderly, intestinal obstruction is usually caused by *strangulated hernias* or *malignancies*. However, in any patient who presents with severe abdominal pain and has a history of prior abdominal surgery, adhesions are the most likely cause of intestinal obstruction.

Pancreatitis occurs most frequently in alcoholics and in patients with gallstones. *Sigmoid volvulus* is more common in males, the mentally retarded, and those with Parkinsonism; *cecal volvulus* is more common in females. *Gallstone ileus* causes small bowel obstruction more often in the elderly and in women. *Mesenteric adenitis* is more common in children. *Peptic esophagitis* is more common in obese patients. The incidence of *diverticulitis* increases with age and is more common after age 60 years.

NATURE OF PAIN

Colicky or crampy pain beginning in the midabdomen that progresses to a constant pain in the right lower quadrant suggests *appendicitis*. Other conditions that may begin in a crampy or colicky fashion and progress to a more constant pain include *cholelithiasis* and *cholecystitis* (which tend to localize in the right upper quadrant), *intestinal obstruction,* and *ureterolithiasis*. This last condition involves excruciating pain that frequently radiates to the groin, testes, or medial thigh.

A constant, often annoying burning or gnawing pain that is located in the midepigastrium and is occasionally associated with posterior radiation is seen with *peptic ulcer*. Peptic ulcer pain may be worse at night, although this is unusual. It is not ordinarily made worse by recumbency. The pain of peptic ulcer in the elderly may be vague and poorly localized. Because of a lack of classic symptoms, an occasional absence of prior symptoms, and a confusing picture of abdominal pain, perforation associated with peritonitis occurs more frequently in the elderly. It is particularly important to note that pain induced by percussion in the epigastrium may be the only physical finding suggesting ulcer disease in a person complaining of typical peptic ulcer pain.

Likewise, severe exacerbation of pain that occurs when the physician percusses over the right upper quadrant strongly suggests the presence of an *inflamed gallbladder.*

The diagnosis of abdominal pain due to an *irritable colon* is fairly easy to make: the pain is usually dull, crampy, and recurrent. It is often assocated with constipation that alternates with diarrhea, small stools, and mucus in the stools. In addition, moderate pain may be elicited when the physician palpates the colon. In the elderly, however, severe diverticulitis may exist with similar symptoms.

Most abdominal pain, even when severe, usually develops over several hours. When the onset of severe abdominal pain is abrupt, it suggests *perforation, strangulation, torsion, dissecting aneurysms,* or *ureterolithiasis.* The most severe abdominal pain occurs with dissecting aneurysms and with ureterolithiasis. The pain of a dissecting aneurysm is often described as a "tearing" or "ripping" sensation and often radiates into the legs and through to the back. Patients with such pain usually present in profound shock. Individuals with the excruciating pain of ureterolithiasis may be writhing in agony but do not experience cardio-vascular collapse. This pain is usually unilateral in the flank, groin, or testicle and is often associated with nausea and occasional vomiting.

LOCATION OF PAIN

The location of the pain is one of the "best tests" for determination of a diagnosis (Fig. 1–1). Right upper quadrant pain is most frequently seen in *cholecystitis, cholelithiasis,* and leaking *duodenal ulcer* (Fig. 1–2). Another clue to gallbladder disease is the radiation of right upper quadrant pain to the inferior angle of the right scapula. Right upper quadrant pain is also seen in patients with *hepatitis* or *congestive heart failure.* In the latter group, the pain is thought to be due to swelling of the liver that results in distention of Glissons's capsule. Less severe right upper quadrant pain may be seen in patients with a *hepatic flexure syndrome* (gas entrapment in the hepatic flexure of the colon). If questioned carefully, these patients will admit to experiencing relief with the passage of flatus.

A gnawing, burning, mid to upper abdominal pain suggests a condition with a peptic etiology—*ulcer, gastritis,* or *esophagitis.* Burning epigastric pain that radiates to the jaw is frequently seen in patients with peptic esophagitis.

Left upper quadrant pain is most frequently seen in patients with *gastroenteritis* or *irritable colon* and less commonly in those with splenic flexure syndrome, splenic infarction, or pancreatitis. The pain from a splenic flexure syndrome can be located in the left upper quadrant or in the chest; therefore, it is also part of the differential diagnosis of chest pain. These pains tend to arise when the individual is bending over or

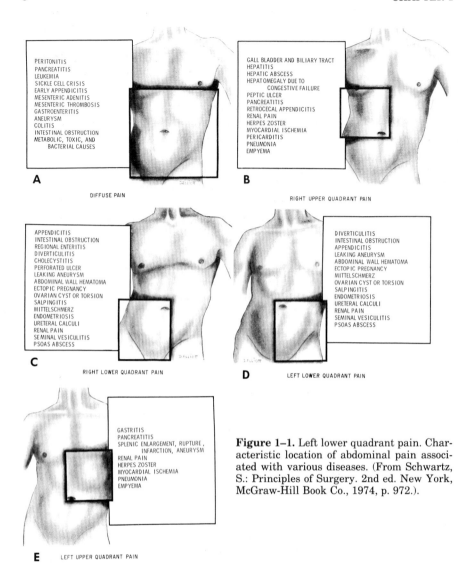

A — DIFFUSE PAIN

PERITONITIS
PANCREATITIS
LEUKEMIA
SICKLE CELL CRISIS
EARLY APPENDICITIS
MESENTERIC ADENITIS
MESENTERIC THROMBOSIS
GASTROENTERITIS
ANEURYSM
COLITIS
INTESTINAL OBSTRUCTION
METABOLIC, TOXIC, AND
    BACTERIAL CAUSES

B — RIGHT UPPER QUADRANT PAIN

GALL BLADDER AND BILIARY TRACT
HEPATITIS
HEPATIC ABSCESS
HEPATOMEGALY DUE TO
    CONGESTIVE FAILURE
PEPTIC ULCER
PANCREATITIS
RETROCECAL APPENDICITIS
RENAL PAIN
HERPES ZOSTER
MYOCARDIAL ISCHEMIA
PERICARDITIS
PNEUMONIA
EMPYEMA

C — RIGHT LOWER QUADRANT PAIN

APPENDICITIS
INTESTINAL OBSTRUCTION
REGIONAL ENTERITIS
DIVERTICULITIS
CHOLECYSTITIS
PERFORATED ULCER
LEAKING ANEURYSM
ABDOMINAL WALL HEMATOMA
ECTOPIC PREGNANCY
OVARIAN CYST OR TORSION
SALPINGITIS
MITTELSCHMERZ
ENDOMETRIOSIS
URETERAL CALCULI
RENAL PAIN
SEMINAL VESICULITIS
PSOAS ABSCESS

D — LEFT LOWER QUADRANT PAIN

DIVERTICULITIS
INTESTINAL OBSTRUCTION
APPENDICITIS
LEAKING ANEURYSM
ABDOMINAL WALL HEMATOMA
ECTOPIC PREGNANCY
MITTELSCHMERZ
OVARIAN CYST OR TORSION
SALPINGITIS
ENDOMETRIOSIS
URETERAL CALCULI
RENAL PAIN
SEMINAL VESICULITIS
PSOAS ABSCESS

E — LEFT UPPER QUADRANT PAIN

GASTRITIS
PANCREATITIS
SPLENIC ENLARGEMENT, RUPTURE,
    INFARCTION, ANEURYSM
RENAL PAIN
HERPES ZOSTER
MYOCARDIAL ISCHEMIA
PNEUMONIA
EMPYEMA

Figure 1–1. Left lower quadrant pain. Characteristic location of abdominal pain associated with various diseases. (From Schwartz, S.: Principles of Surgery. 2nd ed. New York, McGraw-Hill Book Co., 1974, p. 972.).

wearing a tight garment, and they frequently are relieved by the passage of flatus.

Other causes of both right and left upper quadrant pain include supradiaphragmatic conditions with inflammation of the diaphragm, such as pneumonia, pulmonary embolism, pleurisy, and pericarditis.

Right lower quadrant pain is most commonly seen with *muscle strain, appendicitis, salpingitis,* and *diverticulitis* (Fig. 1–3). Diverticulitis pain is more common in the left lower quadrant, however. Less common causes of right lower quadrant pain include ileitis, pyelone-

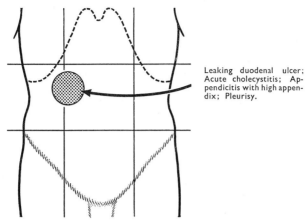

Leaking duodenal ulcer; Acute cholecystitis; Appendicitis with high appendix; Pleurisy.

Tenderness and rigidity in right hypochondrium.

Figure 1–2. Leaking duodenal ulcer; acute cholecystitis; appendicitis with high appendix; pleurisy. (From Cope, Z.: Early Diagnosis of Acute Abdomen. 13th ed. London, Oxford University Press, 1968, p. 43.)

phritis, obturator hernias, carcinoma of the cecum, and colonic obstruction in patients with a competent ileocecal valve.

Other causes of right or left lower quadrant pain include ureterolithiasis, salpingitis, ruptured ovarian cyst, ovarian torsion, ectopic pregnancy, and obturator hernia. The pain of salpingitis usually is unilateral, although it may present bilaterally.

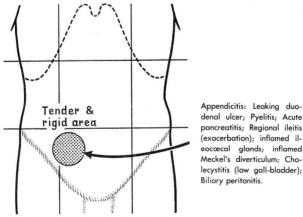

Tender & rigid area

Appendicitis: Leaking duodenal ulcer; Pyelitis; Acute pancreatitis; Regional ileitis (exacerbation); inflamed ileocœcal glands; inflamed Meckel's diverticulum; Cholecystitis (low gall-bladder); Biliary peritonitis.

Tenderness and rigidity in right iliac region.

Figure 1–3. Appendicitis; leaking duodenal ulcer; pyelitis; acute pancreatitis; regional ileitis (exacerbation); inflamed ileocœcal glands; inflamed Meckel's diverticulum; cholecystitis (low gallbladder); biliary peritonitis. (From Cope, Z.: Early Diagnosis of Acute Abdomen. 13th ed. London, Oxford University Press, 1968, p. 45.)

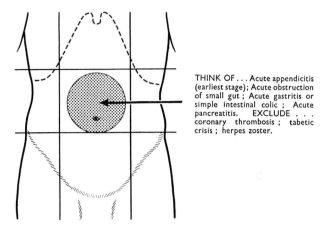

THINK OF . . . Acute appendicitis (earliest stage); Acute obstruction of small gut ; Acute gastritis or simple intestinal colic ; Acute pancreatitis. EXCLUDE . . . coronary thrombosis ; tabetic crisis ; herpes zoster.

Acute central abdominal pain without any other symptom.

Figure 1–4. *Think of* acute appendicitis (earliest stage); acute obstruction of small gut; acute gastritis or simple intestinal colic; acute pancreatitis. *Exclude* coronary thrombosis; tabetic crisis; herpes zoster. (From Cope, Z.: Early Diagnosis of Acute Abdomen. 13th ed. London, Oxford University Press, 1968, p. 38.)

Left lower quadrant pain suggests *irritable colon* and *diverticulitis.*

Common causes of central abdominal pain include early *appendicitis, small bowel obstruction, gastritis,* and *colic* (Fig. 1–4).

PRECIPITATING OR AGGRAVATING FACTORS

The pain of *appendicitis* is aggravated by motion or coughing, as is the pain of *peritonitis,* regardless of its cause. The pain of *gastritis* is worsened by most foods, particularly alcoholic beverages. *Peptic ulcer* pain usually begins an hour or so after eating and is generally relieved by eating. If epigastric pain occurs primarily or is worsened in the recumbent position, *peptic esophagitis* should be suspected. The pain of *salpingitis* and *endometriosis* is often worse during or before menstruation. Although patients may find that this pain is not exacerbated by limited movement in bed, more strenuous activity such as descending a flight of stairs frequently will increase the severity of the discomfort. The symptoms of nonspecific abdominal pain are precipitated and exacerbated by problems in the individual's environment. They may also be part of a long-term psychiatric illness.

AMELIORATING FACTORS

If the patient experiences relief after eating or taking antacids, *peptic ulcer* or *peptic esophagitis* is the probable cause of pain. The pain of *gastritis,* although worsened by ingestion of food and alcoholic beverages, may be relieved by antacids. The pain of peptic esophagitis is often lessened when the patient is in an upright posture.

Pain relieved by defecation or the passage of flatus suggests an *irritable colon* or *gas entrapment* in the large bowel, whereas pain relieved by belching suggests *gaseous distention* of the stomach or esophagus. The pain of *gastroenteritis* is occasionally relieved by vomiting or diarrhea.

ASSOCIATED SYMPTOMS

The abdominal pain seen with a truly *acute abdomen* is usually of such severity that patients overlook any associated symptoms they might have. Thus, it can be said that any additional complaint (e.g., headache) contradicts the dignosis of acute abdomen.

The timing of vomiting in relation to the onset of abdominal pain and associated symptoms may help the physician establish a precise diagnosis. The earlier the vomiting occurs in relation to the onset of abdominal pain, the less the abdominal distention. In lower intestinal obstruction, there is less vomiting and greater distention. Vomiting that precedes the onset of pain reduces the probability of an acute abdomen. Vomiting that begins after the onset of pain is more consistent with the diagnosis of an acute abdomen and frequently is seen in patients with *appendicitis.* The absence of vomiting does not preclude the diagnosis of an acute abdomen.

If vomiting occurs soon after the onset of pain and the vomitus is light in color, the vomitus probably consists of digestive juices and bile; this suggests *gastritis, cholecystitis,* or *obstruction.*

Jaundice, dark urine, and light to acholic stools may be seen in patients with abdominal pain due to *cholecystitis.* These symptoms suggest an obstructive etiology of the jaundice, and complete biliary obstruction should be suspected. **A history of occasional silver-colored stools alternating with normal or light colored stools is virtually pathognomonic of *carcinoma of the ampulla of Vater.*** The production of silver-colored stools is a result of upper gastrointestinal blood from the ampullary carcinoma mixing with acholic stools.

Examination of vomitus from patients with acute abdominal obstruction may provide a clue to the location of the obstruction. Undigested food in the vomitus suggests that the obstruction is proximal to the stomach; this may be due to *achalasia* or *peptic esophagitis.* Occasionally, undigested food may be seen in vomitus from patients with *pyloric obstruction.* This diagnosis is most likely if the vomiting persists and does not contain bile.

Brown vomitus with a fecal odor suggests mechanical or paralytic *bowel obstruction.* The more proximal the obstruction, the more frequent the vomiting.

Constipation with small, dry stools—sometimes alternating with diarrhea or mucus in the stool—is frequently seen in patients experiencing increasing stress and suggests an *irritable colon*.

PHYSICAL FINDINGS

Physical examination of the abdomen in patients presenting with abdominal pain should include inspection, auscultation, palpation, and percussion as well as rectal and pelvic examinations. The physical examination should begin with inspection of the abdomen, with the physician standing at the foot of the patient's bed. This part of the examination often can provide major clues to the diagnosis, as it allows one to note any distention, abnormal pulsations, and abdominal movement with respiration. The second part of the examination should always consist of auscultation; it is preferable for the physician to listen to bowel sounds before beginning a manual investigation. When palpating the abdomen and vaginal area, the physician should be particularly attentive to any lymph node enlargements or hernias and to the quality of femoral pulses.

Specific physical findings in appendicitis, cholecystitis, diverticulitis, and bowel perforation or infarction vary with the disease. If peritonitis is present, however, certain physical findings are common, regardless of disease. The pain of peritonitis is severe, generalized, continuous, and of acute or gradual onset. There is usually abdominal tenderness with guarding, stabbing pain with gentle coughing, and pain to percussion. Abdominal rigidity occasionally is present. There is decreased movement of the abdominal wall with respiration. If rebound pain is present, it usually is found over the area of primary disease. Patients with peritonitis often are in shock, have fever or chills, and present with decreased or absent bowel sounds. The patient usually lies relatively motionless, as movement aggravates the pain. Depending on the severity of the peritonitis and the prior cardiovascular status of the patient, hypotension, tachycardia, pallor, and sweating may also be present. Younger, healthier patients are relatively resistant to hypotension but develop tachycardia easily. In contrast, elderly patients with a decreased cardiovascular reserve become hypotensive more readily. The presence of cardiac disease may impair the development of tachycardia.

Appendicitis. In acute appendicitis there almost always is tenderness over the inflamed appendix. There often is involuntary guarding as well as rebound tenderness over McBurney's point. Classically, there is a disproportionate rise in the pulse rate with respect to the degree of fever.

Cholecystitis. Guarding in the right upper quadrant and tenderness to palpation and percussion suggest cholecystitis. When gallbladder disease is suspected in patients with right upper quadrant pain, the examiner should begin palpation very gently in other parts of the abdomen and end gently over the gallbladder. The goal of this careful palpation is detection of an enlarged (hydrops) gallbladder. An enlarged gallbladder may not be detected by deep palpation or percussion, as such aggressive examination may result in involuntary guarding, which prevents detection of the enlarged gallbladder. In all patients with abdominal pain, the physician should begin palpation away from the painful area and gradually move towards palpation over the most painful spot.

Peptic Ulcer. In patients with symptoms of peptic ulcer disease, there may be no abnormal physical findings except pain to gentle percussion over the midepigastrium or duodenal sweep. When peritonitis develops in patients with peptic ulcer disease, it is secondary to perforation of the involved viscus. If the viscus perforates anteriorly, extreme rigidity of the abdominal wall results. If the viscus penetrates posteriorly, back pain is a major symptom, and the symptoms of peritonitis are minimal. In the early stages of a penetrating or perforated peptic ulcer, bowel sounds may be increased or normal, but as the condition progresses, bowel sounds generally become diminished or absent.

Intestinal Obstruction. Auscultation of the abdomen may help the physician diagnose obstruction. Classically, rushes of high-pitched, tinkling peristalsis are heard. These often are associated with recurring crampy, colicky pain. The physician must listen for a succussion splash in all patients complaining of vomiting. This examination requires the examiner to place the stethoscope over the stomach and to shake the abdomen gently. A succussion splash may be heard over a stomach that is dilated or distended with air and fluid. This finding is normal in infants and in adults immediately after eating. By 30 minutes after eating, however, the sound should not be heard unless there is an obstruction with an air fluid level. Impaired gastric emptying occurs most commonly in patients with *pyloric obstruction* (congenital or acquired); it also occurs in patients with gastric tumors or gastric atony. Atonic gastric dilatation is most commonly seen in postoperative patients and in patients who have severe hyperkalemia or diabetic ketoacidosis.

There is a classic triad of physical findings in patients with acute intestinal obstruction: (1) sudden onset of colicky abdominal pain, (2) vomiting, and (3) obstipation. Bowel sounds are generally hyperactive and high-pitched and occur in rushes; if perforation or peritonitis occurs, the bowel sounds become reduced. When the obstruction is in the large intestine, there may be abdominal distention and general or local distention of the intestine. With *volvulus* there may be gross distention of the entire abdomen; this occurs early in the disease.

Salpingitis. The physical findings of salpingitis include unilateral or bilateral tenderness to palpation in the lower abdomen and increased bowel sounds. Involuntary guarding and rigidity are rare findings. Pelvic examination often elicits pain, particularly with lateral movement of the cervix and adnexal palpation. There is frequently a purulent cervical discharge.

Irritable Colon. Although most patients with an irritable colon have no significant physical findings (the diagnosis is made by careful history), a tender ascending or descending colon occasionally may be palpable.

Acute Diverticulitis. The classic triad for acute diverticulitis is (1) abdominal tenderness, (2) a palpable mass in the left lower quadrant, and (3) fever. The mass or tenderness occasionally may be detected only by rectal examination. Diarrhea and rectal bleeding are uncommon, and bowel sounds are usually decreased.

Ureterolithiasis. Tenderness to percussion in the costovertebral angle and ileus may be the only physical finding in patients with ureterolithiasis. This diagnosis usually is confirmed by the presence of hematuria.

DIAGNOSTIC STUDIES

Although plain or flat abdominal radiographs frequently are ordered in patients with acute abdominal pain, they are diagnostic in less than 50 per cent of cases. If an acute surgical abdomen is suspected and the diagnosis is unknown or dubious, the physician should obtain an electrocardiogram as well as chest and abdominal radiographs and should perform studies of blood count with differential, electrolytes, urea nitrogen, serum amylase (if pancreatitis is suspected), urine, and stool.

Rarely, laparotomy is necesary in patients with recurrent abdominal pain if the diagnosis is not apparent. In one series of 27 laparotomies for unexplained abdominal pain, carcinoma was found in 50 per cent of patients. In patients over 50 years of age presenting with *recurrent nonspecific acute abdominal pain,* the following lab tests should be done to detect cancer: (1) examination of stools for occult blood (this test should be done in all patients over 50 years regardless of the presence of abdominal pain); (2) sigmoidoscopy and, if necessary, colonoscopy; and (3) barium enema.

Specific laboratory tests should be ordered when certain diagnoses are suspected: *appendicitis*—CBC with differential; *cholecystitis*—CBC with differential; isotopic and ultrasonographic scanning; *peptic ulcer*—upper GI radiographs; *perforated peptic ulcer*—radiographs to reveal free air; *acute intestinal obstruction*—abdominal radiographs; *ureterolithiasis*—intravenous pyelogram; microscopic urinalysis; *pancreatitis*—serum amylase. Abdominal computerized axial tomography (CT scans) and abdominal ultrasonography are often helpful, especially when gallbladder, pancreatic, or pelvic disease is suspected.

LESS COMMON DIAGNOSTIC CONSIDERATIONS

Abdominal pain may be due to pneumonia, particularly of a lower lobe. Abdominal pain and vomiting may be the presenting symptoms in diabetes. Right upper quadrant pain can be due to congestive heart failure resulting from stretching of Glisson's capsule. Right upper quadrant pain, jaundice, and anorexia may be the presenting symptoms of hepatitis.

Amebiasis can mimic appendicitis or diverticulitis or both. Abdominal or flank pain or both, when associated with nausea and vomiting, may be the presenting symptoms of a hydronephrosis.

An acute abdomen in a young black patient classically suggests the possiblity of sickle cell crisis. Severe abdominal wall tenderness can result from a spider bite. Rarely, diffuse abdominal pain can be secondary to marked gaseous distention.

Severe pain in the back or flank or vague, poorly localized abdominal pain may be the first presenting symptom in patients with carcinoma of the pancreas. If abdominal pain is associated with thrombophlebitis (in the absence of trauma), migratory thrombophlebitis, or the development of diabetes, carcinoma of the pancreas should be suspected. Carcinoma of the head of the pancreas usually presents with jaundice or abdominal pain early in the course of the illness.

Abdominal pain that may be associated with vomiting and that occurs in the middle of the menstrual cycle is called "mittelschmerz." It represents pain associated with physiologic rupture of an ovarian follicle.

If a child or woman of childbearing age suddenly develops severe, generalized abdominal pain, often associated with syncope or persistent dizziness, ectopic pregnancy must be considered. This is more common in younger women, in those of low parity, and in those with a history of prior pelvic sepsis or infertility. Physical findings include acute abdominal pain with guarding and rigidity, especially in the lower abdomen. Extreme tenderness to cervical manipulation has been reported in 85 per cent of patients with an ectopic pregnancy. Laparoscopy, HCG, and ultrasonography may help the physician establish the diagnosis.

Vascular causes of abdominal pain include mesenteric thrombosis and acute mesenteric occlusion by embolism or torsion. The latter may have no associated signs or symptoms—only severe abdominal pain with bloody stools occurring later. Aortic aneurysm may cause constant low back pain, which may worsen with recumbency; dissection is characterized by severe, excruciating pain.

DIFFERENTIAL DIAGNOSIS OF ABDOMINAL PAIN IN ADULTS

CAUSE	NATURE OF PATIENT	NATURE OF PAIN	LOCATION OF PAIN	ASSOCIATED SYMPTOMS	PRECIPITATING OR AGGRAVATING FACTORS	AMELIORATING FACTORS	PHYSICAL FINDINGS	DIAGNOSTIC STUDIES
Gastroenteritis	Any age	Crampy	Diffuse	Nausea, vomiting, diarrhea, fever	Food	Occasional relief with vomiting or diarrhea	Hyperactive peristalsis	
Gastritis	Especially alcoholics	Constant, burning	Epigastric	Hemorrhage, nausea, vomiting, diarrhea, fever	Alcohol, salicylates, food (occasionally)			
Appendicitis	Any age: peak age 10–20 yrs; M>F	Colicky, progressing to constant	Early in epigastrium or periumbilicus; RLQ later	Vomiting (after the pain has started), constipation, fever	Pain worse with movement and coughing	Lying still	RLQ involuntary guarding; rebound to RLQ	CBC with differential
Cholecystitis and/or cholelithiasis	Adults; F>M	Colicky, progressing to constant	RUQ radiates to inferior angle of right scapula	Nausea, vomiting, dark urine, light stool, jaundice	Fatty foods, drugs, birth control pill, cholestyramine		Tenderness to palpation or percussion in RUQ	Liver function tests, CBC, amylase, ultrasonography
Diverticulitis	More common in elderly	Intermittent cramping	LLQ	Constipation, diarrhea,			Palpable mass in LLQ	
Pancreatitis	More common in alcoholics and patients with cholelithiasis	Steady, mild to severe	LUQ and epigastric; radiates to back	Nausea, vomiting, prostration, diaphoresis	Lying supine	Leaning forward	Abdominal distention, decreased bowel sounds, diffuse rebound	Amylase, ultrasonography

Condition	Population	Onset/Character	Location	Associated Findings	Aggravating	Relieving	Physical Exam	Diagnostic Tests
Intestinal obstruction	Elderly and those with prior abdominal surgery	Colicky, sudden onset		Vomiting, obstipation			Hyperactive peristalsis in small bowel obstruction	Abdominal radiographs
Intestinal perforation (peritonitis)	F>M; elderly	Sudden onset, severe; Sudden or gradual onset	Diffuse	Guarding, rebound	Pain worse with movement or coughing	Lying still	Decreased bowel sounds, guarding, diffuse rebound	
Salpingitis	Menstruating females	Cramplike	RLQ and/or LLQ, nonradiating	Chandelier tenderness of cervix	Pain worse while descending stairs; worse around time of menstruation		Adnexa and cervix tender to manipulation	Ultrasonography, CT scan, HCG to r/o ectopic pregnancy
Ectopic pregnancy	Fertile female with history of menstrual irregularity	Sudden onset, persistent pain	Lower quadrant	Tender adnexal mass (vaginal bleeding)				HCG
Peptic ulcer (with perforation)	M>F; 30–50 yrs.	Gnawing, burning; Sudden onset	Epigastric radiating to sides, back or right shoulder		Empty stomach, stress, alcohol	Food, alkali	Epigastric tenderness to palpation or percussion	
Mesenteric adenitis	Children and adolescents; after respiratory infection	Constant	RLQ	Vomiting, rebound, constipation, diarrhea, fever				CBC with differential

Table continued on following page

DIFFERENTIAL DIAGNOSIS OF ABDOMINAL PAIN IN ADULTS *Continued*

CAUSE	NATURE OF PATIENT	NATURE OF PAIN	LOCATION OF PAIN	ASSOCIATED SYMPTOMS	PRECIPITATING OR AGGRAVATING FACTORS	AMELIORATING FACTORS	PHYSICAL FINDINGS	DIAGNOSTIC STUDIES
Ureterolithiasis		Colicky, occasionally progresses to constant; severe; sudden onset	Lower abdomen; flank radiating to groin	Nausea, vomiting, abdominal distention, chills, fever			CVA tenderness, hematuria	Urinalysis, IVP
Dissection or rupture of aortic aneurysm	Elderly; hypertensive; 40–70 yrs.	Unbearable, sudden onset	Chest or abdomen; may radiate to back and legs	Shock			Shock, decrease or difference in femoral pulses	
Reflux (peptic) esophagitis		Burning, gnawing	Midepigastrium; occasionally radiating to jaw		Recumbency	Antacids		Upper GI radiographs, endoscopy
Irritable colon	More common in young women	Crampy, recurrent	Most common in LLQ	Mucus in stools		Pain occasionally relieved by defecation	Colon tender to palpation	
Incarcerated hernia	More common in elderly	Constant	RLQ or LLQ		Coughing and straining		Hernia or mass	Upper GI radiographs
Mesenteric infarction	Elderly	May be severe	Diffuse	Tachycardia, hypotension			Decreased bowel sounds, blood in stools	Abdominal radiographs

Selected References

Cope, Z.: The Early Diagnosis of the Acute Abdomen. 13th ed. London, Oxford University Press, 1968.

Crouch, M.: The acute abdomen in women. The Practitioner 222:455–463, 1979.

Dombal, F. T.: Picking the best tests in acute abdominal pain. J. Roy. Coll. Phys. Lond. 13:203–208, 1979.

Rogers, A. I.: The acute abdomen. Comp. Ther. 4:25–33, 1978.

Saegesser, F.: The acute abdomen part 1: differential diagnosis. Clin. Gastroenterol. 10:123–144, 1981.

Standeven, A.: The acute abdomen in the elderly. The Practitioner 222:465–469, 1979.

Staneland, J. R., Ditchbarn, J., and de Dombal, F. T.: Clinical presentation of acute abdomen: study of 600 patients. Br. Med. J. 3:393–398, 1972.

Trnka, Y., and Warfield, C. A.: Chronic abdominal pain. Hosp. Pract. 19:201–209, 1984.

Wichern, W. A.: The surgical abdomen: differential diagnosis. Postgrad. Med. 62:145–148, 1977.

Wilson, D. H.: The acute abdomen in the accident and emergency department. The Practitioner 222:480–485, 1975.

ABDOMINAL PAIN IN CHILDREN

Since chronic abdominal pain is rare in children, the main emphasis of this chapter will be the differential diagnosis of acute and recurrent abdominal pain. Because abdominal pain has many causes, a detailed history and a very careful physical examination are necessary. A small number of selected laboratory studies may also be required. Accurate diagnosis is essential because abdominal pain may be a manifestation of a surgical emergency; these cases must be identified promptly. Whenever there is significant concern about the presence of a surgical condition, the patient should be hospitalized to permit serial abdominal examinations and laboratory studies.

Gastroenteritis is the most common cause of acute abdominal pain in children. *Constipation,* another common cause of abdominal pain, may be acute but is more often recurrent. Other common nonsurgical causes of acute abdominal pain include *mesenteric adenitis, nonspecific abdominal pain, urinary tract infection, sickle cell disease, poisoning,* and *diabetes. Recurrent abdominal pain* is defined as three discrete episodes of abdominal pain occurring over 3 or more months. It is quite common over the age of 5 years and often has a psychosomatic etiology.

The most common surgical causes of acute abdominal pain are *appendicitis, hernia strangulation,* and *intussusception.*

NATURE OF PATIENT

Presentation and causes of abdominal pain vary according to three age groups: (1) children under 5 years, (2) patients between 5 and 12 years, and (3) adolescents. The cause of abdominal pain in very young children is difficult to determine unless signs of abdominal tenderness, guarding, doubling up, or vomiting are present. Physical examination is particularly important in this age group. *Intussusception* is likely when signs of intestinal obstruction are found in infants (peak incidence, 6 months). A lead point such as Meckel's diverticulum is rarely found. *Appendicitis* is uncommon in infants and children up to the age of 5 years. Because appendicitis is rarely considered, the diagnosis is often missed or delayed. Perforation is, therefore, more common, and a disproportionately high percentage of deaths due to appendicitis occur in children under 5 years of age. *Poisonings,* most common in children aged 1 to 4 years, are another frequent cause of abdominal pain.

In children between 5 and 12 years, the major dilemma involves *recurrent abdominal pain,* which can be a symptom of either psychosomatic or organic disease; it is usually due to psychologic factors. Among children with recurrent abdominal pain, there is a high frequency of behavioral and personality disorders. These patients tend to be "high strung" perfectionists and are often apprehensive. In this group, many patients have histories of colic and feeding problems in infancy, and there is a high incidence of stressful family and school situations. Unexplained episodes of recurrent abdominal pain occur in 10 per cent of school-aged children, but an organic cause is found in less than 10 per cent of these cases.

Inflammatory bowel disease frequently begins during adolescence and can be a cause of acute or recurrent abdominal pain. Growth failure in adolescents with abdominal pain is an important clue to this diagnosis, although it may also indicate *gluten-sensitive enteropathy. Sickle cell crises* occur almost exclusively in blacks, although they occur occasionally in people of Mediterranean descent. *Acute appendicitis* is most common in children aged 5 to 15 years, with a peak incidence occurring between 10 and 15 years.

NATURE OF PAIN

The timing of the first occurrence of abdominal pain in children may help to identify *psychologic stress* as the cause. For example, abdominal pain that develops at a time of school problems, birth of a sibling, or family discord suggests a psychologic etiology.

In addition to observing the severity, duration, and location of abdominal pain, the examiner must note whether the onset is gradual or sudden. A gradual onset of cramping pain often suggests an intestinal etiology, whereas a sudden onset of noncramping constant pain suggests torsion of a viscus or perforation. The pain of *appendicitis* classically precedes the development of vomiting and anorexia, begins gradually as a crampy epigastric or periumbilical pain, and progresses to a constant pain in the right lower quadrant. In young children, this pain may be mild or discontinuous or both. Because of atypical presentations and decreased incidence in young children, this diagnosis is often missed. The pain of *mesenteric adenitis* often mimics appendicitis, although a child with the former condition is not quite as sick and is not necessarily anorexic. Mesenteric adenitis usually occurs after a viral or bacterial infection. The associated pain may be colicky in younger children and severe and episodic in older children. **There is tenderness and guarding when the pain is present, and usually no guarding when the pain is absent.** This is in contrast to appendicitis, in which the guarding persists despite the absence of pain.

Cramping, diffuse abdominal pain that follows or coincides with the onset of diarrhea, nausea, or vomiting suggests *gastroenteritis*. Cramping pain occurring primarily after meals is often due to *constipation*. This diagnosis should be accepted only when an enema yields a large amount of feces and relieves pain. Sudden onset of severe, crampy, spasmodic pain that causes an infant to scream and draw up his legs should suggest *intussusception*. This spasmodic pain often recurs at 15- to 30-minute intervals, and the child may be normal, lethargic, or sleeping between attacks.

When abdominal pain is severe and colicky and radiates to the groin or flank, *urolithiasis* should be considered. Hematuria may confirm this diagnosis. Hematuria may also be noted when an inflamed retrocecal appendix overlies the ureter. Abdominal pain associated with tenderness to percussion in the costovertebral angle region may indicate *pyelonephritis*.

The abdominal pain of *diabetic acidosis* is often generalized, and ketosis is usually present. The abdominal pain of a *sickle cell crisis* is severe, and there is usually an associated ileus. This diagnosis should be considered in all black children with severe abdominal pain. Certainly, every black child in whom the diagnosis of appendicitis is considered should have a sickle cell test prior to surgery. When appendicitis is suspected in patients with a positive sickle cell test, an appendectomy should not be performed until there is a clear lack of response to medical therapy for sickle cell crisis or there are progressive manifestations of sepsis.

LOCATION OF PAIN

The pain of *gastroenteritis* is poorly localized, whereas the pain of constipation is usually located in the right lower quadrant. The presumed mechanism of right lower quadrant pain in *constipation* involves gaseous distention of the cecum. **Increasing localized tenderness in the right**

lower quadrant associated with rebound to the right lower quadrant is the single most helpful finding favoring the diagnosis of appendicitis. Subsequent to this localization of pain in the right lower quadrant, paralytic ileus may develop. Classic findings often occur with the appendix in its usual location, but atypical symptomatology may result from an unusually located inflamed appendix. It is critical for the physician to perform a rectal examination because pain in the right upper quadrant may be due to a retrocecal appendicitis.

ASSOCIATED SYMPTOMS

A detailed evaluation of associated symptoms often helps establish the diagnosis. Some generally applicable rules concerning the differential diagnosis of acute abdominal pain are as follows:

1. When significant diarrhea is associated with abdominal pain, a surgical lesion is rare.

2. When abdominal distention—particularly with acidosis—is associated with abdominal pain, a surgical emergency is more likely.

3. When vomiting precedes abdominal pain, an extra-abdominal cause is suggested; when abdominal pain precedes vomiting, an abdominal etiology is likely.

When abdominal pain is diffuse and no localizing physical signs are found, associated diarrhea, nausea, or vomiting suggests *gastroenteritis*. A preceding upper respiratory infection (e.g., pharyngitis, tonsillitis, or otitis media), a high fever, nausea or vomiting, and a good appetite suggest *mesenteric adenitis*.

Abdominal pain without systemic signs (e.g., fever or leukocytosis), or localized abdominal findings, especially when there is intense stress at home or school, suggests a *psychosomatic etiology*. Occasionally, children with such findings also have nausea, vomiting, headaches, and diarrhea. Their pain is poorly localized, and there are no peritoneal signs.

A history of polyuria, polydipsia, weight loss, or diabetes in the patient or the family suggests that the abdominal pain may be caused by *diabetic ketoacidosis*.

Growth failure, particularly during adolescence, is an important clue suggesting *inflammatory bowel disease* or a *gluten-sensitive enteropathy*. Weight loss and anemia are other signs of organic disease.

PHYSICAL FINDINGS

For excellent reviews of special techniques useful in pediatric abdominal examination, one should refer to the articles by Jones (1979) and Gryskiewicz (1980). Physical examination should include general observation of the child as well as inspection of the abdomen for signs of distention, masses, or abnormal pulsations. The abdomen should then be auscultated prior to palpation or percussion. Diffuse and generalized hyperperistalsis suggests *gastroenteritis,* whereas rushes of high-pitched peristalsis associated with crampy pains suggest an *obstructive process.*

Patients with *appendicitis* have tenderness over the inflamed appendix. Peritoneal inflammation, present in 97 per cent of children with acute appendicitis, usually results in muscle guarding and rebound tenderness. Other signs of peritonitis include shallow breathing, absent peristalsis, low-grade fever with a disproportionate rise in the pulse rate, and leukocytosis (which may be absent during the first 24 hours). The child may lie quite still or move cautiously and often prefers to lie on his side with the right thigh flexed. With a retrocecal appendix, the child may limp and demonstrate a positive psoas or obturator sign, although these signs are difficult to elicit in very young children. The following features of acute appendicitis have been described as peculiar to children:

1. Surgery should be performed within 24 hours of symptom onset; otherwise, perforation is likely.

2. The pain may be mild and discontinuous.

3. The pain may be atypically located when the appendix is not located in the right iliac area.

Both *mesenteric adenitis* and *nonspecific acute abdominal pain* can mimic appendicitis. It is very difficult for the physician to distinguish mesenteric adenitis from acute appendicitis by physical examination alone. **The value of serial abdominal examinations and serial laboratory tests, often performed in the hospital, cannot be over-emphasized, particularly when the diagnosis is unclear.** With early inflammatory processes, there may be sufficient irritation to make the abdomen diffusely tender, but not enough to produce peritoneal irritation. In these instances, there may be no muscle guarding or rebound tenderness. In mesenteric adenitis, the white blood cell count is usually not elevated, the temperature may be high (even higher than in acute appendicitis), and there is often a history or physical findings of a previous viral or bacterial respiratory infection. Mesenteric adenitis may also follow viral gastroenteritis. In these cases crampy, diffuse abdominal pain with nausea, vomiting, or diarrhea gradually changes to constant right lower quadrant pain.

One long-term study of patients with *recurrent abdominal pain* revealed organic causes in only 2 per cent, a finding that is not very encouraging to the physician who is considering the possibility of early appendicitis. If there is a history of similar pain episodes and if the current episode subsides over 24 hours, the diagnosis of recurrent nonspecific abdominal pain is more likely. Until the diagnosis is clear, active serial observations are essential. Continued pain, tachycardia, anorexia, diarrhea, pain on movement, and especially rebound tenderness all warn that the pain is not nonspecific and that surgical intervention must be seriously considered. When the temperature, blood count, sedimentation rate, urinalysis, and stool examination for occult blood and ova and parasites are normal, recurrent nonspecific abdominal pain is most likely.

A bulge in the inguinal area or the presence of an undescended testicle suggests an *inguinal hernia.* A lump may be palpated either rectally or abdominally in infants with *intussusception.* When intussusception is ileocecal (most common), a lump may be palpated in the right upper quadrant or the epigastrium. Rectal examination classically reveals bloody mucus on the examining finger. The "currant jelly stool" of dark altered blood per rectum is a late sign of intussusception. A barium enema performed carefully not only may reveal the intussusception but also may alleviate it.

Palpation of fecal material in the colon and tenderness over the course of the colon suggest pain due to *obstipation.* A firm inspissated stool may be palpated rectally. This diagnosis is confirmed if an enema yields a large amount of stool and relieves the pain. Occasionally, an enlarged kidney is detected by palpation, suggesting hydronephrosis as the cause of abdominal pain.

Physical findings associated with abdominal pain due to *diabetic ketoacidosis* include Kussmaul respiration, diffuse abdominal pain, and sweet, fruity breath. The presence of Kussmaul respiration and the absence of shallow respiration, usually seen with peritonitis, also suggest diabetic ketoacidosis.

DIAGNOSTIC STUDIES

Many indications for diagnostic studies were reviewed earlier in this chapter. Studies useful in the differential diagnosis of abdominal pain include complete blood count with differential, erythrocyte sedimentation rate, abdominal radiographs, stool examination for occult blood, urinalysis, and urine culture and sensitivity. **Every child should have a blood sugar test and urinalysis prior to abdominal surgery. All black patients should have a sickle cell prep.** Frequent serial tests may be necessary with acute pain. In cases of recurrent abdominal pain, the tests should be repeated, but less frequently. **When recurrent abdominal pain is the chief complaint, when there are no additional symptoms that suggest organic disease, and when a thorough history and physical examination are negative, only simple diagnostic studies should be performed.** In special instances, gastrointestinal barium studies, cholecystography, ultrasonography, intravenous pyelography, computerized tomography, endoscopy, proctoscopy, and small bowel biopsy may be helpful.

LESS COMMON DIAGNOSTIC
CONSIDERATIONS

Congenital intestinal obstruction, Hirschsprung's disease, duodenal atresia, midgut volvulus, and necrotizing enterocolitis may occur in the newborn. Abdominal distention, food refusal, and vomiting are commonly present in all these conditions. Likewise, radiographs are usually diagnostic. Newborns with Hirschsprung's disease fail to pass meconium. Those with duodenal atresia or midgut volvulus often demonstrate visible gastric peristalsis.

A twisted ovarian cyst should be considered in cases of acute lower abdominal pain in girls. A mass ordinarily is palpable, but a thorough rectal examination may be difficult unless it is performed with the patient under general anesthesia. Ultrasonography may help detect an ovarian cyst. A history of mittelschmerz also suggests that the pain may be due to an ovarian cyst. In older girls, salpingitis and pelvic inflammatory disease must be considered whenever a fever is observed in association with lower abdominal pain. The fever is usually higher than that observed with appendicitis, and a vaginal discharge is usually present. If a Gram stain of the vaginal secretion reveals gonococci, the diagnosis is clear.

Complete or incomplete intestinal obstruction resulting from adhesions should be considered as a cause of abdominal pain in any patient with an abdominal scar. This pain is usually cramping in nature and often accompanied by bilious vomiting. Physical examination often reveals abdominal distention, and distended loops of bowel occasionally may be identified clinically or radiographically. In the early phase, there are high-pitched tinkling bowel sounds that often occur in rushes. If the obstruction continues, peristalsis becomes lower in pitch and less frequent.

Peptic ulceration and occasional perforation may develop in children experiencing major stress as the result of serious physical trauma (e.g., burns or severe head injuries). Unfortunately, diagnosis is frequently delayed because of the severity of the other associated problems. Peptic ulceration and perforation should be considered whenever there are abdominal symptoms in children who have suffered major stress. Upright or decubitus radiographs may demonstrate free air in the peritoneal cavity.

Gallstones are rare in children and are most likely to occur in those with hemolytic anemias. Abdominal pain may be the presenting complaint in children with lower lobe pneumonias. Children with migraine headaches also may complain of abdominal pain. Lactose intolerance can cause recurrent abdominal pain in children and should be considered if the onset of pain coincides with heavy lactose ingestion. Before invasive procedures are performed or a psychogenic origin is assumed,

DIFFERENTIAL DIAGNOSIS OF ABDOMINAL PAIN IN CHILDREN

CONDITION	NATURE OF PATIENT	NATURE OF PAIN	LOCATION OF PAIN	ASSOCIATED SYMPTOMS	PHYSICAL FINDINGS	DIAGNOSTIC STUDIES
Gastroenteritis	All ages	Crampy	Diffuse	Diarrhea Vomiting	Hyperperistalsis Low-grade fever	
Intussusception	Under 5 years; peak incidence at 6 months	Severe, crampy			Rushes of high-pitched peristalsis Currant jelly stools Walnut-sized mass, palpated abdominally or rectally	Barium enema
Constipation	Any age; peak incidence at 5–12 years	Recurrent, crampy (especially after meals)	Often RLQ		Feces in rectum Feces may be palpable in colon	Enema yields large amount of feces and relieves pain
Psychosomatic etiology	Frequently 5–12 years High-strung, perfectionist History of colic	Recurrent (3 or more episodes)		Psychologic stress	Absence of systemic signs	Laboratory studies and radiographs within normal limits
Appendicitis	Uncommon in young children Peak incidence 5–15 years	Atypical in children Precedes anorexia and vomiting Worse with movement	Begins gradually in epigastrium or periumbilical area and progresses to a constant RLQ pain	Poor appetite	Serial examinations useful Fever Guarding persists when pain is not present Rebound in RLQ Decreased peristalsis	Leukocytosis
Mesenteric adenitis	As in appendicitis	As in appendicitis	RLQ	Symptoms of recent URI Good appetite	No guarding when pain is not present Fever Similar to appendicitis	CBC with differential Lymphocytosis
Inflammatory bowel disease	Adolescence			Diarrhea	Growth failure Diffuse abdominal tenderness, often without rebound	Upper and lower GI radiographs Elevated ESR
Inguinal hernia			Lower quadrant	Undescended testicle Abdominal distention	Bulge in inguinal area	

a lactose-restricted diet should be attempted. Blunt, nonpenetrating abdominal trauma can cause rupture of the spleen, liver, intestine, or kidney and result in abdominal pain. Crohn's disease should be considered in adolescents who have abdominal pain associated with weight loss, anemia, rectal bleeding, diarrhea, or passage of mucus per rectum. Acute pancreatitis, although rare in children, can be caused by trauma, viral infection (especially mumps), prolonged steroid therapy, or obstruction of the common bile duct due to a stone or an inflammatory process. Patients with this condition usually have marked nausea, vomiting, low-grade fever, and severe constant upper abdominal pain radiating to the back. Allergies to foods and drugs occasionally cause abdominal pain. Lead poisoning should be suspected if there are paroxysms of diffuse abdominal pain alternating with constipation. A history of pica may or may not be obtained from the parents or patient.

Selected References

Galler, J. R., et al.: Clinical aspects of recurrent abdominal pain in children. Adv. Pediatr. 27:31–53, 1980.

Gryskiewicz, J. M., and Huseby, T. L.: The pediatric abdominal examination. Postgrad. Med. 67:126–138, 1980.

Jones, P. F.: The acute abdomen in infancy and childhood. The Practitioner 222:473–478, 1979.

Lake, A. M.: Acute abdominal pain in childhood—finding the cause. Postgrad. Med. 65:119–127, 1979.

Lebenthal, E. B.: Recurrent abdominal pain in childhood. Am. J. Dis. Child. 134:347–348, 1980.

Raffensperger, J. G.: Acute abdominal pain. Comp. Ther. 3:48–53, 1977.

Shrand, H.: Problems in family practice—acute abdominal pain in children. J. Fam. Pract. 2:131–134, 1975.

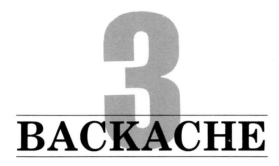

BACKACHE

Certainly all practitioners know that low back pain is an extremely common complaint, but few realize exactly how prevalent it is. Studies show that nearly 80 per cent of Americans experience low back pain sometime during adulthood. As a cause of absence from work, lower back pain is second only to upper respiratory infections. One study conducted in England showed that from 1969 to 1970, time lost from work due to low back pain was three times that lost as a result of employee strikes. Low back pain accounts for approximately 40 per cent of the complaints for which orthopedists and neurosurgeons are consulted. Patients with low back pain that endures longer than 6 months constitute a large segment of permanently disabled individuals. Of those who are disabled for more than 6 months, less than 50 per cent return to the workplace.

Acute lumbosacral strain is the most common cause of low back pain, accounting for 80 per cent of cases. The next most frequent causes are *postural, degenerative arthritis of the lumbosacral spine* and *lumbar disc disease. Gynecologic problems, irritable colon, prostatitis,* and *depression* are also common causes of low back pain.

NATURE OF PATIENT

Backaches in children are relatively uncommon. **In young children, backache represents serious disease more often than in adults, although the most common cause of backache in children is lumbosacral strain.** This type of sprain usually results from participation in sports. Occasionally, a sprained back is caused by *trauma*

29

(e.g., injuries suffered during an automobile accident or during partici-pation in gymnastics). Because low back pain may represent serious illness in children, a thorough history and physical examination should be performed. *Infection* should be a strong diagnostic consideration, especially in suspected intravenous drug users. *Spondylolisthesis* and *spondylolysis* occur more commonly in teenagers than in younger pa-tients. In these patients, pain usually develops after strenuous athletic activity and the cause can best be detected with appropriate radiographs.

Regardless of cause, backache is most common in patients between 20 and 50 years of age. It is more common in people who do heavy manual labor, such as industrial workers and farmers. In young adults who complain of persistent backache, *nonbacterial inflammatory disease,* such as *Reiter's syndrome* and *ankylosing spondylitis,* should be consid-ered. It is particularly important for the examiner to ask these patients about other inflammatory changes that may be associated with Reiter's syndrome (e.g., iritis, pharyngitis, urethritis, and arthritis). Even if the patient has spondylolisthesis, it is important for the physician to rule out inflammatory causes of backache. *Postural backaches* are more common in multigravida patients and in individuals who are obese or otherwise in poor physical condition. *Herniated discs* occur in young adults but are relatively uncommon.

The number of backaches caused by *disc disease* increases as age increases from 25 to 50 years. Disc syndromes are more common in men, particularly older ones. In older patients, backache is a common symptom but not a common chief complaint. When it is the chief complaint in patients over 50 years of age, serious illness must be considered as a possible underlying cause, although the most common cause is *osteoar-thritis of the lumbosacral spine.* It has been said that everyone eventually develops some degenerative joint disease in the low back, but as a rule clinical problems arise only when this degeneration reaches a moderate degree. It is then usually preceded by some traumatic incident, possibly minor, that precipitates the onset of symptoms. **In patients over 50 years who present with backache without significant history of prior backaches, serious conditions such as malignancy and mul-tiple myeloma must be considered.**

NATURE OF SYMPTOMS

To determine the cause of backache, the physician must consider important historical factors such as age, location of pain, possible radiation of pain, effects of motion of back or leg, and previous trauma (Table 3–1).

The pain of *acute lumbosacral strain* is characterized by a sudden onset often related to turning, lifting, twisting, or unusual physical activity. It is usually well localized at the lumbosacral region.

Table 3–1. **Differential Features of Common Causes of Pelvic Girdle Pain**

Cause	Site of Pain	Aggravating and Relieving Factors	Physical Findings	Other Findings
Degenerative disc disease with facet impingement	Buttock, posterior thigh	Worse with spinal extension, relieved by rest in fetal position	Restricted spinal movement, tender spinal segment	Radiographs abnormal
Degenerative disc disease with nuclear prolapse	Buttock, posterior thigh	Worse with spinal extension; relieved by rest in fetal position	Restricted spinal movement, tender spinal segment, nerve root dysfunction	Radiographs abnormal; prolapse shown on film
Sacroiliitis	Buttock, posterior thigh	Worse at rest; relieved with activity	Often associated restriction of spinal movement	Radiographs abnormal
Osteoarthritis of hip	Groin, occasionally buttock or knee	Worse with activity; relieved with rest	Restricted hip movement	Radiographs abnormal
Meralgia paresthetica	Lateral thigh paresthesia	Worse at night	Tenderness just below anterior superior iliac spine	Relieved by local infiltration of anesthetic and steroids
Trochanteric bursitis	Lateral thigh	Worse at night and with activity	Tenderness over greater trochanter	Relieved by local infiltration of anesthetic and steroids

(From Little, H.: Trochanteric bursitis. Can. Med. J. *120*:456–458, 1979.)

The pain of a *musculoskeletal strain* and a *postural backache* is often described as dull and persistent and associated with stiffness. Patients have difficulty locating a precise point of maximum pain. After trauma, this pain may have an immediate or delayed onset. Patients may state that they felt something "give way." The pain typically radiates across the lower back and occasionally into the buttocks, but rarely into the lower extremity.

The low back pain of *degenerative lumbosacral arthritis* has a gradual onset, is not usually precipitated by physical activity, and is usually associated with a history of morning stiffness. Patients with this condition often complain that their lumbosacral motion is limited by pain and stiffness that is often worse in the morning but that improves an hour or so after arising. Radiation of pain to the knee, calf, or lower leg is uncommon.

Patients with a *herniated disc syndrome* often have a history of previous, less severe episodes. The pain usually has a sudden onset and often radiates into the buttock, down the posterolateral aspect of the leg, and sometimes to the foot. The pain of a disc syndrome has been compared with a toothache—sharp, lancinating, radiating pain that may be associated with paresthesias and muscle weakness (caused by nerve root pressure). Remitting pain usually indicates a posterolateral disc protrusion, but an intermittent backache also can be caused by a disc that does not produce significant root irritation. More than 90 per cent of lumbar disc herniations occur at L4–L5 or L5–S1. If root irritation is present, neurologic findings (sensory loss, motor weakness, or hyporeflexia) are diagnostic. There also may be tenderness to palpation in the sciatic notch.

The qualitative characteristics of low back pain can be of considerable practical diagnostic importance. Variable, diffuse, and intense sensations of pressure often occur in patients without demonstrable organic disease. When the pain is described consistently and specifically, it is easier for the physician to demonstrate organic disease. If pain is related to posture, trauma, or overly strenuous activities; if it is episodic and intermittent; if it is aggravated by action; and if it is relieved by rest and recumbency, inflammatory disease (e.g., ankylosing spondylitis) and infectious processes (e.g., tuberculosis) are not likely.

Back pain in *sacroiliac syndromes* tends to be localized over the posterior superior iliac spine. In *sacroiliitis* (an inflammatory arthritis of the sacroiliac joints), the pain may alternate from side to side, although it is usually felt in the low back and buttocks, and may radiate into the posterior thigh.

Occasionally, low back pain may be a manifestation of the *irritable bowel syndrome*. In these cases, there often is an associated midback pain, abdominal pain, and a history characteristic of an irritable colon. This pain does not radiate into the leg. The low back pain from *prostatitis* is usually a vague ache that is not affected by movement or coughing and is not associated with muscle spasm or limited mobility.

Rarely, the acute pain of *renal colic* presents with excruciating pain in the back rather than in the flank or groin. In these cases, there is a gradual shift in the location of pain to the flank with radiation into the groin. With renal colic, the straight leg-raising test usually is negative, and the urinalysis generally shows hematuria.

Some patients with *depression* may experience chronic low back pain. It is often described as diffuse, accompanied by a sensation of severe pressure. When somatic pain is a manifestation of depression, the severity of the pain varies with the mental state: Pain increases with anxiety and depression and often decreases with extreme fear. If an elderly patient describes a burning or aching back pain, particularly if the pain is described as superficial and unilateral, *herpes zoster* should be suspected, since this pain often precedes the herpetic skin lesions.

ASSOCIATED SYMPTOMS

With *osteoarthritis of the lumbar spine,* patients often have pain in other joints. Patients with a *herniated disc syndrome* usually have neurologic symptoms such as sciatica, paresthesias, dysesthesias, hypoesthesias, anesthesias, paresis, sphincter problems, or impotence. **Pressure on the unmyelinated fibers may cause cauda equina syndrome, a rare surgical emergency whose signs include central back pain associated with weakness of the leg muscles, impotence, urinary frequency, urinary retention (sometimes with oveflow), incontinence, saddle anesthesia, and loss of sphincter tone.** Low back pain that is associated with vaginal discharge suggests a *gynecologic* etiology. In men, back pain associated with burning on urination, difficulty in urination, or fever suggests *prostatitis.* If herpes zoster is associated with back pain, underlying *malignancy* should be strongly considered.

PRECIPITATING AND AGGRAVATING FACTORS

Acute lumbosacral strain usually is precipitated by lifting, twisting, unusual physical activity or position, or trauma. Patients often are older and overweight and have not been physically active. When acute lumbosacral strain occurs in athletes, it may be due to poor equipment, inadequate coaching, insufficient warm-up or conditioning, or any body position that unnecessarily exaggerates lordosis. Acute lumbosacral strain in adolescent athletes may be precipitated or aggravated during periods of rapid growth, since the soft tissues, ligaments, and musculo-tendinous units do not keep up with bone growth. It should be noted that patients with acute lumbosacral strain experience pain with motion but not with coughing and straining. *Postural backaches* worsen as the day progresses.

In patients with a *herniated disc syndrome,* pain can be precipitated by trauma or certain types of movement (particularly twisting in the bent back position, as when starting a lawn mower or outboard engine). Aging also facilitates the development of this syndrome; herniation of the nucleus pulposus is the result of degenerative changes that occur with aging of the disc. The pain of a disc syndrome may be exacerbated by coughing, laughing, straining at stool, sneezing, sitting, and lateral bending; in acute cases it may be aggravated by almost any activity that results in the movement of the lower back, particularly hyperexten-sion. The pain caused by *degenerative lumbosacral arthritis* also may be increased by lateral bending and extension of the lumbar spine. Back-aches that worsen during or just after menstruation suggest a *gynecologic* etiology.

AMELIORATING FACTORS

Patients with an *acute lumbosacral strain* often state that lying prone and motionless relieves the pain. Most acute back pain, which is relieved by rest, is of mechanical origin. This can be a significant point in differential diagnosis if the malingerer, neurotic, or patient with strong secondary gain can be ruled out. Patients with low back pain due to *osteoarthritis* often state that their pain diminishes when they lie on the floor or on a firm mattress. Likewise, some patients with a disc syndrome are relieved by lying down. This variable, therefore, is not a truly helpful factor in the differential diagnosis of low back pain. What is helpful is that some patients with *disc syndrome* will inform the physician that they feel better when walking or lying on their sides with their knees flexed (fetal position). This latter finding strongly suggests that the pain is due to disc disease. If disc pain is unrelieved within 10 to 14 days of conservative nonoperative procedures (including rest), surgery may be required.

The back discomfort due to *irritable colon* may be relieved by defecation.

PHYSICAL FINDINGS

The following is an outline for a satisfactory examination of a patient presenting with low back pain. History should include a general medical, personal, sociologic, occupational, and sexual history. Special attention should be paid to previous backaches and factors that precipitate, aggravate, or ameliorate the pain, as well as to a history of trauma or heavy physical activity. **Physical examination should include a rectal and a pelvic evaluation, especially in patients over the age of 40 years and in those without a history or physical findings characteristic of the common causes of backache.** Particular attention should be paid to observations made during examination of the breast, prostate, thyroid, lymph nodes, and peripheral pulses. Any evidence of systemic inflammatory disease such as iritis, urethritis, or arthritis should be noted. Examination of the spine should include determination of range of motion anteriorly, posteriorly, and laterally.

Examination of the back also should include observation of the patient in the anatomic position, determination of range of motion of both the trunk and lumbar spine, cervical flexion with and without trunk flexion, and gait. With the patient sitting, knee and ankle reflexes should be checked, as should extension of each leg. The examiner also should determine the strength of dorsiflexion of toes and ankles, sensation to touch and pinprick in the lower extremity, and integrity of proprioception (Figs. 3–1 to 3–3) while the patient is in this position.

With the patient supine, five tests should be performed: straight leg-raising, Lasègue's compression (Fig. 3–4), bow string, knee compression, and pelvic pressure. The range of motion of hip joints must be established, and painful areas of extremities must be palpated. With the

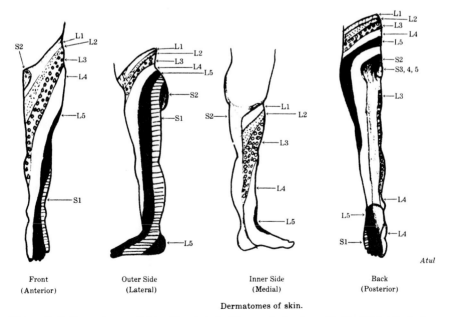

Dermatomes of skin.

Figure 3–1. Dermatomes of skin. (Reprinted with permission from *Medical Trial Technique Quarterly* [pp. 456–466, 1980 Annual], edited by Fred Lane, J. D., published by Callaghan & Co., 3201 Old Glenview Rd., Wilmette, IL 60091.)

Quadriceps Femoris

Tibialis Anterior

Extensor Digitorum Longus

Extensor Hallucis Longus

Tibialis Posterior

Long Flexor of Toes

Gastrocnemius & Soleus

Hamstrings

Gluteus Maximus

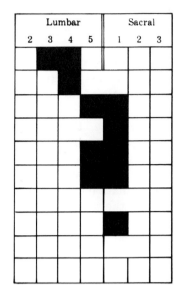

Figure 3–2. Nerve supply of various muscles (the main nerve roots are shaded). (Reprinted with permission from *Medical Trial Techniques Quarterly* [pp. 456–466, 1980 Annual], edited by Fred Lane, J. D., published by Callaghan & Co., 3201 Old Glenview Rd., Wilmette, IL 60091.)

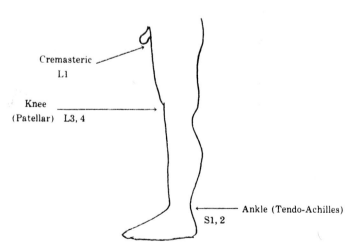

Cremasteric
L1

Knee
(Patellar) L3, 4

Ankle (Tendo-Achilles)
S1, 2

Figure 3–3. Root origin of reflexes. (Reprinted with permission from *Medical Trial Techniques Quarterly* [pp. 456–466, 1980 Annual], edited by Fred Lane, J. D., published by Callaghan & Co., 3201 Old Glenview Rd., Wilmette, IL 60091.)

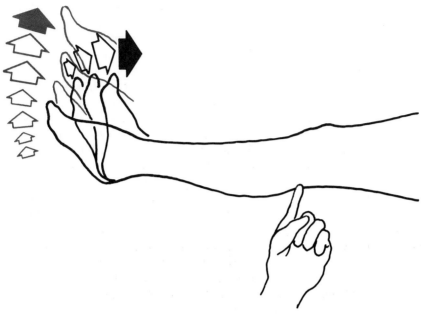

Figure 3–4. Sciatic nerve stretch test. The examiner uses the Lasègue test to invoke pain down the leg by raising the limb with knee extended. If this fails to induce pain, compression of the posterior tibial nerve in the lateral popliteal space is painful if there is nerve root involvement, or pain may be provoked by sharp dorsiflexion of the foot (Bragard test). (From Jacobs, B.: American Family Physician Monograph, Oct. 1978, p. 13.)

patient prone, the spine should be palpated, as should the sacroiliac joints; the hips should be hyperextended and the knees flexed.

Physical findings in patients with *acute lumbosacral strain* generally are limited to the lower back, which demonstrates some limitation of motion. There may be local swelling and tenderness to palpation as well as spasm of the paraspinal muscles. The neurologic examination is negative, unlike in cases of herniated disc, with which there often are associated spasm of the hamstring muscles and neurologic findings in the lower leg. During palpation over the sciatic notch, there may be pain or tenderness with some radiation to the knee or upper calf, but sensory and motor examination is intact. Often there is an increase in the lumbar lordotic curve; this lumbar curve may change very little with bending. There frequently is limited range of motion of the lower back, particularly anteriorly and posteriorly, but not as much laterally. Although a straight leg-raising test may cause back pain, it does not induce pain with a sciatic distribution.

When *osteoarthritis* causes low back pain, there may be symmetric restriction of movement, unlike in cases of *herniated disc,* which usually causes asymmetric limitation of motion. There may be tenderness to palpation in the lumbosacral region or at L4, L5, or S1.

When low back pain results from a *disc syndrome,* the physical findings often are markedly different from those of a *lumbosacral strain* or *osteoarthritis.* Instead of increasing the lumbar lordotic curve, a disc syndrome usually reverses the lumbar curve often with forward and/or lateral tilt. As with osteoarthritis and lumbosacral strain, there is limitation of spinal movement with a disc syndrome. The distinguishing features are the production of sciatic pain after hyperextension or lateral tilt and diminished or absent knee jerks in patients with disc syndrome. As with the other causes of low back pain, there may be spasm of the paraspinal muscles and tenderness to palpation in the sciatic notch.

Restricted straight leg-raising implies root irritation and is suggestive, but not diagnostic, of a herniated disc. Positive crossed, straight leg-raising usually indicates a massive or central herniated disc or a mass lesion. The location of pain elicited by straight leg-raising often suggests the area of nerve root irritation. Pain in the back or lumbosacral region suggests a higher lesion than pain in the calf or along the distribution of the sciatic nerve. Another clue to a ruptured disc may be asymmetric hamstring tightness.

Patients with sciatic nerve root irritation, regardless of its cause, usually experience pain in the calf with straight leg-raising. They generally demonstrate a positive Lasègue sign as well.

It should be noted that only rarely is a surgical emergency present in patients with a herniated disc syndrome. **There are three basic factors that influence the outcome of pressure on a nerve root: the amount of pressure on the nerve root; the duration of pressure; and the amount of myelin surrounding the nerve axon.** Mild pressure with local edema and inflammation causes nerve root irritation with some pain and paresthesias. Stretching the root aggravates the pain, as is the case with a positive straight leg-raising or a Lasègue sign. With increased pressure there is impaired conduction, motor weakness, reflex diminution, and some sensory loss in addition to pain. Severe pressure produces marked motor paralysis, loss of reflexes, and anesthesia. Mild to moderate pressure for short periods of time is tolerated fairly well by myelinated fibers. Prolonged pressure, however, is poorly tolerated, particularly by minimally myelinated nerves. *If paralysis following compression of myelinated fibers persists for 24 hours, it may be irreversible.* Myelin protects nerves from compression; the central parasympathetic nerve fibers to sphincters, however, are unmyelinated. **Therefore, loss of sphincter tone or urinary retention is a surgical emergency. If pressure on these unmyelinated fibers is not relieved immediately, permanent damage may ensue.**

DIAGNOSTIC STUDIES

In patients with osteoarthritis or a mechanical etiology of their low back pain, the sedimentation rate (ESR) and alkaline phosphatase are within normal limits. The ESR is elevated in *multiple myeloma, infectious spinal disease,* and *ankylosing spondylitis.* The alkaline phosphatase is elevated in patients with *Paget's disease.*

Radiographic examination is normal or may show increased lumbar lordosis in patients with an acute lumbosacral strain or low back strain. When osteoarthritis causes low back pain, radiographs frequently show narrowing of the lumbar spaces with spurring and often sclerosis of the vertebra. Radiographs may assist in the diagnosis of compression fractures, malignancy, Paget's disease, and multiple myeloma. CT scans (with or without contrast media) are helpful in locating herniated discs and spinal tumors.

LESS COMMON DIAGNOSTIC CONSIDERATIONS

Although most backaches are due to lumbosacral strain, disc disease, osteoarthritis, or postural backache, there are innumerable less common causes. Backaches can result from disease of almost any system and have been classified as viscerogenic, vascular, neurogenic, psychogenic, spondylogenic, genitourinary, musculoskeletal, and secondary to metastatic or primary tumors of bone or soft tissue. They also may be due to functional-mechanical derangement in the musculoskeletal system, resulting from poor posture or obesity. Back pain in children is a rare complaint and may have a serious, organic etiology. In older patients in whom back pain is a major complaint, particularly if it is the first attack, it is necessary for the physician to consider serious diseases such as metabolic disorders (osteoporosis, osteomalacia, chondrocalcinosis, and Paget's disease), malignancy, compression fractures, and infections.

Ankylosing spondylitis most often occurs in young to middle-aged males. It has an insidious onset and lasts at least 3 months. Classically, it is associated with marked morning stiffness. In contrast to more common causes of backache, ankylosing spondylitis is associated with a significantly elevated sedimentation rate and, rarely, with fever. There may be a family history of the same illness. Other joints may be involved, and the pain is frequently worse at night. The HLA-B27 antigen test rarely is positive. Fifty per cent of patients with ankylosing spondylitis develop transient arthritis of larger peripheral joints; sometimes they develop conjunctivitis or urethritis.

DIFFERENTIAL DIAGNOSIS OF BACKACHE

CONDITION	NATURE OF PATIENT	NATURE OF SYMPTOMS	ASSOCIATED SYMPTOMS	PRECIPITAT-ING AND AG-GRAVATING FACTORS	AMELIO-RATING FACTORS	PHYSICAL FINDINGS	DIAGNOSTIC STUDIES
Acute lumbos-acral strain	*Adults (20–50):* especially those who do strenuous work *Children:* often due to trauma or sports	*Sudden onset* Pain usually localized to the lumbosacral region		Precipitated by lifting, twisting, unusual physical activity Aggravated by motion but not by coughing or straining	Lying prone and motionless	*Neurologic examination negative* Paraspinal muscle spasm and pain Straight leg-raising causes back but not leg pain Limitation of motion of L–S spine region anteriorly and posteriorly Increased lumbar lordosis	Radiographs show increased lumbar lordosis

Postural backache (low back strain)	Obese, physically unfit adults	Vague low back pain / Difficult to locate point of maximum pain / Occasional radiation into buttocks		Worsens as day progresses		Neurologic examination negative / Limitation of motion (LOM) anteriorly and posteriorly / Increased lumbar lordosis / Straight leg-raising causes back pain, not leg pain	
Degenerative lumbosacral arthritis	>50 years	Gradual onset, not precipitated by physical activity, L–S spine motion limited / Pain worse in morning / Pain radiation into leg is uncommon	Often arthritis in other joints	Aggravated by lateral bending and extension of lumbar spine	Lying on back on floor / Better 2 hours after arising	Symmetric restriction of movement / *Neurologic examination negative*	Radiograph shows disc space narrowing and spurring

Table continued on following page

DIFFERENTIAL DIAGNOSIS OF BACKACHE *Continued*

CONDITION	NATURE OF PATIENT	NATURE OF SYMPTOMS	ASSOCIATED SYMPTOMS	PRECIPITAT-ING AND AG-GRAVATING FACTORS	AMELIO-RATING FACTORS	PHYSICAL FINDINGS	DIAGNOSTIC STUDIES
Lumbar disc disease	More common in males age 40 and older Rare in children	Sudden onset, previous less severe episodes Pain often radiates down posterolateral aspect of leg Buttock pain or paresthesia, pain can be lancinating or like a severe toothache	Hypesthesia Dysesthesia Weakness of some leg muscles	Coughing Sneezing Hyperextension of lumbar spine	Lying on side with knees flexed	Neurologic signs in lower leg Asymmetric limitation of motion Hamstring spasm Tender to palpation in sciatic notch Reversal of lumbar lordotic curve Forward or lateral tilt Pain of sciatic distribution after hyperextension or lateral tilt Restricted straight leg-raising	CT scan of spine

Condition							
Gynecologic disorders			Vaginal discharge	Worse around menstruation or ovulation	Lying supine with knees flexed	Abnormal pelvic examination	
Prostatitis	Older men	Constant low back pain	Urinary hesitancy	Change in sexual frequency		Prostate tender to palpation No LOM of back No muscle spasm	WBCs in prostatic secretion
Irritable colon	Young female adults Stressed individuals	Pain occurs in mid-back	Mucus in stools Abdominal pain	Stress	Defecation	Colon tender to palpation	
Depression	Adults	Severity of pain varies with mental state Diffuse, pressure-like pain	Early morning wakefulness Fatigue Constipation Anorexia	"Loss"		Depressed affect	
Neoplasm (usually backache caused by metastases)	History of cancer, especially of breast and prostate First episode of backache occurs after age 50	Gradual onset of pain	Weight loss	May be worse lying down		Rectal, pelvic, or breast examination may reveal primary tumor	Radiograph and CT scan of spine
Herpes zoster	Elderly	Burning superficial pain	Herpetic lesions appear after onset of pain			Herpetic vesicles	

Vertebral fractures ("compression fractures") may occur with severe trauma or, more commonly, with osteoporosis of the vertebrae in elderly patients. In these patients, vertebral fracture may occur following minor trauma. It also can occur after prolonged immobilization or steroid use. The back pain usually is at the level of the fracture and radiates locally across the back and around the trunk, but rarely into the lower extremities. Vertebral fractures occur more frequently in the mid and lower dorsal spine. Radiographs are useful in the confirmation of the diagnosis.

Infectious diseases of the spine, more common in children and intravenous drug users, also cause backaches. Patients with such infections often have an elevated sedimentation rate and may be febrile. An infectious cause of backache should be considered in cachectic individuals or patients undergoing prolonged steroid or immunosuppressive therapy. Uncommon causes of disc space infection include actinomycosis, tuberculosis, brucellosis, and fungal infections.

Neoplastic disease can cause backache, particularly in the elderly. Although primary neoplasms are rare, myeloma and metastatic disease are more common. In a patient with a known malignancy, the onset of back pain should suggest spinal metastases. Metastatic carcinoma is more common in older patients and should be particularly suspected if they have a history of malignancy. There often is an insidious onset of a waist-level or midback pain that becomes progressively more severe and persistent. The pain usually is unrelieved by lying down and frequently is worse at night. Unexplained weight loss with severe back pain aggravated by rest should suggest metastatic carcinoma in the spine. Multiple myeloma can cause severe, unremitting backaches; these are present at rest and may be worse with recumbency. This diagnosis can be confirmed with radiographs of the spine, pelvis, and skull; elevated sedimentation rate; and abnormal serum protein electrophoretic patterns.

The back pain of *acute pancreatitis* is invariably associated with marked gastrointestinal symptoms. Chronic low-grade pancreatitis, however, may cause vague back pain without noticeable abdominal symptoms. Patients with posterior penetrating ulcers may present with pain in the high midback as their chief complaint. This pain usually is not in the lumbar area and occasionally is relieved by antacids. Frequently, there is tenderness to epigastric palpation. Pain can be referred to the back from the urinary tract, uterus, prostate, and retroperitoneal structures.

Spinal stenosis can cause central low back pain that may radiate into one or both legs. The pain has the character of intermittent claudication: the patient is forced to rest after walking one or two blocks. An important diagnostic feature is that the pain also is relieved by flexion of the spine. It may occur at night, and the patient may find relief by walking, especially in a stooped position.

Spondylolisthesis and spondylolysis occur infrequently in the general population but are common causes of back pain in growing individuals. These conditions are caused by repetitive flexion and extension forces, particularly in congenitally predisposed individuals. They are more common in gymnasts and in football linemen. The pain is severe, worse with activity, and relieved by rest. Diagnosis is confirmed by appropriate radiographic studies.

Selected References

Belken, S. C., and Quiglers, T. B.: Finding the cause of low back pain. Med. Times 105(7):59–63, 1977.

Bunnell, W. P.: Back pain in children. Orthop. Clin. North Am. 13:587–604, 1982.

Clancy, W. G.: Low back pain in athletes. Am. J. Sports Med. 7(6):361–369, 1979.

Grabias, S. L., and Maukin, H. J.: Pain in the lower back. Bull. Rheu. Dis. 30(8):1040–1045, 1979–1980.

Gunn, C. C., and Milbrandt, W. E.: Early and subtle signs in low-back sprain. Spine 3(3):267–281, 1978.

Hoppenfeld, S.: Back pain. Pediatr. Clin. North Am. 24(4):881–887, 1977.

Kaushal, S. P.: The aching back—the history and physical examination. Med. Trial Tech. Q. 26(4):456–466, 1980.

Kirkaldy-Willis, W. H.: Five common back disorders: how to diagnose and treat them. Geriatrics, December, 1978, pp. 32–41.

Quinet, R. J., and Hadler, N. M.: Diagnosis and treatment of backache. Semin. Arthr. Rheum. 8(4):261–287, 1979.

Waddell, G., and Hanblen, D. L.: The differential diagnosis of backache. Practitioner 227:1167–1175, 1983.

Winter, R. B., and Lupscomb, P. R.: Back pain in children. Minnesota Med. 61(3):141–147, 1978.

4
BELCHING, BLOATING, AND FLATULENCE

In this chapter, *belching* is defined as the eructation of gas through the mouth; *bloating* is gaseous abdominal distention; and *flatulence* is the passage of intestinal gas per rectum.

BELCHING

Belching is not a symptom of organic disease. There is only one cause of belching, which is swallowing of air *(aerophagia)*. Air is swallowed or, more accurately, sucked into the stomach and released in the form of a belch. Air-swallowing may occur with eating or drinking; more air is swallowed with liquids than with solids. Aerophagia also occurs as a conscious or, more often, as an unconscious nervous habit unassociated with food ingestion. It also can be associated with mouth-breathing, gum-chewing, orthodontic appliances, and ill-fitting dentures. Chronic, repetitive, "unintentional" belching usually is caused by repetitive inhalation of air and regurgitation of it from the stomach or esophagus in the form of a belch. Some patients who demonstrate these findings consciously or unconsciously relax the upper esophageal sphincter during inspiration.

NATURE OF PATIENT

Excessive belchers tend to be nervous, anxious and tense. Belching often is normal in infants, although excessive belching may be the result of excessive air-swallowing during feeding. If there is an inadequate seal of the infant's lips around the real or artificial nipple, air may be ingested during nursing. This may be exaggerated if during feeding the child is held in a position that is too horizontal.

In some instances, patients with gastric or biliary disorders develop a habit of trying to relieve abdominal discomfort by swallowing (sometimes unconsciously) air and belching it up again; they feel that this provides some relief of their abdominal discomfort.

If associated pathology can be confidently ruled out, patients must be reassured that nothing serious is wrong. It may help to describe how a patient with a laryngectomy can be trained to swallow air; accordingly, a patient with a belching problem can be untrained. Simply instructing some patients not to belch when they feel the urge to do so may gradually stop their habit of swallowing air and belching it back. The use of antifoaming agents has not been shown to be particularly helpful. Rather, patients should be instructed to avoid chewing gum, eating quickly, smoking, and drinking carbonated beverages.

ASSOCIATED SYMPTOMS

The most common associated symptom is abdominal distention, representing gas in the stomach. Most swallowed air that is not belched up is reabsorbed in the small intestine. Usually, intestinal gas is derived by fermentation of intestinal contents. Some patients who swallow large amounts of air may experience or perceive abdominal discomfort until they belch. An urge to belch accompanied by chest pain on belching is a rare finding that may indicate an inferior wall myocardial infarction.

PRECIPITATING AND AGGRAVATING FACTORS

The most common precipitating factor is air-swallowing and subsequent relaxation of the esophageal sphincter to produce a belch. Nervous concern about belching can initiate a vicious cycle of unconscious air-swallowing and more belching. For some individuals, a supine position prevents swallowed gastric air from escaping into the esophagus, and an upright position faciliates belching. *Emotional stress* increases the likelihood of air-swallowing.

DIAGNOSTIC STUDIES

Although belching is invariably caused by swallowing air, this does not rule out coexisting unrelated pathology. If other symptoms warrant it, a cholecystogram, upper GI studies, and a chest radiograph should be considered.

LESS COMMON DIAGNOSTIC CONSIDERATIONS

Rarely, there is oral eructation of intestinal gas. In these instances, the odor is offensive, resembling that of methane or hydrogen sulfide. This suggests fermentation in stagnating gastric contents secondary to pyloric obstruction from ulcer, tumor, or previous vagotomy.

BLOATING AND FLATULENCE

Bloating and flatulence are two common complaints reported to physicians. The problem has been recognized since the time of Hippocrates, who taught that "passing gas is necessary to well being." In the days of early Rome, it was noted that "all Roman citizens shall be allowed to pass gas whenever necessary." Since swallowed air is reabsorbed in the small bowel, most of the gas in the distal small bowel and colon is produced within the bowel by fermentation. In most instances, flatulence is not of any clinical significance, but since various pathologic conditions may be associated with it, their presence should be investigated if the flatulence is excessive.

Flatulence is usually caused by excessive production of gas in an otherwise normal individual or increased discomfort from normal amounts of abdominal gas in healthy individuals. If bloating and flatulence have persisted for several years without the development of signs of serious organic pathology (e.g., weight loss, ascites, or jaundice), the patient can be reassured that the flatulence is not of great clinical significance. It must always be remembered, however, that some patients with *gallbladder disease, colon carcinoma, diverticulitis,* and *diverticulosis* may present with a chief complaint of abdominal discomfort, bloating, and occasionally flatulence. Patients wih colon carcinoma may present with vague abdominal discomfort or distention.

NATURE OF PATIENT

Flatulence is particularly common in infants up to age 3 months. This is referred to as "3-month colic" and is due to immature nervous control of the gut, which permits gas to become trapped in bowel loops. *Malabsorption* may lead to excessive fermentation of unabsorbed nutrients; this may produce an increase in flatulence. This can occur in patients with pancreatic insufficiency, pancreatic carcinoma, biliary disease, celiac disease, or bacterial overgrowth in the small intestine. A patient, particularly of African or Mediterranean descent, complaining of excess bloating or flatulence may have malabsorption and subsequent fermentation due to an *inherited lactose intolerance*. This diagnosis is confirmed if diarrhea develops or if the bloating or flatulence is exacerbated after ingestion of a lactose load (found in milk, ice cream, or other dairy products). Flatulence also may be seen in patients with *diverticulitis* or *diverticulosis*.

NATURE OF SYMPTOMS

Most gas that passes from the rectum has an unpleasant, foul odor. The gases that cause this odor are produced by intestinal bacteria. Because of their odor, these gases are detectable in minute quantity.

ASSOCIATED SYMPTOMS

Flatulence, of no clinical significance, may be associated with abdominal distention, bloating, borborygmi, abdominal discomfort, and cramping pain. When flatulence or bloating occur, moderate abdominal pain may be associated, even in the absence of organic disease. Patients may be unable to obtain relief by passing flatus. In some individuals, this is due to disodered motility of the gut; it cannot propel the gas forward through the bowel. This is not due to an increased volume of gas, but to the patient's inability to propel the gut gas forward. Some individuals have an exaggerated pain response to bowel distention despite a normal volume of intestinal gas. *Diverticulitis* should be suspected if flatulence is accompanied with lower abdominal pain, constipation, or diarrhea. *Giardiasis* should be suspected as the cause of flatulence, particularly if it is accompanied by foul-smelling, watery, or semisolid stools or abdominal distention.

PRECIPITATING AND AGGRAVATING FACTORS

The symptoms of bloating and flatulence are exacerbated by the ingestion of unabsorbable carbohydrates; these provide a substrate for the intestinal bacterial production of carbon dioxide and hydrogen. Constipation may also aggravate the symptoms of abdominal distention. This can be explained by the increased smooth muscle spasm in the colon around the gas bubbles. **It should be noted that although constipation may aggravate abdominal bloating, diarrhea usually does not relieve such distention.**

Patients with *gas entrapment syndromes* often experience a worsening of the pain when bending over to tie their shoes or when wearing a tight garment. Occasionally, this pain is exacerbated by flexion of the leg on the abdomen.

AMELIORATING FACTORS

Factors that may be associated with decreasing symptoms are diets low in undigestable carbohydrates or in lactose, failure of the patient to recline after meals, exercise, and ingestion of buttermilk or broad-spectrum antibiotics. Passage of flatus often relieves the sensation of abdominal bloating, at least temporarily. Any abdominal pain syndrome that is markedly relieved by passage of flatus should suggest gas entrapment.

PHYSICAL FINDINGS

When gas is trapped in the splenic flexure, palpation of the left upper quadrant can cause abdominal pain or pain in the chest ("pseudoangina"). With hepatic-flexure gas entrapment, the pain most frequently is in the right upper quadrant, and gallbladder discomfort may be simulated.

DIAGNOSTIC STUDIES

The physician should consider the following studies when appropriate: upper and lower gastrointestinal radiographic examination, proctosigmoidoscopy, cholecystogram, and stool analysis for fat and occult blood. If these tests do not reveal organic disease, the patient should be reassured, and dietary modification recommended. Likewise, a therapeu-

DIFFERENTIAL DIAGNOSIS OF BELCHING, BLOATING, AND FLATULENCE

CONDITION	NATURE OF PATIENT	NATURE OF SYMPTOMS	ASSOCIATED SYMPTOMS	PRECIPITATING AND AGGRAVATING FACTORS	AMELIORATING FACTORS	PHYSICAL FINDINGS	DIAGNOSTIC STUDIES
Belching Aerophagia	Nursing infants Nervous, anxious, and tense children and adults	Occurs with eating or drinking Conscious or unconscious nervous habit	Abdominal distention	In infants: nursing while in a position that is too horizontal Mouth-breathing Gum-chewing Orthodontic appliances Emotional stress Ill-fitting dentures Supine position Gastric or biliary disorders	Behavior modification: Avoidance of gum-chewing, eating quickly, smoking and drinking carbonated beverages Upright position	Those of gas in stomach	
Bloating and Flatulence Excessive intestinal bacterial fermatation causing increased gas Increased awareness of normal amount of gas	Most common cause at any age, especially in elderly adults	Flatulence Bloating	Abdominal discomfort or pain	Ingestion of nonabsorbable carbohydrates	Avoidance of all carbohydrates, particularly the nonabsorbable ones Passage of flatus		

Malabsorption	Patients with pancreatic insufficiency, pancreatic carcinoma, biliary disease, celiac disease, and bacterial overgrowth in the small intestine	Increased flatulence	Diarrhea	Nonabsorbable carbohydrates		Greasy, foul-smelling stools	Stool analysis GI radiographs
Lactase deficiency	Common in patients of African or Mediterranean descent	Bloating Excess flatulence	Diarrhea	Lactose load (i.e., from dairy products)	Avoidance of lactose Lactase supplement		Mucosal biopsy Lactose load
Giardiasis	Campers and hikers at higher risk	Increased flatulence	Abdominal distention Watery diarrhea, often foul-smelling	Drinking water infected with *Giardia*			Stool analysis for *Giardia*
Gas entrapment Splenic flexure			"Pseudo-angina"	Abdominal pain worsened by bending or wearing tight garments	Passage of flatus	LUQ pain on palpation Pain worsened by flexion of left leg on abdomen	Fluoroscopy for trapped gas
Hepatic flexure			Pain resembling gallbladder discomfort		Passage of flatus	RUQ pain on palpation Pain worsened by flexion of right leg on abdomen	

tic trial of a lactose load can be used to determine, presumptively, if a lactase deficiency is present. If this exacerbates bloating, flatulence, or diarrhea, the patient should avoid foods with lactose.

More complicated tests can be performed, such as D-xylose absorbtion, mucosal biopsy, and the analysis of flatus for the volume and composition of the various intestinal gases. Large quantities of carbon dioxide or hydrogen suggest malabsorption and fermentation of unabsorbable carbohydrates such as fruits and beans. Lactase deficiency also can lead to excessive quantities of hydrogen in the flatus. Flatulogenic foods include milk, onions, dry beans, celery, carrots, raisins, bananas, apricots, prune juice, apple juice, pretzels, bagels, wheat germ, brussel spouts, and ice cream. There is a tremendous individual variation with regard to the flatulogenic properties of these foods.

LESS COMMON DIAGNOSTIC CONSIDERATIONS

Incomplete or intermittent bowel obstruction, malabsorption syndromes, small bowel diverticula, maldigestion due to pancreatic or biliary disease, and short bowel syndrome may cause bloating or flatulence.

Selected References

Bond, J. H., and Levitt, M. D.: Gaseousness and intestinal gas. Med. Clin. North Am. 62:155–164, 1978.
Bouchier, I. A. D.: Flatulence. The Practitioner 224:373–377, 1980.
Hightower, N. C.: Intestinal gas and gaseousness. Clin. Gastroenterol. 6:597–606, 1977.
Levitt, M. D., and Bond, J. H.: Flatulence. Annu. Rev. Med. 31:127–137, 1980.
Raskin, J. B.: Intestinal gas. Geriatrics 38(12):77–93, 1983.

5

CHEST PAIN

Chest pain is one of the most common complaints of adult patients. Regardless of whether they admit it, they are usually concerned that this pain is due to some type of cardiac disease. Therefore, the physician must be thoroughly familiar with the differential diagnosis of chest pain. Although the physician must realize that it is in the patient's interest not to overlook any acute cardiac illness, it is just as essential that cardiac disease not be incorrectly diagnosed or inferred since such misdiagnosis may cause some patients to become "iatrogenic cardiac cripples."

Common causes of chest pain include *angina pectoris, myocardial infarction, nonspecific myositis, trauma, cervicodorsal arthritis, psychoneurosis, esophagitis, esophageal spasm, pleuritis,* and *mitral valve prolapse* (Table 5–1). Less common causes of chest pain include lung tumors, costochondritis, gas entrapment syndromes, pulmonary hypertension, pulmonary embolus, and pericarditis. Persons with biliary disease including cholelithiasis, cholecystitis, and common duct stones may also present with pain in the chest.

NATURE OF PATIENT

Chest pain due to coronary artery disease is least likely in young individuals. In children, chest pain is most likely to be due to *musculoskeletal system trauma* (e.g., myositis or costochondritis) or to an *inflammatory disease* (e.g., pleurisy). When pain similar in quality to angina pectoris occurs in a child or adolescent, *peptic esophagitis* or *mitral valve*

Table 5–1. **Noncardiac Causes of Chest Pain**

Resembles Angina Slightly	Not Typical of Angina
Psychoneurosis*	Psychoneurosis*
Pulmonary hypertension*	Costochondritis
Esophagitis and esophagospasm*	Nonspecific myositis
	Radiculitis
	Cervicodorsal arthritis
	Bursitis
	Shoulder disease
	Pericarditis
	Pneumonia
	Aneurysm
	Gastrointestinal distention with gaseous entrapment*
	Peptic ulcer
	Gallbladder disease*
	Diaphragmatic or paraesophageal hernia*

*Relieved by nitroglycerin
(From Seller, R. H. In Rakel, R. E., and Conn, H. F.: Family Practice. 2nd ed. Philadelphia, W. B. Saunders Co., 1978.)

prolapse should be suspected. Rarely, children with congenital anomalies of the coronary arteries may have ischemic pain. Although *pulmonary embolism* is uncommon in children, it should be suspected in any postoperative, immobilized, or bedridden patient. Likewise, females of any age are at increased risk for pulmonary embolism if they are taking oral contraceptives.

In an adult population, all causes of chest pain may occur. In older patients, *coronary artery disease, cervicodorsal arthritis, tumors, esophagitis,* and *pulmonary embolism* are the most common causes.

NATURE OF PAIN

Although it is important for the physician to differentiate chest pain of cardiac origin from other types of pain, it is not sufficient to establish whether or not the pain is of cardiac origin. Patients with pain of cardiac origin should receive varying forms of therapy and will have a different prognosis, depending on whether their pain was due to *angina pectoris, Prinzmetal's angina, hypertrophic cardiomyopathy, mitral valve prolapse,* or *pericarditis.* An accurate diagnosis usually can be made by a precise history. In eliciting the history of chest pain, the examiner should note five specific characteristics of the discomfort: the location of pain, the quality of pain, the duration of pain, the factors that precipitate or exacerbate the pain, and ameliorating factors.

The distinctive clinical characteristics of *angina pectoris* are that the pain is paroxysmal (lasting 30 seconds to a few minutes), dull, pressing, squeezing, or aching; it is located substernally; and it may radiate to the precordium, upper extremities, neck, or jaw. The term *anginal salute* refers to the way patients hold a clenched fist over their sternum to describe their pain. Some anginal patients experience no chest pain, but only neck, arm, or jaw discomfort. The location of pain in patients with angina pectoris may vary a great deal from person to person, but it differs little with recurrent episodes in the same patient. Thus, if the patient complains of chest pain in different locations during separate episodes, the pain is probably not due to angina pectoris. Pain of biliary tract or esophageal origin is likely to be substernal, whereas the pain of pericarditis is likely to be precordial.

Patients with angina pectoris describe their pain as a tightness, pressure, or heaviness, and, infrequently, as a burning sensation. Burning is relatively uncommon; if present, it suggests the possibility of *peptic esophagitis,* the most frequent imitator of coronary artery disease. **Rarely, if ever, is anginal pain described as knife-like, sharp, or sticking. Although some patients describe the pain as "sharp," they usually mean that it is severe in intensity rather than knife-like in quality.** The pain of *pulmonary hypertension,* which often occurs in patients with mitral stenosis or primary pulmonary disease, may be indistinguishable from the pain of *angina pectoris.* It is usually described as a dull, pressing, substernal pain, precipitated by exertion, and relieved by rest or administration of nitroglycerin. Although this pain may radiate to either arm, it has been said to radiate more frequently to the right arm. It must be recognized that patients with pulmonary hypertension and coronary artery disease may experience chest pain as a result of pulmonary hypertension, coronary artery disease, or both.

Dull, achy, or burning chest pain also may be experienced by patients with *peptic esophagitis* or *esophagospasm, pulmonary hypertension, cervicodorsal arthritis, gallbladder disease, diaphragmatic* or *paraesophageal hernias,* and *mitral valve prolapse.* In these cases the associated exacerbating or ameliorating factors are most helpful in establishing the diagnosis.

Sharp sticking pains, especially if only of a few seconds duration, are more characteristic of *psychoneurosis, costochondritis, cervicodorsal arthritis, mitral valve prolapse, chest wall syndrome, pericarditis,* and *pleuritic processes.* The location of the pain usually is not helpful in differentiating the cause of the chest pain in these conditions, with a few exceptions. Pain on the side of the chest, particularly if it is exacerbated by respiration, is more likely to be pleuritic. Pain localized to the costochondral junction or specific intercostal spaces is most likely due to *costochondritis* or *intercostal myositis.* The pain of *chest wall syndrome* may occur during exercise or at rest; occasionally, it is nocturnal. The pain not uncommonly is described as "sticking" in nature, but it may also be described as "dull" and "pressing." The most critical finding in the diagnosis of chest wall syndrome is detection of chest wall

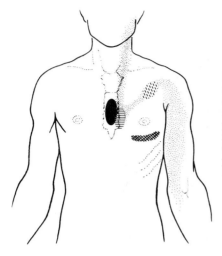

Figure 5–1. Regions of anterior chest where spontaneous pain was most frequently experienced and where tenderness could be elicited. Circumscribed areas represent primary site of pain and of tenderness; stippled areas represent radiation of pain. (From Epstein, S. E., et al.: Chest wall syndrome: A common cause of unexplained cardiac pain. J.A.M.A. *241*:2793–2797, 1979.)

tenderness on physical examination. It is frequently located substernally, at the left parasternal region, near the shoulder, and in the fourth or fifth left intercostal space (Fig. 5–1).

It is important to remember that the presence of cervicodorsal arthritis or reflux esophagitis does not rule out the possibility that chest pain is due to coronary disease. Patients may have two conditions, each of which contributes to their chest pain. For example, a patient may have pain due to esophagitis as well as pain due to angina pectoris. Not uncommonly, when two conditions coexist the patient may be able to distinguish between the two different types of chest pain. For instance, if questioned carefully, a patient may describe a dull substernal pain often induced by exercise and relieved by nitroglycerin but not antacids as well as another dull substernal pain radiating to the neck and arms that is not as thoroughly relieved by nitroglycerin but that is occasionally ameliorated by antacids. When further investigated, this type of patient may have documented coronary artery disease and reflux esophagitis.

ASSOCIATED SYMPTOMS

The pain of *mitral valve prolapse* occasionally may be indistinguishable from that observed in patients with coronary artery disease in that it may occur with exertion and rarely be relieved by nitroglycerin. More often, the chest pain of mitral valve prolapse has features not typical of angina that should alert the physician to the fact that the pain is not of coronary origin. The chest pain of mitral valve prolapse usually occurs during rest. Although it may last for a few minutes, it may also last for several hours. It often is described as "sticking" and not substernally located. It frequently is alleviated by lying down; the pain of *angina pectoris* often is worsened by recumbency, as is the pain of *reflux esophagitis*. **If atypical chest pain is associated with arrhythmias (particularly tachyarrhythmias) and lightheadedness or syncope, mitral valve prolapse should be suspected.**

Patients with *pneumonia* or *pulmonary embolism* may have chest pain, but they usually also have fever, cough, or hemoptysis. Patients who have protracted or vigorous coughing may experience chest pain resulting from intercostal muscle or periosteal trauma. In these instances, however, local chest wall tenderness usually is present.

Patients with *hypertrophic cardiomyopathy* (HCM) may have typical angina pectoris, but their chest pain is not necessarily due to coronary artery disease. **In patients with HCM, the most common symptom is dyspnea, which usually precedes the development of chest pain.** In any individual with angina pectoris who has coexisting or antecedent dyspnea, a careful search for HCM should be made.

Although the pain due to *esophagitis* often is similar to anginal pain, the associated symptoms are helpful in establishing the differential diagnosis. The pain of esophagitis usually is not related to exertion but is related to overeating and recumbency. The pain frequently awakens the patient at night. This symptom is rare in patients with angina pectoris unless they have angina decubitus. Patients with angina decubitus usually have congestive heart failure, and their pain often is precipitated by minimal exertion.

Cervical dorsal arthritis may produce chest pain. This pain is rarely similar to angina pectoris. More often, it is sharp and piercing, although the pain occasionally may be described as a deep, boring, dull discomfort. The major characteristics of *root pain* are (1) pain with movement of the body, (2) pain on coughing and sneezing, and (3) pain after prolonged recumbency. The pains may occur in any part of the chest or shoulder girdle and radiate down the arms. The pains may be bilateral or unilateral. Chest pain may be precipitated by bending or hyperextension of the upper spine or neck. Usually, the pain is not related to exercise and is fleeting in nature and thus is not truly relieved by rest.

The chest pain associated with *pericarditis* may be pleuritic or heavy and steady.

AMELIORATING FACTORS

Nitroglycerin usually relieves *angina pectoris* within 2 to 4 minutes; rest alone usually brings relief in less than 10 minutes. Unfortunately, a positive response to nitroglycerin does not confirm coronary artery disease as the cause of pain. Nitroglycerin works primarily by relaxing

smooth muscle. **It also may relieve chest pain due to peptic esophagitis and esophageal spasm, biliary dyskinesia and cholelithiasis,
gas entrapment syndrome, pulmonary hypertension, mitral valve
prolapse, and occasionally psychoneurotic chest pain.** However,
pain can be due to coronary artery disease and yet not be relieved by
nitroglycerin. The pain may be too severe or the nitroglycerin may be
outdated or administered improperly. If the symptoms suggest coronary
artery disease and sublingual nitroglycerin does not provide relief, the
physician should determine whether the patient is taking the medication
properly. A helpful method is to take a tiny piece of paper, crumple it
into the size of a nitroglycerin tablet, and have the patient place it
under his tongue. The patient should be instructed to let the nitroglycerin dissolve and remain under his tongue unswallowed. He should be
told to expect a warm, flushing feeling and to keep the saliva under his
tongue until the pain is relieved. At this point, the patient may either
swallow the saliva or expectorate it. **The Valsalva maneuver also may
give prompt relief of angina pectoris, but it does not usually
relieve the chest pain of obstructive HCM.** Occasionally, patients
with HCM get relief of chest pain by squatting, which decreases outflow
obstruction.

If antacid relieves a patient's chest pain, this strongly suggests that
the discomfort is due to *reflux esophagitis.* Relief of chest pain by
recumbency suggests *mitral valve prolapse,* whereas relief by squatting
suggests *hypertrophic cardiomyopathy.* Relief of chest pain by passage of
flatus suggests *gas entrapment* in the hepatic or splenic flexure.

PRECIPITATING AND AGGRAVATING FACTORS

Anginal pain often is precipitated by physical exertion, emotional
stress, sexual activity, exposure to cold, and occasionally by eating
(Table 5–2). *Prinzmetal's angina* occurs at rest. Chest pain due to
pulmonary hypertension also is induced by exertion.

Chest pain due to *peptic esophagitis* often is precipitated by overeating and recumbency. It frequently awakens the patient at night. Chest
pain due to *esophageal spasm* can be precipitated by swallowing certain
substances, particularly cold liquids and anything that stimulates the
production of endogenous gastrin. Thus, chest pain that follows ingestion
of alcohol should suggest the possibility of esophageal spasm.

If the pain is exacerbated or reproduced when pressure is applied
over the painful area, *costochondritis, Tietze's syndrome, rib fractures,
chest wall syndrome,* and *nonspecific myositis* are more likely. Reproduction or exacerbation of pain with chest wall pressure does not usually
occur in patients with ischemic cardiac pain.

Table 5–2. Diagnosis of Chest Pain

Condition	Chest pain		Dizziness, vertigo, syncope	Response to		Cardiac auscultation	Abnormal EKG		Stress EKG	Sx reproduced at bedside
	Typical	Atypical		Nitrates	Propranolol		QRS	ST–T		
Coronary heart disease	+++	+	Rare	++++	++++	–To+++	Common	Common	+++	–
Angina with normal coronary arteries	++	++	Rare	++	++	–	Occasional	Common	+++	–
Hypertrophic cardiomyopathy	+++	+	++	+	+++	–To+++ Variable	Common	Common	+++	Rare
Mitral valve prolapse	+	+++	++	+	+++	–To+++ Variable	Rare	Common	++	Rare
Hyperventilation syndrome	+Rare	++	++	–	+	–	–	Rare	+	++
Esophageal disease	+(?)	+++	–	+	–	–	–	–	–	–
Radicular syndromes	+	+++	+	+(?)	–	–	–	–	–	+++
Chest wall syndromes	–	+++	–	–	–	–	–	–	–	+++

(From Levine, H. J.: Differential problems in the diagnosis of chest pain. Am. Heart J. *100*:108–117, 1980.)

Although a few patients with chest pain due to *HCM* obtain relief with nitrates, the pain of HCM usually is exacerbated and the murmur is intensified by nitroglycerin. **Just as chest pain associated with dyspnea should alert the physician to the possibility of HCM, chest pain made worse by nitrates should likewise alert the physician to the possibility of HCM, as should the association of lightheadedness, dizziness, or syncope.**

PHYSICAL FINDINGS

There are few physical findings diagnostic of *angina pectoris*. A sinus tachycardia or a bradycardia may coincide with anginal pain. Signs of *congestive heart failure* in patients with chest pain suggest that the pain probably is due to myocardial ischemia. If a careful examination performed during an episode of ischemic heart pain reveals a palpable systolic bulge near the apex, paradoxical splitting of the second sound, a diastolic filling sound (S3 or S4), or a transient mitral regurgitant murmur, this strongly suggests that ischemic heart disease is the cause of chest pain. Likewise, the presence of cutaneous manifestations of atherosclerosis such as *xanthomas, hypertension,* and *diabetic retinopathy* increase the probability of coronary artery disease as the cause of chest pain.

Squatting decreases outflow tract obstruction and thus diminishes the characteristic midsystolic murmur of *HCM*. The systolic murmur of HCM is increased with the patient in the upright position and during the Valsalva maneuver. Atrial and ventricular arrhythmias are common in hypertrophic cardiomyopathy and occasionally may be the earliest manifestation. Chest wall tenderness to palpation or auscultation of a pericardial friction or a pleural friction may help in diagnosis.

Tenderness in the region of spontaneous pain, especially if the quality of pain can be reproduced by pressure on the area, strongly suggests *chest wall syndrome*. In addition to application of pressure on various areas of the chest, certain maneuvers—including horizontal flexion of the arm and the so-called "crowing rooster" maneuver—also may cause the pain of chest wall syndrome. *Mitral valve prolapse (MVP)* is suggested by auscultation of a midsystolic "click," late systolic murmur, or both. It should be remembered, however, that patients may have MVP with absent or transient auscultatory findings.

DIAGNOSTIC STUDIES

Resting electrocardiograms may be normal in 50 per cent of patients with angiographically confirmed coronary artery disease. An electrocardiogram obtained during a bout of chest pain is more likely to be abnormal. Some studies have revealed that even during an episode of chest pain, ST segment depression occurs in only 50 per cent of the patients. **An appropriately administered exercise electrocardiogram is probably the single most useful and noninvasive test in the diagnosis of coronary artery disease.**

Myocardial perfusion scanning and radionuclide cineangiography have greatly enhanced our ability to diagnose coronary artery disease using noninvasive tests. Coronary angiography should be reserved for those patients who will probably need, and who consent to have, coronary artery surgery as well as for certain other selected patients.

The electrocardiogram of *mitral valve prolapse* may show changes similar to those of coronary artery disease. If electrocardiographic changes are present, they usually include ST segment depression and T-wave inversion or abnormalities in leads II, III, and AVF and occasionally in the precordial leads. The ST–T wave changes of MVP may be differentiated from those of coronary artery disease by the oral administration of 40 mg of propranolol. The ST–T wave abnormalities seen in some patients with mitral valve prolapse (and in some athletes) may diminish or disappear 1 to 2 hours after propranolol administration, whereas patients with angina pectoris are unaffected.

The electrocardiogram usually is abnormal in patients with *obstructive hypertrophic cardiomyopathy,* although a normal electrocardiogram may be obtained. The most common electrocardiographic abnormalities include those of left ventricular hypertrophy, intraventricular conduction defects, and nonspecific ST–T wave changes. The electrocardiographic findings (P wave abnormalities) most helpful in the diagnosis of hypertrophic cardiomyopathy are those that are not generally seen in patients with coronary artery disease. These P wave abnormalities suggestive of atrial enlargement are common in patients with hypertrophic cardiomyopathy and uncommon in patients with coronary artery disease. An electrocardiographic picture of transmural infarction (Q waves in the anteroseptal or inferior leads) also may be seen in some patients with HCM.

The echocardiogram is most useful in the diagnosis of both mitral valve prolapse and hypertrophic obstructive cardiomyopathy.

LESS COMMON CAUSES OF CHEST PAIN

The pain ot costochondritis and costochondrodynia usually is localized to the costochondral junction. The pain may be constant or may be exacerbated by movement of the chest wall, including respiratory motion. One may confirm the diagnosis by applying pressure over the painful area, thus replicating the pain.

DIFFERENTIAL DIAGNOSIS OF CHEST PAIN

CONDITION	NATURE OF PATIENT	NATURE OF PAIN	ASSOCIATED SYMPTOMS	AMELIORATING FACTORS	PRECIPITATING AND AGGRAVATING FACTORS	PHYSICAL FINDINGS	DIAGNOSTIC STUDIES
Angina pectoris	Adult	Achy, dull, tight, severe, pressing, not usually sharp or sticking Substernal		Nitroglycerin Rest Valsalva maneuver	Exertion, cold exposure, emotional stress	Sinus tachycardia, bradycardia, apical systolic bulge coincident with pain Xanthomas Signs of heart failure	Exercise EKG Coronary arteriography Radionuclide tests
Prinzmetal's angina	Adult	Achy, dull, tight, severe, pressing, not usually sharp or sticking Substernal		Nitroglycerin Rest	Often occurs at rest		EKG during attack Coronary arteriography
Esophagitis	Any age	Burning Tightness May be identical to that of angina	Water brash "Heartburn" after alcohol	Antacids	Overeating Recumbency (may awaken from sleep) Not precipitated by exertion		Esophagoscopy Infusion of dilute acid into the esophagus (Bernstein test)
Esophageal spasm	Especially obese adults	May be identical in quality to angina		Occasionally relieved by nitroglycerin	Often induced by ingestion of alcohol or very cold liquids		Esophageal manometry

Mitral valve prolapse	Any age	Usually not substernal Often has a sticking quality May last several hours Not typical of angina	Palpitations Arrhythmias Often occurs at rest Syncope	Beta-blockers Recumbency		Click and/or late systolic murmur	Echocardiogram Phonocardiogram
Hypertrophic cardiomyopathy	Any age	Pain may be similar to that of angina	Dyspnea Arrhythmias Lightheadedness	Beta-blockers Squatting	Pain may be aggravated by nitroglycerin	Murmur intensified by nitroglycerin and Valsalva maneuver Decreased by squatting	Echocardiogram
Intercostal myositis	Any age	May be sticking in quality			May intensify with inspiration	Localized tenderness to palpation No pleural friction	
Cervicodorsal arthritis	Adult	May be sharp or sticking Duration only a few seconds			May be precipitated by certain movements (e.g., neck exercises and twisting) Not related to stress		Radiographs of cervicodorsal spine

Table continued on following page

DIFFERENTIAL DIAGNOSIS OF CHEST PAIN *Continued*

CONDITION	NATURE OF PATIENT	NATURE OF PAIN	ASSOCIATED SYMPTOMS	AMELIORATING FACTORS	PRECIPITATING AND AGGRAVATING FACTORS	PHYSICAL FINDINGS	DIAGNOSTIC STUDIES
Chest wall syndrome	Adult	Often sharp and sticking Fleeting			May be aggravated by recumbency and certain positions	Local tenderness to palpation "Crowing rooster" maneuver may precipitate pain	
Pericarditis	Any age	Sharp or dull Protracted duration	Fever Recent viral infection			Pericardial friction	EKG Echocardiogram CBC
Myocardial infarction	Adult	Severe Crushing Precordial Protracted duration	Sweating Fatigue Nausea	Not relieved by nitroglycerin			EKG Enzymes Radionuclide studies
Gas entrapment syndrome	Any age Often obese	Dull, achy	Flatulence	Passage of flatus Nitroglycerin	Aggravated by bending and tight garments	Flexing thigh and palpation of colon may elicit pain	Gas in hepatic or splenic flexure on radiographs

Gas entrapment syndromes (gas trapped in the hepatic or splenic flexure) are suggested by a history of chest pain when the patient bends over or wears a tight garment. The pain may be exacerbated by bending, flexing the thigh on the chest, or palpation of the colon. The pain may be relieved by passage of flatus or by ingestion of sublingual nitroglycerin.

The pain of pulmonary hypertension may be indistinguishable from that due to angina pectoris and other causes of exercise-induced chest wall pain. It also can be relieved by sublingual nitroglycerin. It should be suspected in patients with mitral stenosis or other causes of pulmonary hypertension, pulmonary disease, an accentuated pulmonary second sound, or electrocardiographic signs of right atrial disease (peaked P waves) or right ventricular overload. The pain of a pulmonary embolus in the acute phase may be due to pulmonary hypertension. Subsequently, the pain is related to pulmonary infarction with associated pleurisy. The pain usually is not related to exercise and tends to become more constant (often with a pleuritic component) in the later stages.

Pericarditis should be suspected in the presence of continual chest pain associated with diffuse electrocardiographic changes. This pain tends to be aggravated by changes in position. A pericardial friction rub confirms this diagnosis.

Lung and mediastinal tumors often present with chest pain, which tends to be constant, especially in the later stages. **Whenever the diagnosis of chest pain is not clear, particularly in adult patients, one should obtain a chest radiograph to detect any tumors that may be present.**

Selected References

Diehl, A. M.: Chest pain in children: Tip-offs to cause. Postgrad. Med. *73(6)*:335–337, 340–342, 1983.

Editorial: Diagnosis of chest pain. Lancet *1*:129–130, 1977.

Epstein, S. E., Gerber, L. H., and Borer, J. S.: Chest wall syndrome—a common cause of unexplained cardiac pain. J.A.M.A. *241*:2793–2797, 1979.

Hecht, H. S., et al.: Reproducibility of equilibrium radionuclide ventriculography in patients with coronary artery disease: response of left ventricular ejection fraction and regional wall motion to supine bicycle exercise. Am. Heart J. *104*:567–584, 1982.

Levine, H. J.: Difficult problems in the diagnosis of chest pain. Am. Heart J. *100*:108–117, 1980.

Schroeder, J. S., Lamb, I. H., and Hu, M.: The prehospital course of patients with chest pain. Analysis of the prodromal, symptomatic, decision-making, transportation and emergency room periods. Am. J. Med. *64*:742–748, 1978.

Zoob, M.: Differentiating the causes of chest pain. Geriatrics *33*:95–101, 1978.

6
COLDS, FLU, AND STUFFY NOSE

It might appear that the differential diagnosis of colds, flu, and stuffy nose is unimportant, as most of these conditions have no specific cures. However, because upper respiratory infections are the most common affliction of adults and children, the sheer case volume requires the physician to be particularly expert in the diagnosis and symptomatic treatment of these conditions.

Many different *viruses* are responsible for causing colds, upper respiratory infections, and flu. It is important that the physician be able to differentiate these viral infections from *allergic rhinitis* (both perennial and seasonal), *vasomotor rhinitis,* and the common complications of these viral infections, which include *sinusitis, otitis media, bronchitis,* and *pneumonia.* These last four complications usually are secondary to superimposed bacterial infections, which will respond to appropriate antibiotic therapy. The constitutional complaints often associated with upper respiratory infection also may represent the prodrome of other viral infections, such as *infectious mononucleosis, measles,* and *mumps.*

NATURE OF PATIENT

Children often experience more severe constitutional symptoms with upper respiratory infections or colds than do adults. After a *common cold,* adults with a history of bronchitis, allergies, asthma, heavy cigarette smoking, or immune incompetence and children with a history of recurrent bronchitis, allergies, or cystic fibrosis develop lower respiratory tract infections more frequently than other individuals. *Influenza* tends to be milder in neonates and children; severity increases with the age of the patient. Elderly patients often develop a superimposed *bacterial pneumonia.* Over 70 per cent of deaths recorded during known influenza epidemics have occurred in patients over 65 years of age. Other high-risk groups include patients with chronic cardiorespiratory disease, chronic renal disease, diabetes, and third trimester pregnancies. *Rhinitis medicamentosa* should be suspected in patients who frequently use nasal drops, sprays, or inhalers. It is most important for the physician to be alert for the development of complications of common upper respiratory infections. *Sinusitis* is more likely to occur in a patient with a history of recurrent sinusitis; *otitis media* is more common in young children; *bronchitis* is more common in smokers and those with underlying *pulmonary disease*; and *pneumonia* is more common in older and diabetic patients.

NATURE OF SYMPTOMS

Symptoms of common *viral upper respiratory infections* are well known. These symptoms, however, largely depend on the particular infective viral agent, the patient's age, and the underlying medical conditions. The incubation period is 1 to 3 days. Usually, there is a profuse nasal discharge and congestion with complaints of stuffy nose, sneezing, postnasal drip, cough, and sore throat. Patients may complain of headache, fever, malaise, and hoarseness. They also may note pharyngeal exudates, oropharyngeal vesicles, and lymphadenopathy. In children, there may be vomiting, diarrhea, abdominal pain, and wheezing. Although an upper respiratory infection is the most frequent cause of nasal airway obstruction, less common causes must be considered, including polyps, foreign body, herpes simplex, furuncle (folliculitis of nasal vibrissae) and less common infections. In neonates, unilateral nasal obstruction may be caused by a congenital abnormality (e.g., choanal atresia). In a child with unilateral nasal obstruction as the presenting symptom, the physician should consider the possibility of a foreign body.

Although the symptoms of influenza and common upper respiratory infection may be similar, *influenza viral infections* often can be differentiated from the symptoms of a common cold by the sudden onset of typical signs of flu: shivering, chills, malaise, insomnia, marked aching of the limb and back muscles, dry cough, retrosternal pain, and loss of appetite. Patient with *type A influenza* may not have coryza.

It is particularly important for the physician to recognize *allergic* and *vasomotor rhinitis* as causes of nasal stuffiness. There are two types of allergic rhinitis—*perennial* and *seasonal*. Patients who have perennial rhinitis usually complain of nasal airway blockage with a persistent watery mucoid drainage. Their nasal turbinates are pale and boggy. Patients who have seasonal rhinitis usually complain of sneezing, itching eyes, lacrimation, and a watery discharge from the nose. They usually have a seasonal variation in their symptoms. The perennial group does not.

Vasomotor rhinitis, or idiopathic rhinitis, is not known to have a specific etiology. Patients with this condition usually have persistent engorgement of the nasal turbinates, which leads to nasal obstruction and a profuse watery rhinorrhea. Their symptoms are exacerbated by allergy, stress, hormonal changes (e.g., those associated with menstruation and menopause), marked temperature variations, and chemical irritants. These patients often complain of persistent nasal obstruction that may alternate from side to side. Sneezing is not as common as it is in allergic rhinitis.

When symptoms of a cold and cough persist longer than the patient's fever, the upper respiratory infection may have subsided, and the persistent symptoms may be due to a sinusitis of bacterial origin.

AMELIORATING FACTORS

Ameliorating factors are not particularly helpful in differential diagnosis.

PHYSICAL FINDINGS

The physical examination is most helpful in the detection of complications such as otitis media, sinusitis, pneumonia, and other bacterial infections. The physician should suspect something more serious than a simple upper respiratory infection if the temperature is greater than 102° F. If there is severe sore throat, exudative pharyngitis, earache, severe head or neck pain, or wheezing, it is particularly important for the physician to exclude complications such as *streptococcal pharyngitis, otitis media, sinusitis, meningitis,* and *bacterial pneumonia,* since these conditions respond well to appropriate antibiotic therapy.

Patients with acute *sinusitis* often have pain over the involved sinuses that usually is unilateral and dull in the early stages but that may become bilateral and more severe later. Coughing, sneezing, and percussion over the involved sinuses often exacerbate the pain. Percussion of the teeth may produce pain when the maxillary sinuses are infected. In fact, some individuals may present with a toothache as an early manifestation of sinusitis. Patients with ethmoid sinusitis often experience retro-orbital pain on coughing or sneezing. They also may demonstrate chemosis, proptosis, extraocular muscle palsy, or orbital

DIFFERENTIAL DIAGNOSIS OF COLDS, FLU, AND STUFFY NOSE

CONDITION	NATURE OF PATIENT	NATURE OF SYMPTOMS	COMPLICATIONS	PRECIPITATING AND AGGRAVATING FACTORS	PHYSICAL FINDINGS	DIAGNOSTIC STUDIES
Common cold/viral upper respiratory tract infection	Anyone	Constitutional symptoms worse in children; Incubation period 1–3 days; Profuse nasal drainage; Nasal congestion; Sneezing; Postnasal drip; Cough; Sore throat; Headache; Fever (<102° F); Hoarseness; General malaise	Lower RTI,* especially in adults with history of bronchitis, allergies, asthma, heavy cigarette smoking, immunoincompetence; Sinusitis, especially in patients with history of recurrent sinusitis; Bronchitis in smokers and patients with pulmonary disease; Pneumonia in elderly and diabetics; Nasal airway obstruction; Streptococcal pharyngitis; Meningitis		Mucopurulent nasal discharge; Nasopharyngeal mucosal infection and swelling; Temperature usually <102° F; Pharyngeal exudates less frequent than with bacterial infections; Lymphadenopathy	Throat culture (to rule out streptococcal infection and pharyngitis); Monospot (to rule out infectious mononucleosis)
	Children	Vomiting; Diarrhea; Abdominal pain; Wheezing	Lower RTI in children with history of recurrent bronchitis, allergies, cystic fibrosis; Otitis media		Fever, may be >102° F; Wheezing when bronchiolitis is associated	
Allergic rhinitis Perennial	Onset before 20 years; Family history of allergic disease	Nasal airway blockage; Persistent watery nasal discharge; No seasonal variation			Pale/boggy nasal turbinates; Watery nasal discharge	Nasal smear shows eosinophils

Condition	Predisposing factors	Symptoms	Complications	Precipitating factors	Signs	Laboratory
Seasonal		Sneezing Itchy eyes Lacrimation Watery, nasal discharge Seasonal variation		Allergens such as dust, pollen, spores	Pale/boggy nasal turbinates	
Vasomotor (idiopathic rhinitis)		Persistent nasal obstruction May alternate sides Profuse watery rhinorrhea Sneezing not common		Allergy Stress Hormonal changes Marked temperature changes Chemical irritants	Swollen nasal turbinates	
Sinusitis	Prior history of sinusitis	Often recurrent pain over sinuses Early: unilateral dull Later: bilateral severe May present as toothache		Coughing Sneezing Percussion of involved sinuses		Sinus radiographs Transillumination of sinuses
Maxillary					Pain with percussion of tooth	
Ethmoid		Retro-orbital pain Mucopurulent nasal discharge (may be bloody)	Visual loss Cavernous sinus thrombosis Brain abscess	Coughing and sneezing may cause retro-orbital pain	Chemosis Proptosis Extraocular muscle palsy Orbital fixation	
Rhinitis medicamentosa	Frequent users of nasal drops, sprays, or inhalants Hypertensive patients taking certain antihypertensive drugs	Congestion Nasal stuffiness		Nasal medications Reserpine Beta-blockers Clonidine Hydralazine Methyldopa Prazosin	Mucosa injected	No eosinophils on nasal smear

*RTI = respiratory tract infection.

fixation. A mucopurulent nasal discharge, with or without blood, frequently is present. Examination should include not only palpation and percussion over the sinuses but also careful observation of the pharynx, cranial nerves, eyes (including evaluation of visual acuity), ears, nose, and mouth. Visual loss, cavernous sinus thrombosis, and brain abscesses are serious sequelae to be avoided. When correctly performed, transillumination may be helpful in the diagnosis of frontal and maxillary sinusitis.

DIAGNOSTIC STUDIES

Throat cultures may be useful in cases of streptococcal pharyngitis. The Monospot test is helpful in the diagnosis of infectious mononucleosis. Nasal smears allow one to detect eosinophils in allergic rhinitis. Sinus radiographs help one detect sinusitis. Computerized atrial tomography permits one to visualize intracranial lesions.

LESS COMMON DIAGNOSTIC CONSIDERATIONS

Frequent respiratory infections should alert the physician to the possibility of an anatomic abnormality, immune incompetence, or mucoviscidosis. Less common causes of nasal blockage include nasal polyps, tumors, foreign body, collagen vascular disorders, and congenital malformations in neonates.

Selected References

Beare, A. S.: Upper respiratory infections. Practitioner 227:953–961, 1983.
Bickmore, J. T.: Vasomotor rhinitis: an update. Laryngoscope 91:1600–1605, 1981.
Busse, W. W.: Chronic rhinitis—a systemic approach to diagnosis and treatment. Postgrad. Med. 73:325–335, 1983.
Newman, R. K., and Johnson, J. T.: Nasal airway obstruction—approach to diagnosis and management. Postgrad. Med. 68:184–191, 1980.
Reed, S. E.: The common cold. Practitioner 223:753–757, 1979.
Stevenson, J.: Influenza. Practitioner 223:759–763, 1979.
Stott, N. C. H.: Management and outcome of winter upper respiratory tract infections in children aged 0–9 years. Br. Med. J. 6:29–31, 1979.

7

CONSTIPATION

Constipation is common in Western society. The frequency with which physicians diagnose constipation depends on both the patient's and the physician's definition of the problem. One bowel movement each day is what most patients consider normal. Many physicians, however, may accept two to three hard and dry stools a week as normal if this is usual and customary for the individual. Some experts in the field believe that anyone who strains to defecate or who does not effortlessly pass at least one soft stool daily is constipated. By this definition, constipation is very common.

Constipation has been attributed to the deficiency of dietary fiber in the customary Western diet. Dietary fiber has been replaced by excessive ingestion of refined carbohydrates. Constipation may also be defined as a change in the individual's normal bowel pattern to less frequent or more difficult defecation. In this chapter, constipation will be defined as straining with bowel movements or bowel movements that occur less than five times per week.

Constipation usually is not due to a serious disease. In most instances, it can be corrected by decreasing the amount of refined carbohydrate and increasing the amount of fiber ingested. It is particularly important for the examiner to ask whether the constipation is of recent onset and constitutes a change in previous bowel habits, as such findings may indicate serious disease.

The most common causes of constipation are *laxative habit, diets high in refined carbohydrates and low in fiber, change in daily habits or environment, drug-induced, irritable bowel syndrome,* and *painful defecation due to a local anorectal problem.* Less common causes include bowel tumors, fecal impaction, pregnancy, and metabolic disorders (e.g., hypothyroidism, diabetes, and hypercalcemia). The common causes of constipation can be divided into three categories—simple, disordered motility, and secondary constipation. *Simple constipation* usually results from a diet that contains excessive refined carbohydrates and is deficient in fiber. It may be influenced by environmental factors such as uncomfortable lavatories, suppression of the urge to defecate, and travel. *Disordered motility,* the next most common category, is seen with idiopathic slow transit (most common in the elderly), idiopathic megacolon and megarectum (more common in children), irritable bowel syndrome, and uncomplicated diverticular disease. *Secondary constipation,* the third common form of constipation, can be a response to drugs (e.g., codeine, morphine, analgesics, phenytoin, aluminum-containing antacids, anti-Parkinsonian drugs, cough mixtures, and antidepressants), chronic laxation, prolonged immobilization, and organic disease of the anus, rectum, or colon (anal fissures, strictures, and carcinoma).

NATURE OF PATIENT

Constipation is uncommon in neonates; if it occurs, it is usually due to *anal fissures* or *feeding problems.* In children, the most common cause of constipation is a change in their daily habits or environment. The earlier in childhood constipation begins, the greater the likelihood of an organic cause.

Disorders of defecation in children are common, difficult to manage, and negatively perceived by the family. Approximately 85 to 95 per cent of constipation in children is functional. In children from 6 months to 3 years, it frequently results from some psychologic cause. Early diagnosis of psychologic causes of constipation in children facilitates treatment. In some cases, toilet training may have occurred recently, or constipation may have developed because the child had a condition, such as a rectal fissure, that caused painful defecation. Fearing painful defecation, the child suppresses the urge to defecate, perpetuating the production of hard, dry stools, which continue to irritate the rectal fissure.

In adults, most constipation is due to *dietary fiber deficiency* or *laxative habit.* Laxative use is more common in women. Constipation is a common complaint in the elderly, although 80 to 90 per cent of patients over the age of 60 years have one or more bowel movements per day. Despite this, 50 per cent of patients over the age of 60 years use laxatives. This apparent discrepancy may be due to the fact that older patients have a greater preoccupation with bowel function than do younger individuals. Constipation in elderly patients most often is due to inappropriate diet, decreased activity, poor dentition, use of constipating medications, and impaired motility. Constipation ranks with joint

Betty L. McMullen

pain, dizziness, forgetfulness, depression, and bladder problems as one of the major causes of misery in older patients.

Obstipation (the regular passage of hard stools at 3- to 5-day intervals) and *fecal impaction* are most common in elderly patients. Patients with fecal impaction occasionally will have continuous soiling (liquid passing around hard stools), which they describe as diarrhea. Elderly patients who are confined to bed, drink small amounts of fluid, or take constipating drugs are particularly vulnerable to fecal impaction. Although fecal impaction is more frequent in the elderly, the physician must be aware that it can occur in any patient subjected to sudden immobility, bed rest, or a marked change in diet or fluid consumption.

Tumors of the bowel are uncommon in children and young adults, but their frequency increases after age 40 years. **In any patient over 40 years who presents with recent constipation or marked change in bowel habit, carcinoma of the colon and rectum must be ruled out.**

NATURE OF SYMPTOMS

The most important factor in determining when constipation should be investigated for a serious cause or treated symptomatically and by dietary modification is whether the constipation is chronic or of recent onset. Patients who have long-standing constipation and those whose constipation developed with a recent depressive illness, change in diet, recent debility, or ingestion of constipating medicine can be treated symptomatically. Their clinical status should be reassessed after a few weeks of appropriate therapy. **Patients with unexplained constipation of recent onset or a sudden aggravation of existing constipation associated with abdominal pain, passing of blood or mucus, a progressive decrease in the number of movements per day, or a substantial increase in laxative requirements should be investigated even in the absence of abnormal physical findings.** These patients should have a sigmoidoscopic examination as well as a barium enema, and stools should be tested for occult blood. **It is notable that constipation occurs in less than one third of patients with carcinoma of the colon and is less common than diarrhea in these patients.**

Ribbon-like stools suggest a motility disorder. They can also be caused by an organic narrowing of the distal colon or sigmoid. A progressive decrease in the caliber of the stools suggests an organic lesion. If the patient complains of stools that have a "toothpaste-like" caliber, a fecal impaction should be suspected.

Tumors of the descending colon are more frequent in older adults. Right-sided lesions increase in frequency as the patient get older. One third of colon cancers in patients older than 80 years are right-sided, and less than one-half of these patients have altered bowel habits. They usually present late with an anemia or a palpable mass on the right side of the colon.

ASSOCIATED SYMPTOMS

In children, simple constipation often is associated with abdominal distention, decreased appetite, irritability, reduced activity, and soiling. Children who are obstipated (i.e., those who pass hard, dry stools every 3 to 5 days) also may have overflow soiling. If soiling persists after the constipation or obstipation has improved, the physician should search for some *psychologic disturbance*; fecal impaction is relatively rare in children. When children have abdominal distention associated with constipation, it usually is caused by improper diet or decreased motility; intestinal obstruction is a rare cause of constipation in children. When observed in children, signs of psychologic disturbances (e.g., acting out, school problems, and difficulties with interpersonal relationships) should suggest that the constipation has a psychologic etiology.

If constipation is associated with steatorrhea and greenish-yellow stools, a *small bowel* or *pancreatic lesion* should be suspected. Constipation with early morning rushes, hypogastric cramps, tenesmus, and passage of blood per rectum all suggest that the constipation is of colonic origin.

In adults, colicky pain, abdominal distention, anemia, decreased effectiveness of laxatives, weight loss, anorexia, and blood, pus, or mucus in the stool should suggest a *colonic tumor*. It should be remembered that weight loss, anorexia, and anemia usually are observed only in the late phases of colonic tumors. Rectal discomfort, leakage of stool, bleeding, urgency, and tenesmus, diarrhea alternating with constipation, and rectal prolapse all suggest a *rectosigmoid tumor*. In contrast, abdominal distention and sudden onset of obstipation suggest a more proximal colon lesion.

Constipation—particularly if it alternates with diarrhea or is accompanied by passage of hard scybala or intermittent left- or right-sided iliac pain that occasionally radiates through to the back—is likely due to the *irritable bowel syndrome*. A change in stool frequency or consistency, associated with abdominal pain, also suggests an irritable colon as do abdominal distention and mucus in the stools.

Fecal incontinence (which some patients actually describe as diarrhea) should suggest a *fecal impaction*. Usually, patients with this condition must strain at stool; do not have normal, formed stools; often have a "toothpaste-like" stool; and often have continuous soiling. Rectal examination usually reveals large quantities of hard feces in the rectal ampulla.

Constipation that develops after painful *hemorrhoids* suggests that the constipation is secondary to suppression of defecation because it induces pain. Patients with this condition, as well as others with local anorectal problems, often report blood in the bowel movements. When questioned, they usually recognize that the blood is on the surface of their stool, on the toilet paper, or in the toilet bowl rather than mixed in with the stool.

PRECIPITATING AND AGGRAVATING FACTORS

Patients and their family members should be questioned about stressful problems such as divorce, death of a spouse, or loss of a job. It is interesting to note that 20 per cent of children have moderate constipation when they begin to become effectively toilet-trained. Functional constipation may be precipitated by admission to the hospital, traveling, suppression of the urge to defecate, uncomfortable lavatory environment (such as a latrine), and immobilization. Reduction in laxative dose or change in brand of laxative occasionally precipitates constipation.

In elderly patients, constipation can be aggravated by limited variety in meals, decreased fiber intake, poor dentition, increased costs of fresh, high-fiber foods (e.g., fruits and vegetables), impaired motility, decreased fluid intake, debilitating illnesses, confinement to bed, and frequent ingestion of constipating drugs.

Certain drugs commonly cause constipation. These include antacids that contain aluminum hydroxide or calcium, anticholinergics, anti-Parkinsonian drugs, diuretics, tricyclic antidepressants, opiates, phenytoin, codeine (in analgesics or cough medicine), morphine-containing drugs, calcium channel blockers, iron-containing compounds, and certain antihypertensive and antiseizure drugs.

AMELIORATING FACTORS

A diet that is high in fiber (whole grain cereals, bran or vegetable fiber) and low in refined sugar often alleviates constipation. Many patients find that weight-reduction diets that are low in carbohydrates and high in fiber relieve constipation. Increased fluid intake, particularly in patients who do not drink enough fluids or who take diuretics, often is helpful. Relief of painful anorectal problems frequently alleviates constipation. If a change in daily routine (e.g., rushing off to work or giving up the morning cigarette) has caused constipation, instructing the patient to readjust daily activities to permit bowel movements at the time of the urge to defecate often is effective.

PHYSICAL FINDINGS

A rectal examination should be performed in all patients with a significant complaint of constipation. This examination allows the physician to determine whether the rectum is full or empty, whether there is an anorectal problem (e.g., fissure or hemorrhoids), and whether there is a rectal mass, and it allows him to obtain a stool specimen that will be observed for occult blood. The physician should conduct an abdominal examination, with special attention to the colon, to detect palpable masses (fecal or otherwise) or abdominal tenderness. Normally, the colon is neither palpable nor tender. If the colon can be palpated and if it is tender—particularly over the descending or ascending regions—an irritable or spastic colon is probable. Stigmata of myxedema and abdominal distention should suggest that the constipation is secondary to hypothyroidism. Anemia, manifested by tachycardia and conjunctival pallor, should suggest a right-sided colonic lesion.

DIAGNOSTIC STUDIES

Examination of stools for occult blood, hematocrit or hemoglobin, and a sedimentation rate are appropriate, inexpensive, and noninvasive tests that the physician should utilize to evaluate constipation. Anoscopy, sigmoidoscopy, colonoscopy, and barium enema also are helpful.

LESS COMMON DIAGNOSTIC CONSIDERATIONS

In neonates, Hirschsprung's disease (aganglionic megacolon) is the most prevalent of the less common causes of constipation. It is important that it be diagnosed early. To differentiate between Hirschsprung's disease and chronic constipation one should be aware that each condition is associated with characteristic symptoms. In Hirschsprung's disease, symptoms usually date from birth, soiling is absent, and the rectum is empty. In cases of chronic constipation, the onset may occur from 6 months to 3 years, soiling is common, and the rectum is usually full of feces. Other less common causes of constipation in children include anorectal stenosis, chronic lead poisoning, hypothyroidism, hyperparathyroidism, medication, anal fissures, allergy to cow's milk, and neurologic abnormalities such as spina bifida.

If constipation is associated with nausea, polyuria, fatigue, and, sometimes, a history of kidney stones, hypercalcemia, although uncommon, may be the cause of the constipation. Other metabolic and endocrinologic causes of constipation include diabetes, pregnancy, and hypo-

DIFFERENTIAL DIAGNOSIS OF CONSTIPATION

CONDITION	NATURE OF PATIENT	NATURE OF SYMPTOMS	ASSOCIATED SYMPTOMS	AMELIO-RATING FACTORS	PRECIPITATING AND AGGRAVATING FACTORS	PHYSICAL FINDINGS	DIAGNOSTIC STUDIES
Simple Constipation Low dietary fiber	Most common cause of constipation in adults	Dry, hard stools Stool frequency less than 5 times/week Straining at stool	In children: May be associated with abdominal distention	Increased dietary fiber Decreased intake of refined carbohydrates	Excessive intake of refined carbohydrates		
Functional (environmental/daily-habit changes)	Most common cause of constipation in children Common cause in adults	Vague abdominal discomfort	In children: Abdominal distention Decreased appetite Irritability Decreased activity Soiling	Resume prior habits	Toilet-training Traveling Uncomfortable lavatories Immobilization		
Disordered Motility Irritable bowel syndrome	Any age, especially young adults	Change in stool frequency and consistency Constipation alternates with diarrhea Mucus in stools	Abdominal distention Abdominal pain	Increased dietary fiber Decreased environmental stresses	Stress	Colon tender to palpation	

Table continued on following page

DIFFERENTIAL DIAGNOSIS OF CONSTIPATION *Continued*

CONDITION	NATURE OF PATIENT	NATURE OF SYMPTOMS	ASSOCIATED SYMPTOMS	AMELIORATING FACTORS	PRECIPITATING AND AGGRAVATING FACTORS	PHYSICAL FINDINGS	DIAGNOSTIC STUDIES
Disordered Motility *Continued* Obstipation/fecal impaction	Most common in elderly or those subject to sudden immobility, bed rest, or decreased fluid consumption	Regular passage of hard stools at 3- to 5-day intervals Possible continuous soiling that patients describe as "diarrhea" "Toothpaste" caliber stools Fecal incontinence Straining at stool				Large quantities of hard feces in rectal ampulla	
Idiopathic slow transit	Most common in elderly	Dry, hard stools Decreased stool frequency		Increased exercise Increased dietary fiber Increased fluids Improved dentition	Decreased exercise Decreased dietary fiber Decreased fluid intake		
Hirschsprung's disease (aganglionic megacolon)	Rare cause of constipation in children	Present from birth Soiling is absent				Rectum is empty	Barium enema
Secondary Constipation Anal fissure	Affects any age	Patient suppresses painful defecation Hard stools	Blood "on surface" of feces, on toilet paper, or in toilet			Anal fissure	Anoscopy

Hemorrhoids	Adults	Patients suppress painful defecation	Blood "on surface" of feces, on toilet paper, or in toilet	Pregnancy Prior hemorrhoid problems	Hemorrhoids	Anoscopy
Drug-induced condition	Chronic laxative users Patients taking other medications Most common in elderly patients		Laxatives Codeine Morphine Analgesics Aluminum-containing antacids Anti-Parkinsonian drugs Cough mixtures Antidepressants			
Bowel tumors	Uncommon in children Frequency increases after age 40 years	Constipation occurs in less than 1/3 of patients with colon cancer (diarrhea is a more common symptom) Early morning rushes Decreased effectiveness of laxatives Blood, pus, or mucus in stool	Elderly patients with right-sided lesions may present late with anemia Weight loss, anorexia Colicky, abdominal pain Abdominal distention		Possible palpable mass	Rectal examination Stool examination for occult blood Colonoscopy Barium enema
Rectosigmoid tumor		Rectal discomfort Stool leakage Urgency, tenesmus Progressive narrowing of stool caliber	Rectal bleeding Rectal prolapse			
Proximal colon tumors		Sudden onset Obstipation	Abdominal distention		Anemia	

thyroidism. Constipation may be the presenting symptom in patients with classic myxedema. Myxedematous patients frequently have an adynamic bowel with moderate abdominal distention. Adynamic bowel also occurs with senility, scleroderma, and spinal cord injuries and diseases. Idiopathic megacolon and megarectum also can produce severe constipation.

Psychiatric causes of constipation include depressive illness and anorexia nervosa. Occasionally, constipation is induced in depressed patients as the result of the anticholinergic effect of antidepressant drugs. Marked prostatic enlargement may contribute to constipation. Disease or weakness of the abdominal muscles, neurologic diseases, diverticular diseases, occult rectal prolapse, pancreatic carcinoma, and lead poisoning are all rare causes of constipation.

Selected References

Banks, S., and Marks, I. N.: The etiology, diagnosis and treatment of constipation and diarrhea in geriatric patients. South Am. Med. J. *51*:409–414, 1977.

Bramble, M. G., and Record, C. O.: Drug-induced gastrointestinal disease. Drugs *15*:451–463, 1978.

Lloyd-Still, J. D.: Constipation in children. Comp. Ther. *3(9)*:35–39, 1977.

Nivatvongs, S., and Hooks, V. H.: Chronic constipation: Important aspects of work-up and management. Postgrad. Med. *74*:313–323, 1983.

Painter, N. S.: Constipation. Practitioner *224*:387–391, 1980.

Steinheber, F. U.: Interpretation of gastrointestinal symptoms in the elderly. Med. Clin. North Am. *60*:1141–1157, 1976.

Thompson, W. G., and Heaton, K. W.: Functional bowel disorders in apparently healthy people. Gastroenterology *79*:283–288, 1980.

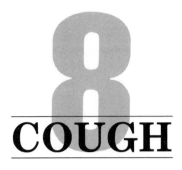

COUGH

When evaluating patients with a cough, the physician should remember that (1) most healthy people rarely cough, and (2) the main function of coughing is airway clearance. The complaint of cough should be taken seriously, since it is one of the few ways by which abnormalities of the respiratory tree manifest themselves. Cough can be initiated by irritation of upper or lower airways. The most common causes of an acute cough are *infections* (most commonly *viral upper respiratory tract infection, bronchitis,* and *laryngitis*), *allergies* (often seasonal), and *postnasal drip.* The common causes of a chronic cough include *bronchitis, postnasal drip, chronic obstructive pulmonary disease (COPD), heart failure, tuberculosis, lung tumor,* and *habit.* The most common causes of recurrent cough in children are *asthma, viral bronchitis,* and *allergies.*

NATURE OF PATIENT

Viral infections are the most common cause of acute cough at all ages. This is particularly true of preschool children and even more likely if they are in close daily contact with many other children. In school-age children, *Mycoplasma pneumoniae* is quite common. Because its incubation period is long (approximately 21 days), infection spreads slowly. *Bacterial pneumonias* also cause coughing and have their highest incidence in winter months. **Recurrent viral bronchitis is most prevalent in preschool and young school-age children and is the most common cause of a persistent cough in children of all ages.** There may be a genetically determined host susceptibility to frequently recurring bronchitis. Young patients with recurrent cough often are asthmatic. Physicians should be suspicious of underlying asthma contributing to a recurrent cough when there is a family history of allergies, atopy, or asthma.

A chronic cough in children frequently is due to *allergic rhinitis, chronic sinusitis,* or *enlarged adenoids.* Although rare, chronic cough in very young children (under 12 months) should suggest congenital malformations or neonatal infections, including viral and chlamydial pneumonias. Other relatively rare causes of chronic cough in young infants include recurrent aspiration of milk, saliva, or gastric contents and cystic fibrosis. A chronic cough in children between 1 and 5 years of age should suggest bronchiectasis or cystic fibrosis after the more common causes have been ruled out.

Chronic cough in adults most commonly is due to *chronic bronchitis* (especially in smokers), *asthma, environmental irritants, allergies, postnasal drip,* and *habit.* In older adults, any chronic cough without an obvious explanation should suggest *tumor* or *tuberculosis.*

NATURE OF SYMPTOMS

When the cough is of sudden onset and associated with fever or symptoms of an acute infection, a *viral* etiology is most likely. In these cases, the cough is noisy, produces minimal sputum, and often is worse at night. With *bacterial and mycoplasma infections,* cough often is the most prominent symptom. Its onset may occur over hours or days, and the sputum produced is usually thick and yellowish. In *Mycoplasma* infections, the cough may be severe and persist for 1 to 4 months, although all other signs and symptoms abate within 7 to 10 days.

The cough caused by a viral upper respiratory infection or viral bronchitis usually lasts for 7 to 10 days. If the cough persists for longer than 14 days, there may be a secondary bacterial infection. If the cough is associated with shortness of breath and bilateral wheezing, asthma is likely. The cough of asthma usually is nonproductive; if it is productive, there is a minimal amount of clear mucoid secretions.

Patients with an acute or chronic cough secondary to a *postnasal drip* may not be aware of this condition. They should be questioned about whether they are aware of swallowing mucus, frequent throat-clearing, hawking, or a cough that is worse in the morning. Oral examination may reveal mucoid secretions in the posterior pharynx.

A nocturnal cough associated with shortness of breath should suggest *paroxysmal nocturnal dyspnea* or *congestive heart failure.* A nocturnal cough without associated dyspnea indicates an *allergic origin.* A cough that recurs in late afternoon or early evening also often is of allergic origin. This type of cough may occur in people who work in the city (where the pollen count is low) and then return in late afternoon or evening to their suburban home (where the pollen count is higher). A seasonal incidence of cough is highly suggestive of an allergic etiology.

In smokers, a chronic minimally productive cough, often worse in the morning, probably is related to the irritant effect of *inhaling tobacco smoke*. Although this is more common in cigarette smokers, it also can occur in cigar and pipe smokers who inhale.

The evaluation of all patients whose chief complaint is cough should include a complete history, with particular attention given to duration and character of the cough, smoking history, environmental and occupational experiences, antecedent allergies, asthma, sinusitis, symptoms of upper respiratory tract infections, heartburn, or shortness of breath or fainting while coughing ("tussive syncope").

ASSOCIATED SYMPTOMS

If a runny nose, a sore throat, or generalized aches and pains are present, an *infectious* etiology of the cough is most probable. The presence of fever, chills, exudative or nonexudative pharyngitis, conjunctivitis, otitis, abdominal pain, headache, or pleuritic chest pain suggests the presence of *bacteria* or *Mycoplasma*. Since a *postnasal drip* (one cause of cough) may coexist with other conditions that produce chronic cough, such as *bronchiectasis, heart failure, bronchogenic carcinoma* and *tuberculosis,* the physician should not automatically assume that the postnasal drip is the only cause of the cough.

If sneezing, a boggy edematous nasal mucosa, conjunctivitis, tearing, itching of the roof of the mouth, or itching of the eyes is present, an *allergic* etiology of an otherwise unexplained cough is most likely.

Elderly patients, whose physical activity may be restricted by arthritis or other associated disease, may not present with the usual symptom of dyspnea on exertion. The chief complaint instead may be a chronic unexplained cough that may occur only at night while the patient is recumbent or that may worsen at night. **Therefore, any unexplained nocturnal cough in elderly patients should suggest congestive heart failure.**

PRECIPITATING AND AGGRAVATING FACTORS

In all cases of unexplained cough (particularly in children) when exercise precipitates the cough, an asthmatic etiology should be suspected, even when there is no typical wheezing. Some coughs are precipitated by exposure to very dry, superheated air. This frequently is the case in patients whose homes are heated with forced hot air. This cough may be exacerbated by sensitivity to spores in the dry, super-heated air.

Chronic debilitating conditions such as alcoholism, malnutrition, diabetes uremia, leukemia, and antitumor therapy may facilitate the development of infections that produce coughing. Long-term *cigarette smoking,* chronic exposure to *industrial irritants,* or *chronic respiratory disease* in childhood predispose the patient to the development of lung disease and cough.

Patients with *allergic rhinitis* and *chronic sinusitis* are predisposed to postnasal drip and its resultant cough. This cough may be worse at night, when the patient is recumbent, because more mucus drips into the throat when one is in this position. **Other coughs that are worse when the patient is in the recumbent posture or at night include those caused by allergies, paroxysmal nocturnal dyspnea, asthma, reflux esophagitis, and breathing dry, hot air.**

AMELIORATING FACTORS

In patients with allergic rhinitis, antihistamine therapy may ameli-orate coughing by reducing secretions in the nose and paranasal sinuses. If smokers with chronic cough stop smoking, the cough usually abates. In one study of 200 patients, "smokers cough" stopped in 77 per cent of patients who ceased smoking, and a marked reduction in coughing was noted in 13 per cent. The majority of the 77 per cent in whom the cough disappeared lost their cough after 1 month of no smoking.

PHYSICAL FINDINGS

Special attention should be paid to examination of the ears, nose, mouth, throat (including indirect laryngoscopy), sinuses, neck, lungs, and cardiovascular system. The patient should always be asked to cough so that the cough characteristics may be heard and the sputum examined. A mucopurulent sputum suggests *infection,* although some *allergic* coughs are productive. If a large number of eosinophils are observed in a stained sputum specimen, an allergic etiology is probable.

In patients with an acute cough secondary to infection, the chest examination often is normal, but the pharynx may be injected or pale, boggy, and swollen. The sinuses should be palpated, percussed, and transilluminated for evidence of *sinusitis.* When the mucosa of the nose and oropharynx has a cobblestone appearance (from chronic stimulation of submucosal lymphoid follicles) *postnasal drip* probably is causing the cough. If the lung fields are hyperresonant to percussion and auscultation reveals distant breath sounds, scattered rhonchi or wheezes, or prolonged expiration, *chronic obstructive pulmonary disease* should be suspected.

It should be noted that cough may be the earliest symptom of *heart failure,* particularly in patients with pulmonary hypertension or mitral stenosis. Cough may occur before the usual findings of chronic congestive heart failure (rales, edema, tachycardia, gallop) are evident.

DIAGNOSTIC STUDIES

Tests used to determine the etiology of cough include complete blood count, an eosinophil count, sinus and chest radiographs, and cytologic and microscopic sputum examination. Pulmonary function tests, bronchoscopy, and cardiovascular studies may help in some cases.

The chest radiograph may be negative in some patients with diffuse infiltrative lung disease. Approximately 5 per cent of patients with *sarcoidosis* have normal chest films. Likewise, patients with cough due to a tracheobronchial lesion may have a normal chest radiograph.

If an asthmatic cough is suspected and wheezing is absent, pulmonary function tests that measure response to isoproterenol should be performed. In rare instances, bronchial provocation tests may be performed, but only with extreme care. If these tests are positive, asthma is the most likely cause of the cough.

A simple outpatient diagnostic test for a cough due to congestive heart failure is the administration of a potent oral diuretic for 2 to 3 days. If the patient diureses several pounds and at the same time demonstrates marked improvement of the cough, one may assume that the cough was due to pulmonary congestion secondary to heart failure.

LESS COMMON DIAGNOSTIC
CONSIDERATIONS

Most people who complain of cough do not have bronchogenic carcinoma. However, 70 to 90 per cent of patients with bronchogenic carcinoma develop a cough at some time during the course of their disease. Various studies have documented that cough was the presenting symptom in 21 to 87 per cent of patients with bronchogenic carcinoma. The possibility of bronchogenic carcinoma is especially strong in chronic cigarette smokers who develop a cough that lasts for months or who demonstrate a marked change in the character of their cough. Pulmonary tumors often are characterized by change in the cough pattern, hemoptysis, chest pain, or enlarged supraclavicular nodes.

In patients with a lung abscess, cough is the dominant symptom more often than bloody sputum, pain, or dyspnea. The cough observed in patients with bronchiectasis usually is of long duration; productive of loose, moist, purulent sputum; and occasionally associated with hemoptysis. The cough of tuberculosis often is chronic (although it may be acute), and associated with hemoptysis, fever, night sweats, apical rales, and weight loss.

The physician should be particularly suspicious of disorders of the trachea or larynx in patients with inspiratory stridor or a dry, brassy, high-pitched, and unproductive cough. If the cough is associated with marked dyspnea, tachypnea, tachycardia, calf tenderness, prolonged immobility, atrial fibrillation, pleural friction, or hemoptysis, pulmonary embolism should be suspected.

Patients ranging in age from 3 months to 6 years may develop croup (laryngotracheal bronchitis). This cough has a barking quality. Intercostal retraction with inspiration, inspiratory or expiratory wheezing, hoarseness, and difficulty with air movement all suggest this potentially critical condition. Hospitalization for intensive therapy may be necessary. In young children, the possibility of an inhaled foreign body also must be considered as the cause of coughing.

A rare, frequently written about, and usually unrecognized cause of chronic cough is impaction of cerumen, foreign body, or hair in the ear canal, which stimulates a cough through a reflex (ear-cough) mechanism. This cough is triggered by irritation of the external auditory canal or tympanic membrane.

Exposure to noxious gases, dusts, industrial pollutants, and smog can produce cough. This is particularly true in people who have underlying lung disease.

Reflux esophagitis does not usually present with cough, but patients with this condition may cough when recumbent if they aspirate small quantities of fluid.

Ornithosis, although rare, should be considered in patients who have a dry, hacking, unproductive cough with fever and who are in contact with fowl or pet birds. These patients often have a normal physical examination except for fever and cough. Coccidioidomycosis should be suspected if cough develops after the patient has visited an endemic area such as the San Joaquin Valley.

When complete history and thorough physical and laboratory examinations reveal no cause of cough, a subdiaphragmatic process (abscess or tumor) should be considered. If no organic cause for a chronic cough is found, a psychogenic etiology may be strongly considered. In such cases, patients do not cough at night and often can stop coughing if so instructed. This cough is rarely productive. In children, it may be an attention-getting device; in adults, it may be associated with other signs of hysterical behavior.

DIFFERENTIAL DIAGNOSIS OF COUGH

CONDITION	NATURE OF PATIENT	NATURE OF SYMPTOMS	ASSOCIATED SYMPTOMS	AMELIO-RATING FACTORS	PRECIPITATING AND AGGRAVATING FACTORS	PHYSICAL FINDINGS	DIAGNOSTIC STUDIES
Acute Cough Viral upper respiratory tract infections	Most common cause of acute cough in all ages	Acute onset of noisy cough (over hours or days) Cough is worse at night and may persist for 7 to 10 days Sputum is thick and yellowish, but minimal amount is produced	Fever Runny nose Sore throat General aches and pains			Pharynx may be injected or pale, boggy and swollen Coarse rhonchi	
Mycoplasma Bronchitis or pneumonia	Common cause of acute cough in school-aged children Frequent cause of persistent cough in adults	Long incubation period (approximately 21 days) Severe cough may persist for 1 to 4 months Other symptoms (fever, etc.) abate within 10 days	Same as for bacterial pneumonia but not usually as severe			Scattered rales Signs of pneumonia	Chest radiograph
Viral bronchitis	Recurrent infections are the most common cause of persistent cough in children who are often asthmatic	Cough may persist for 7 to 10 days	Fever				
Allergies	History of allergy in family	Minimally productive May be nocturnal Recurrent cough without dyspnea May have seasonal incidence	Sneezing Conjunctivitis Tearing Itching of eyes and roof of mouth Postnasal drip	Antihistamine		Boggy, edematous nasal mucosa	Stained sputum smear for eosinophils

Table continued on following page

DIFFERENTIAL DIAGNOSIS OF COUGH *Continued*

CONDITION	NATURE OF PATIENT	NATURE OF SYMPTOMS	ASSOCIATED SYMPTOMS	AMELIORATING FACTORS	PRECIPITATING AND AGGRAVATING FACTORS	PHYSICAL FINDINGS	DIAGNOSTIC STUDIES
Acute Cough *Continued* Bacterial pneumonia		Noisy cough Incidence highest in winter Acute onset Cough is worse at night	Fever, chills Signs of acute infection Pharyngitis Conjunctivitis Otitis Abdominal pain Headache Pleuritic chest pain		Chronic debilitating conditions	Signs of pneumonia	Chest radiograph Sputum and blood cultures
Chronic or Recurrent Cough Postnasal drip	May not be aware of condition	Frequent throat-clearing and hawking Cough worse in morning			Recumbency Allergic rhinitis Chronic sinusitis	Mucoid secretions seen in posterior pharynx Palpation, percussion, and transillumination of sinuses reveal sinusitis Mucosa of nose and oropharynx has cobblestone appearance	

Asthma	May have family history of allergies, atopy, or asthma	Recurrent cough that is minimally or not at all productive (if productive, secretions are clear and mucoid)	Shortness of breath		Exercise May be worse during seasonal allergies	Bilateral wheezing	Pulmonary function tests Response to isoproterenol
Chronic obstructive pulmonary disease (COPD)	Elderly		Shortness of breath			Lungs are hyperresonant to percussion Auscultation reveals distant breath sounds, scattered rhonchi, wheezes, or prolonged expiration	Pulmonary function tests
Chronic bronchitis	Most common cause of chronic cough in adults (especially smokers)	May be minimally productive Often worse in morning		Smoking		Scattered rhonchi	
Congestive heart failure	Elderly patients present differently May have only chronic, unexplained cough	Cough often is nocturnal	Dyspnea on exertion Paroxysmal nocturnal dyspnea	Diuresis	Recumbency Exercise	Rales Pitting edema Tachycardia Gallop	Chest radiograph Potent diuretic for 2 to 3 days should improve patient's symptoms

Selected References

Brashear, R. E.: Cough: diagnostic considerations with normal chest roentgenograms. J. Fam. Pract. *15*:979–985, 1982.

Fedson, D. S., and Rusthaven, J.: Acute lower respiratory disease. Primary Care *6*:13–41, 1979.

Irwin, R. S., and Demers, R. R.: Management of the patient with cough. Comp. Ther. *5*:43–49, 1979.

Irwin, R. S., Rosen, M. J., and Braman, S. S.: Cough: a comprehensive review. Arch. Int. Med. *137*:1186–1191, 1977.

Loudon, R. G.: Cough: a symptom and a sign. Basics of RD. Am. Thorac. Soc. Vol. 9, No. 4, 1–6, March, 1981.

Mellis, C. M.: Evaluation and treatment of chronic cough in children. Pediatr. Clin. North Am. *26*:553–564, 1979.

DIARRHEA

In this chapter, *diarrhea* is defined as an increase in frequency, fluidity, or volume of bowel movements relative to the usual habit for an individual. It is notable that acute diarrhea is second in frequency only to acute respiratory tract disease in American families. Diarrhea most commonly is due to *acute gastroenteritis* caused by a virus or, less commonly, by bacteria or protozoans. Other common causes of diarrhea include *irritable bowel syndrome* (also called irritable colon, mucous colitis, or functional diarrhea) and ingestion of *antibiotics, antiinflammatory agents, magnesium-containing substances, alcohol,* and excessive (intolerable) amounts of *lactose.* Patients with *diabetes* also frequently suffer with diarrhea.

When evaluating a patient's complaint of diarrhea, the physician must question the usual frequency and pattern of bowel movement; the current pattern of bowel movements; the presence of nocturnal diarrhea; the presence of blood or mucus in the stool; travel within the United States or abroad; recent diet changes; exacerbation of diarrhea by particular foods such as dairy products; recent drug ingestion; change in nature of food intake; and any significant previous medical or surgical history.

NATURE OF PATIENT

In all age groups, *viral gastroenteritis* is the most common cause of acute diarrhea. This usually is a benign, self-limited condition in adults; it can, however, result in severe dehydration in infants and children. In infants under 3 years of age, *rotovirus* is responsible for about 50 per cent of wintertime, nonbacterial gastroenteritis. This winter peak is even greater in temperate climates, such as that found in the United States. *Salmonella,* as a cause of gastroenteritis, is more common in children aged 1 to 4 years. Epidemics of *Shigella* have been noted in children aged 1 to 4 years and in people living in closed environments, particularly those with substandard sanitation (e.g., prisons and custodial institutions for children and retarded individuals).

Giardiasis is not common in children, but infants are susceptible. Infants may be quite ill in contrast to adults, who are often asymptomatic. However, acute or subacute diarrhea with marked symptomatology also may occur in some adults with giardiasis. Reports of symptomatic giardiasis have increased, primarily among hikers and campers, who are most likely to drink *Giardia*-infected water.

Whenever diarrhea in infants less than 1 year of age corresponds to increased ingestion of dairy products, *lactose intolerance* (lactase deficiency) should be suspected. This form of diarrhea is not limited to infants and young children: It is being reported with increasing frequency in adults, particularly those of Mediterranean extraction. Although these individuals may not have previously demonstrated lactose intolerance, it should be remembered that lactase production normally decreases with age; in some people, this decrease is more pronounced. In these individuals, diarrhea seems to follow acute or chronic ingestion of large quantities of lactose, as found in milk, cheeses, ice cream, and other dairy products. A transient lactase deficiency is common following infectious gastroenteritis.

Middle-aged women with chronic diarrhea are more likely to have functional diarrhea or an *irritable colon.* This condition seems to have a predilection for young women who are raising children, especially if they have the added responsibility of a job outside the home. It affects other stressed individuals as well. Another form of diarrhea reported to be more frequent among middle-aged women is the misuse or surreptitious use of purgatives. Patients who use laxatives surreptitiously often demonstrate other features of hysterical behavior. The addition of NaOH to the stool provides a simple test for some forms of laxative abuse. Ex-Lax, Feen-a-Mint and Correctol contain phenolphthalein, which turns the stool red when alkali (NaOH) is added to the stool.

Diabetics with associated neurologic dysfunction also may suffer with chronic diarrhea. Some diabetics have gastric stasis and poor bowel motility. This permits bacterial overgrowth in the small bowel, which may produce an uncontrollable, explosive, postprandial diarrhea. In some instances, patients with this condition refrain from eating before leaving their homes to avoid uncontrollable diarrhea at an inconvenient time. A therapeutic trial with tetracycline may effectively stop the diarrhea by combatting the bacterial overgrowth.

Although acute diarrhea usually is benign and self-limited, the following patients are particularly prone to serious complications from acute and, certainly, from chronic diarrhea: neonates, elderly people, patients with sickle cell disease, and those who are immunocompromised (by underlying disease or chemotherapy).

NATURE OF SYMPTOMS

A useful approach to the differential diagnosis of diarrhea is to separate *acute diarrhea* (which has an abrupt onset, lasts less than 1 week, and may be associated with nausea, vomiting, or fever) from *chronic diarrhea* (in which the initial episode lasts longer than 2 weeks or symptoms continue to recur over months or years). **The acute onset of diarrhea in a previously healthy patient, without signs or symptoms of other organ system involvement, suggests an infectious etiology that most commonly is viral.**

Chronic diarrhea most frequently is caused by the irritable bowel syndrome. Irritable bowel syndrome may present as chronic or intermittent diarrhea (which classically alternates with constipation) or as flareups of diarrhea that occur during stressful periods. A history of hard, often marble-like stools alternating with soft bowel movements, especially if associated with mucus in the toilet bowel or on the surface of the stool, also suggests *irritable bowel syndrome*. It is important to remember that although a patient suffers from a chronic irritable colon, the possibility of a superimposed case of viral gastroenteritis, salmonellosis, or giardiasis must still be considered. In such patients, a new etiology of diarrhea should be sought if there is a change in the character of, or exacerbation of, the usual diarrhea associated with their irritable colon.

Persistent diarrhea with frothy, foul-smelling stools that sometimes float suggests a *pancreatic* or *small bowel* etiology. Foul-smelling, watery, explosive diarrhea with mucus often is seen in *giardiasis*. The latency period may be 1 to 3 weeks. The onset of diarrhea due to giardiasis may be acute or gradual; it may persist for several weeks or up to 6 months.

Functional diarrhea almost never occurs at night and rarely awakens the patient. It is, however, commonly present in the morning. There may be copious amount of mucus, but there is rarely blood in the stool, except that from hemorrhoidal bleeding. If questioned, the patient may admit to noticing undigested food in the stool and rectal urgency.

ASSOCIATED SYMPTOMS

It often is diagnostically helpful for one to classify acute diarrhea into two groups: *toxin-mediated diarrhea* (or "small bowel" diarrhea) and *infectious diarrhea* ("colonic diarrhea"). Patients with a toxin-mediated ("small bowel") diarrhea have an abrupt onset (often a few hours after eating potentially contaminated foods) of large volume, watery diarrhea associated with variable nausea, vomiting, increased salivation, crampy abdominal pain, general malaise, but little or no fever. The onset of neurologic symptoms in association with diarrhea suggests *Clostridia toxin (botulism)*. Diarrhea of an infectious etiology should be suspected if there is a history of prior good health, acute onset of diarrhea, and no signs or symptoms of involvement of systems other than the gastrointestinal tract. This type of diarrhea is due to *colonic mucosal invasion* and has also been referred to as a *dysentery syndrome.* The presence of fever, vomiting, nausea, abdominal cramps, headaches, general malaise, and myalgia along with a watery diarrhea suggests a *viral, Salmonella,* or *Campylobacter gastroenteritis*. Diarrhea of *colonic origin* should be suspected if fever, early morning rushes, hypogastric cramps, tenesmus, blood in the stools, or soft stools mixed with copious mucus are associated with diarrhea. Patients with fever and symptoms of small bowel or colonic diarrhea may have *shigellosis;* this is more common in summer. Diarrhea due to *Salmonella* may have an acute or subacute onset, or may even present as chronic diarrhea. When a patient known to have intermittent chronic diarrhea due to an irritable colon presents with an increase in diarrhea, the cause may be additional stress or a superimposed infectious diarrhea (e.g., *Salmonella*) superimposed on an irritable colon. *Campylobacter jejuni* has recently been implicated in a large number of cases of foodborne diarrhea. It is usually associated with fever, bloody diarrhea, and abdominal pain.

Blood on the surface of stools or on toilet paper suggests blood of anal origin, most often a bleeding hemorrhoid or small anal fissure, particularly if the bleeding occurs after hard stools. Copious bleeding or blood mixed with the stools, however, suggests a more serious cause, such as *ulcerative colitis*. Marked weight loss associated with persistent diarrhea and frothy, foul-smelling stools that sometimes float suggests a pancreatic or small bowel cause of *steatorrhea* and diarrhea. When acute diarrhea and severe vomiting (out of proportion to the diarrhea) begin 2 to 4 hours after eating potentially contaminated foods (especially milk products or meats), a *toxic staphylococcal gastroenteritis* should be suspected. The diagnosis is confirmed presumptively if these symptoms also developed in several other people who ate the same foods.

In addition to foul-smelling, watery, explosive mucoid stools, patients with giardiasis may have increased flatulence, nausea, and, in severe cases, anorexia and weight loss. Some patients complain of abdominal distention and occasionally greasy stools.

Diarrhea associated with perianal excoriation (related to acidic stools), abdominal distention, occasional vomiting, fever, anorexia, and, in children, failure to thrive indicates *lactose intolerance*.

The presence of muscle weakness, lassitude, or hypokalemia can be seen in all patients with protracted, copious diarrhea but should make the physician suspicious of surreptitious *laxative abuse,* particularly if other components of a hysteric personality are present.

PRECIPITATING AND AGGRAVATING FACTORS

Drug-induced diarrhea should be suspected if diarrhea develops after the administration of antibiotics or other drugs. The most commonly implicated antibiotics are ampicillin, tetracycline, lincomycin, clindamycin, and chloramphenicol. The diarrhea ranges from mild and watery with nonspecific crampy abdominal pain and low-grade fever to a severe colitis with pseudomembrane formation. *Pseudomembranous enterocolitis* is life-threatening and is of the colonic or dysentery type. It is more common if several different antibiotics have been administered but classically is due to a clindamycin-permitted *Clostridium difficile* superinfection. Symptoms may begin during or after the course of antibiotic therapy. In addition to antibiotics, magnesium-containing antacids, guanethidine, methyldopa, digitalis, beta blockers, systemic anti-inflammatory agents, iron-containing compounds, laxative abuse, high dosage of salicylates, colchicine, quinidine, and phenothiazine agents can cause diarrhea.

If the onset of diarrhea is temporally related to acute stress, particularly *emotional,* a functional etiology is probable. In these instances, the onset of diarrhea may be gradual or acute, and the duration may be protracted.

Ingestion of *contaminated water* or *food* may occur at any time, but especially during travel abroad or camping, thus producing "traveler's diarrhea."

AMELIORATING FACTORS

The diarrhea of *lactose intolerance* abates with fasting or avoidance of foods that contain lactose. Functional diarrhea is alleviated with decreased stress.

PHYSICAL FINDINGS

Physical examination must include a careful abdominal examination and, in some instances, a rectal examination. Fever in association with acute diarrhea suggests an infectious etiology. The colon may be tender to palpation in patients with the irritable bowel syndrome. Stools should be examined with the naked eye for blood or mucus and microscopically for fecal leukocytes, ova, and parasites.

DIAGNOSTIC STUDIES

Studies have shown that a specific etiologic agent cannot be isolated in approximately 60 per cent of patients with acute gastroenteritis. Examination of patients with persistent, unexplained diarrhea should include colonoscopic examination with particular attention to the colonic mucosa. Frequently, this helps establish the cause of diarrhea when radiographs and routine sigmoidoscopy are negative. Patients with invasive (so-called colonic) diarrhea have an erythematous colonic mucosa that may have ecchymoses, friability, excess mucus, and small ulcerations. These ulcerations must be differentiated from the ragged ulcers of *ulcerative colitis* and the discrete, punched out ulcers that are almost pathognomonic of *amebic colitis.*

In addition to obtaining a precise history, the physician must examine the stool for fecal polymorphonuclear or mononuclear leukocytes. It is a simple test: A fleck of mucus or liquid stool is placed on a microscope slide, mixed with an equal volume of Loeffler methylene blue, and examined after 2 or 3 minutes with the "high, dry" objective. Since fecal leukocyte production is stimulated by bacteria that invade the colonic mucosa, these leukocytes are frequently seen in infections caused by *Salmonella, Shigella, Yersinia,* and invasive *Escherichia coli.* If fecal leukocytes are present, the stool should be cultured; blood should be cultured if high fever is present. Fecal leukocytes also are seen with disorders associated with colonic mucosa inflammation, such as *ulcerative colitis,* when blood and stool cultures are not remarkable.

Organisms that cause diarrhea by toxin production *(Escherichia coli, Clostridium perfringens, Vibrio cholera,* and *Staphylococcus)* or by induction of small bowel lesions *(Giardia* and viruses) may cause a watery stool without fecal leukocytes. Amebic dysentery usually is not associated with fecal leukocytes.

Microscopic examination of the stools reveals *Giardia* cysts in 50 per cent of patients with giardiasis. If negative, a string test, jejunal biopsy, and jejunal or duodenal aspiration also may reveal *Giardia* cysts.

In patients with diarrhea caused by laxative abuse, proctoscopic examination may reveal melanosis coli, urine and stool tests may be positive for phenolphthalein, and a barium enema may show increased haustral markings.

The stool pH is less than 6, and the stool sugar is greater than 1 gram per cent in patients with lactose intolerance.

LESS COMMON DIAGNOSTIC
CONSIDERATIONS

Less common causes of diarrhea include amebiasis, bacterial over-growth after abdominal surgery, achlorhydria, gastric stasis (in diabetes), carcinoid syndrome, blind loop syndrome with bacterial overgrowth, inflammatory bowel disease, Crohn's disease, and ulcerative colitis.

Antidiarrheal drugs can result in obstipation. With obstipation and fecal impaction (which is more common in the elderly), there may be frequent small, loose, and watery bowel movements without much solid stool. Fecal impactions usually can be diagnosed by rectal examination. In inflammatory bowel disease there usually are frequent small stools or diarrhea with passage of blood, mucus, and occasionally pus. Patients with this disease frequently have rectal leakage, nocturnal diarrhea, pain, urgency, and early morning rushes. In the acute form, patients may appear toxic and have malaise, fever, dehydration, and tachycardia. With chronic inflammatory bowel disease, there may be weight loss, anemia, joint pains, and skin lesions (e.g., erythema nodosum).

Malabsorption conditions other than lactose intolerance include adult nontropical sprue (actually a gluten sensitivity); intolerance to carbohydrates, cow's milk, or protein; and loss of absorptive surface due to bowel resection, sprue, or pancreatic insufficiency.

Pancreatic islet cell tumors and colorectal carcinoma may present initially with diarrhea. The latter is more common in middle-aged than in elderly patients. It may present with any change in bowel habits, most commonly in diarrhea alternating with constipation. Diarrhea may be the only presenting symptom, particularly if the lesion is in the cecum or ascending colon.

CHRONIC DIARRHEA IN CHILDREN

The term "chronic" is used generally to refer to prolonged diarrhea; the specific time that must elapse to be considered chronic is a matter of controversy. Although there is some agreement that persistence for two weeks justifies diagnosing chronic diarrhea in adults, the prevalent feeling is that diarrhea in a child must persist for 1 month or more to be considered chronic. In addition, the child must have either lost weight or failed to gain weight during that period for the situation to be considered clinically significant.

It is particularly important for the physician to have a concept of normal stool patterns in children. Under 4 months, breastfed infants pass 2 to 4 stools daily; their color is yellow to golden, they are soft in consistency, and they have a pH near 5. Formula-fed infants under 4 months have 2 to 3 stools daily that are firm and have a pH around 7. From 4 to 12 months, most children pass 1 to 3 stools per day. These are darker yellow and firmer in consistency. After one year, children's stools are formed and resemble adult stools in odor and color.

One approach of the differential diagnosis of chronic diarrhea in children is to clarify them by type of stool: watery stools, fatty stools, or bloody stools. Watery stools are most commonly seen in the following

Text continued on page 106

DIFFERENTIAL DIAGNOSIS OF DIARRHEA

CONDITION	NATURE OF PATIENT	NATURE OF SYMPTOMS	ASSOCIATED SYMPTOMS	PRECIPITATING AND AGGRAVATING FACTORS	AMELIORATING FACTORS	PHYSICAL FINDINGS	DIAGNOSTIC STUDIES
Acute Diarrhea Viral or bacterial gastroenteritis	All ages	Abrupt onset lasts for <1 week. No symptoms of other organ involvement Most common cause of diarrhea In adults: benign, self-limited condition In children: may lead to severe dehydration	Nausea and vomiting Fever Crampy abdominal pain			Hyperactive peristalsis Fever	Stool culture
Rotavirus	Most common in infants under 3 years	Symptoms have peak incidence in winter					
Salmonella *Shigella*	Peak incidence in children ages 1–4 years					Stool culture	

Drug induced laxatives	Mostly women	Diarrhea Muscle weakness Lassitude			Proctoscopic examination Stool NaOH test for phenolphthalein Barium enema Hypokalemia
Antibiotics	Taking antibiotics	Mild, watery diarrhea	Nonspecific crampy, abdominal pain Low-grade fever	Ampicillin Tetracycline Lincomycin Chloramphenicol Clindamycin	
Pseudomembranous enterocolitis	Taking antibiotics especially clindamycin	Severe colitis with pseudomembrane formation Life-threatening diarrhea of colonic or dysenteric type		Use of several different antibiotics Classically, clindamycin permitted Clostridia difficile superinfection	
Other drugs				Iron or magnesium-containing compounds, high doses of salicylates, quanethidine, quinidine, anti-inflammatory agents, β-blockers, methyldopa, digitalis, phenothiazines	

Table continued on following page

DIFFERENTIAL DIAGNOSIS OF DIARRHEA *Continued*

CONDITION	NATURE OF PATIENT	NATURE OF SYMPTOMS	ASSOCIATED SYMPTOMS	PRECIPITATING AND AGGRAVATING FACTORS	AMELIORATING FACTORS	PHYSICAL FINDINGS	DIAGNOSTIC STUDIES
Acute Diarrhea *Continued*							
Toxin-mediated ("small bowel diarrhea")		Abrupt onset of large volume, watery diarrhea	Nausea and vomiting Increased salivation Crampy abdominal pain General malaise Little or no fever	Contaminated food			
Clostridia toxin (botulism)			Neurologic symptoms	Contaminated food			
Staphylococcus toxin		Severe vomiting and diarrhea begins 2–4 hours after eating contaminated food (especially meat or dairy products)		Contaminated food			
Dysentery syndrome ("infectious or colonic diarrhea)	Has history of prior good health	No symptoms other than GI involved Acute, watery diarrhea	Fever Nausea and vomiting Abdominal cramps Headache General malaise Myalgias				Microscopic stool examination for fecal leukocytes If leukocytes are present, obtain stool culture If high fever is present, obtain blood culture
Chronic Diarrhea							
Inflammatory bowel disease In adults:		Initial episode is >2 weeks May recur over months or years	Weight loss Bloody stools Fever Arthralgia			Fever Anemia	Proctoscopy Colonoscopy Gastrointestinal radiographs
In children:		Diarrhea must persist for >1 month	Failure to gain weight	Enteritis Intestinal infections			

Irritable bowel syndrome (irritable colon, mucous colitis, functional diarrhea)	Most common in young women with children and other stressed individuals	Chronic or intermittent diarrhea, which classically alternates with constipation Hard, marble-like stools alternating with soft bowel movements Rarely occurs at night or awakens patient Commonly present in morning May have rectal urgency	Mucus in bowl or on stool surface	Stress	Reduction in stress	Colon tender to palpation
Lactase deficiency	Infants <1 year old Adults, especially those of African and Mediterranean descent	Diarrhea	Flatulence Perianal excoriation Abdominal distention Vomiting Fever Anorexia In children: failure to thrive	Lactose load Infectious gastroenteritis		Lactose tolerance test Mucosal biopsy
Diabetes	Diabetics	Uncontrolled, explosive postprandial diarrhea	Neurologic dysfunction	Meals	Antibiotics	Blood sugar Colony count of gastric contents
Giardiasis	Symptoms more severe in children Adults may be asymptomatic Hikers and campers at higher risk	Foul-smelling, watery, explosive diarrhea Latency period of 1–3 weeks Onset may be acute or gradual and may persist from a few weeks to 6 months	Mucus in stool Increased flatulence Nausea Anorexia and weight loss Greasy stools Abdominal distention	Drinking water, infested with *Giardia lamblia*		Microscopic stool examination for *Giardia* "String" test

situations: (1) *persistent post enteritis* diarrhea (with or without secondary carbohydrate intolerance); (2) *intestinal infections* from viruses, bacteria *(Shigella, Salmonella, Escherichia coli, Yersinia),* and *parasites* (particularly *Giardia)*; and (3) *disaccharidase deficiency.* A *lactase deficiency* secondary to an acute gastroenteritis is much more common than a primary lactase deficiency. A sucrase-isomaltase deficiency is rare. Allergic gastroenteropathies, in which the child is allergic to cow's milk protein or soy-protein, may also cause watery diarrhea in infants and children. Other, much less common, causes of watery diarrhea include *Hirschsprung's disease, short bowel syndrome,* primary immune defects and diarrhea associated with endocrine disorders.

Fatty stools suggest *cystic fibrosis, pancreatic insufficiency, celiac disease,* or *allergic gastroenteropathy.* Rarely, drugs like neomycin may induce steatorrhea.

Chronic bloody diarrhea suggests *Shigella* or *Salmonella, dysentery, inflammatory bowel disease* (including ulcerative colitis and Crohn's disease), *amebic dysentery,* or, less commonly, antibiotic-induced pseudomembranous colitis.

Selected References

Arau, T. S., Wyliie, R., and Fitzgerald, J. F.: Chronic diarrhea in infants and children. Am. Fam. Phys. *19*:87–94, 1979.

Bramble, M. G., and Record, C. O.: Drug-induced gastrointestinal disease. Drugs *15*:451–463, 1970.

DuPont, H. L.: Enteropathogenic organisms. New etiologic agents and concepts of disease. Med. Clin. North Am. *62*:945–960, 1978.

Kane, J. A., and Blachlow, N. R.: Infectious diarrhea. Primary Care *6*:63–80, 1979.

Matseshe, J. W., and Phillips, S. F.: Chronic diarrhea—practical approach. Med. Clin. North Am. *62*:141–154, 1978.

Satterwhite, T. K., and DuPont, H. L.: The patient with acute diarrhea—an algorithm for diagnosis. J.A.M.A. *236(23)*:2662–2664, 1976.

10
DIZZINESS/ LIGHTHEADEDNESS AND VERTIGO

When a patient complains of dizziness, the physician must first determine whether the patient has true vertigo or dizziness/lightheadedness. True vertigo is classified as objective or subjective. Objective vertigo is the illusion that one's surroundings are moving. Subjective vertigo is the feeling that, with eyes closed, one's body or head is moving or turning in space. In contrast, lightheadedness, dizziness, and giddiness represent a sensation of being about to faint; this is not accompanied by true syncope or a feeling of rotation or movement. Some patients describe lightheadedness as a lack of strength or a generalized weakness and may state that they feel they would pass out if they did not lie down; this symptom usually improves rapidly with recumbency.

TRUE VERTIGO

Nature of Patient

Most vertiginous episodes in children are benign and self-limiting, except those associated with a seizure disorder. Although true vertigo is uncommon in children, they may complain of vertigo after an *upper respiratory tract infection* or an acute *viral infection* in which hearing was also disturbed. Vertigo may be secondary to an acute *viral labyrin-*

thitis. Children with *serous otitis media* usually do not complain of dizziness or vertigo but may have nondescript balance disturbances. Vertigo or headaches may develop in children several weeks after a *head injury.* Some physicians feel that when paroxysmal vertigo occurs in children with a family history of migraine, it may represent a *migraine equivalent.* Vertigo rarely is the initial symptom of a seizure; when it is, it may be followed by transitory unconsciousness or amnesia of the event.

In adults, true vertigo frequently is caused by *benign positional vertigo, Meniere's syndrome,* and *labyrinthitis.* Ototoxic and salt-retaining drugs, acoustic neuroma, and brainstem dysfunction are less common causes.

Nature of Symptoms

Although the clinical differential diagnosis of vertigo is best made on the basis of associated symptoms, physical findings, and diagnostic studies, there are some distinguishing features about the nature of vertigo. Recurrent attacks often occur with *benign positional vertigo* and *Meniere's syndrome. Labyrinthitis* usually is not recurrent. The vertigo associated with *otitis media* has a gradual onset and may persist after the otitis subsides. If the vertigo has been continuous and progressive for several weeks or months, a *mass lesion* should be suspected.

Benign positional vertigo, Meniere's syndrome, and labyrinthitis have varying duration of symptoms. In positional vertigo, symptoms last from minutes to hours; in Meniere's syndrome, from hours to days; in toxic labyrinthitis or brainstem lesion, from days to weeks.

In many instances, prior episodes of vertigo may have been correctly diagnosed. However, if the previous physician did not obtain a precise history and perform an appropriate physical examination, prior episodes of vertigo may have been misdiagnosed as "nerves," "tension," or "low blood pressure."

Associated Symptoms

Tinnitus, ear fullness, and other hearing disturbances usually are present with Meniere's syndrome, are rare in labyrinthitis, and are absent in benign positional vertigo. Nausea and vomiting may be present in all. If vertigo is associated with an acute onset of unilateral weakness, uncoordination, diplopia, or numbness, the vertigo is due to *brainstem disease.* In these cases, hearing usually is normal, although there are other signs of brainstem dysfunction (e.g., vertical, lateral, or rotatory nystagmus). These signs also are observed in *Meniere's syndrome* and *benign positional vertigo.* If there has been a chronic, progressive, unilateral hearing deficit with tinnitus, facial numbness or weakness, an *acoustic neuroma* should be suspected. "Cafe au lait" spots or neuro-fibromatosis also may be observed in patients with acoustic neuromas.

Precipitating and Aggravating Factors

By definition, positional changes such as head-turning precipitate or aggravate benign positional vertigo; this usually is not so in Meniere's syndrome. The latter is thought to have its onset around *menstruation* as well as during times of excessive *emotional stress. Ototoxic drugs* (e.g., ethacrynic acid, aminoglycosides, and, rarely, furosemide) also may cause vertigo. Recurrent vertigo may occur when salt-retaining drugs (e.g., steroids or phenylbutazone) are ingested.

An acute onset of isolated vertigo suggests a viral infection or *lesion of the middle or inner ear;* repeated vertigo episodes associated with nausea and vomiting of many years duration suggest *Meniere's syndrome* or *benign positional vertigo.*

Ameliorating Factors

During attacks of benign positional vertigo, patients may be comfortable when they are still. Vertigo persists in patients with Meniere's syndrome, otitis, labyrinthitis, and acoustic neuroma even if they do not move.

Physical Findings

The symptoms caused by benign positional vertigo can be replicated with caloric stimulation, Barany testing, or certain postural maneuvers. Nystagmus occurs in benign positional vertigo, Meniere's syndrome, and labyrinthitis. Vertical nystagmus occurs only with central causes of nystagmus, and its presence excludes the aforementioned (labyrinthine) causes of vertigo.

The typical lateral nystagmus of benign positional vertigo occurs within a few seconds after the patient assumes a provocative posture or performs a provocative maneuver. The nystagmus abates after a few seconds and also fatigues (does not occur) with serial repetition of the maneuver.

There is no latency or fatigue when the nystagmus is caused by a central lesion.

Diagnostic Studies

For detailed discussions of the utilization of diagnostic studies, the reader is referred to the articles listed in the references at the end of this chapter, particularly those by Drachman and Hart (1972), Torok (1980), and Singleton (1978).

Less Common Diagnostic Considerations

Less common otologic causes of vertigo include tumors of the middle and inner ear, cholesteatoma, and impacted cerumen. Less common neurologic causes of vertigo include cerebellopontine angle tumors, brainstem tumors, multiple sclerosis, and vertebrobasilar insufficiency (more common in elderly patients). Vertigo may be a migraine equivalent.

LIGHTHEADEDNESS/DIZZINESS AND GIDDINESS

Patients often describe these symptoms as a sensation of generalized, nonspecific weakness or as the feeling that they are going to faint without actually fainting. Patients may feel that this symptom abates when they recline. The most common causes of lightheadedness include *psychologic problems, circulatory problems* (sometimes related to *hypotensive drugs), arrhythmias,* and *hyperventilation.*

Nature of Patient

When this symptom occurs in children, especially in those who are at or near puberty, a *psychologic etiology* (e.g., stressful home or school environments) should be suspected. Syncope and orthostatic lightheadedness occasionally occur during the adolescent growth spurt. Although much less common in children than in adults, *hyperventilation syndrome* may produce symptoms of lightheadedness.

When episodes of dizziness are associated with syncope or palpitations, the patient (child or adult) may be suffering from a "sick sinus syndrome." Some children and adults experience symptoms of lightheadedness during the rapid tachycardia of a *Wolff-Parkinson-White syndrome.* If the child is old enough, he should be asked whether he is aware of any rapid or irregular heartbeat during the episode of lightheadedness.

Patients may complain of lightheadedness or unsteadiness due to *drug ingestion.* Antihypertensive agents of all types, particularly the more potent drugs, can produce orthostatic hypotension. Phenytoin and psychotropic agents can produce feelings of unsteadiness. Ototoxic drugs (e.g., gentamycin, streptomycin, neomycin, quinine, and salicylates in high doses) may cause lightheadedness without true vertigo.

An initial onset of lightheadedness in elderly patients suggests a *cardiovascular disturbance* or *cerebrovascular insufficiency;* vascular insufficiency secondary to cervical arthritis is less common. Postural dizziness related to *unstable vasomotor reflexes* is more common in the elderly but can be seen at any age. When a patient who frequently visits the doctor complains of transient lightheadedness and no specific cause can be found after a reasonably complete history and physical, the lightheadedness most likely is of psychogenic origin. However, when a patient who rarely sees a doctor complains of lightheadedness, a more thorough history and physical should be done so that a specific cause can be ascertained. In this case, psychogenic etiology should be a diagnosis of exclusion. When lightheadedness occurs in a patient with a significant psychiatric disorder, *hyperventilation syndrome* or a *reaction to psychotropic agents* should be considered.

Nature of Symptoms

Psychogenic dizziness may be recurrent but often is persistent. Drug-induced giddiness also is persistent. Orthostatic hypotension, reactive hypoglycemia, and arrhythmias cause recurrent episodes of lightheadedness. Psychogenic dizziness and that due to hypoglycemia are not particularly related to position.

Associated Symptoms

There often are many "functional" complaints in patients with *psychogenic dizziness.* If circumoral or digital paresthesias are present, the dizziness probably is due to hyperventilation. An irregular or rapid heartbeat suggests an *arrhythmia* as the etiology of the lightheadedness. Nervousness and sweating indicate *hypoglycemia.*

Precipitating and Aggravating Factors

If giddiness occurs while the patient is standing, *orthostatic hypotension* should be suspected. This most commonly is induced by antihypertensive drugs. Some patients who have significant systolic pressure reduction, especially elderly individuals, experience lightheadedness when they assume the erect posture, despite systolic levels of greater than 120 mm Hg, particularly if the blood pressure has been reduced rapidly with antihypertensive agents. Orthostatic hypotension also may be secondary to severe diabetic or alcoholic neuropathy.

If dizziness has a temporal periodicity (mid to late morning, mid to late afternoon, or approximately 2 to 4 hours after eating) *reactive hypoglycemia* should be suspected. The dizziness can be due either to the hypoglycemia itself or to hypoglycemia-induced paroxysmal tachycardia. Dizziness on arising in the morning should suggest orthostatic hypotension or hypoglycemia, particularly if the patient is receiving a long-acting insulin.

If transient episodes of lightheadedness (without syncope) have been occurring for many years, and a reasonably complete history and physical examination do not suggest a specific etiology, the patient should be reassured that he probably has no serious illness. In such a case, the symptom may be a manifestation of tension, and the patient should be instructed to record associated signs and symptoms as well as precipitating factors until his next visit.

Ameliorating Factors

If lightheadedness abates with recumbency, *orthostatic hypotension* should be suspected. If recurrent lightheadedness and dizziness abate when the patient is on vacation or removed from stressful situations, a *psychogenic etiology* should be suspected. If ingestion of carbohydrates or rebreathing in a paper bag alleviates the symptom, hypoglycemia or hyperventilation should be considered, respectively.

Physical Findings

There usually are no abnormal physical findings with psychogenic dizziness. Occasionally, the patient can replicate the symptoms of hyperventilation syndrome (dizziness, circumoral numbness) by hyperventilating voluntarily. Patients with reactive hypoglycemia may manifest excessive sweating and a tachycardia. Intermittent tachycardia or bradycardia may be observed in patients with WPW or "sick sinus syndrome," respectively. Orthostatic hypotension may be secondary to drugs but also may be secondary to a diabetic or alcoholic neuropathy.

Less Common Diagnostic Considerations

Less common diagnostic considerations include cardiac arrhythmias such as bradyarrhythmias, paroxysmal atrial fibrillation, complete heart block, paroxysmal atrial tachycardia, and WPW syndrome (especially in

DIFFERENTIAL DIAGNOSIS OF DIZZINESS/LIGHTHEADEDNESS AND VERTIGO

CONDITION	NATURE OF PATIENT	NATURE OF SYMPTOMS	ASSOCIATED SYMPTOMS	AMELIORAT-ING FACTORS	PRECIPITAT-ING AND AGGRAVAT-ING FACTORS	PHYSICAL FINDINGS	DIAGNOSTIC STUDIES
True Vertigo Benign positional vertigo	Adults Uncommon in children	Recurrent over many years *Not* associated with tinnitus or hearing loss Episodes are of short duration (minutes to hours)	Nausea and vomiting No neurologic defect	Some relief if patient is motionless	Positional changes (e.g., head-turning)	Nystagmus and vertigo occur a few seconds after assumption of a provocative posture Lateral or rotatory nystagmus	Symptoms can be replicated by caloric stimulation, Barany testing, or certain postural maneuvers Electronystagmography
Otitis media	More common in children	Persistent vertigo	Earache		Upper respiratory infection	Those of otitis media (acute or chronic)	Audiometric testing Tympanogram
Meniere's syndrome	Adults	Sudden onset of vertigo Not precipitated by sudden movement Recurrent Duration hours to days	Tinnitus Hearing loss Ear fullness Nausea and vomiting		Menstruation Emotional stress	Lateral or rotatory nystagmus No nystagmus between attacks Hearing deficit	Audiometric testing
Labyrinthitis (peripheral vestibulopathy)	Any age	Sudden onset of vertigo Lasts hours to days	Rarely associated with tinnitus Nausea and vomiting Hearing loss possible		May be precipitated by viral infection		Caloric and postural maneuvers Electronystagmography

Table continued on following page

DIFFERENTIAL DIAGNOSIS OF DIZZINESS/LIGHTHEADEDNESS AND VERTIGO *Continued*

CONDITION	NATURE OF PATIENT	NATURE OF SYMPTOMS	ASSOCIATED SYMPTOMS	AMELIORATING FACTORS	PRECIPITATING AND AGGRAVATING FACTORS	PHYSICAL FINDINGS	DIAGNOSTIC STUDIES
True Vertigo *Continued*							
Acoustic neuroma	Adults	Gradual onset Persistent vertigo	Chronic, progressive unilateral hearing deficit Tinnitus Facial numbness Weakness Café-au-lait spots			May be café-au-lait spots Hearing loss Other neurologic problems	CT scan
Drugs: ototoxic		Persists days to weeks		Stop drug	Ethacrynic acid Aminoglycosides Furosemide Steroids Phenylbutazone		
salt-retaining		Vertigo recurs when patient is taking drugs					
Brainstem dysfunction (vertebrobasilar insufficiency or tumors)	Elderly	Acute onset of vertigo Normal hearing Recurrent Progressive with mass lesions	Blurred vision Diplopia Slurred speech Paresthesia Uncoordination Usually no nausea and vomiting			Vertical, lateral, or rotatory nystagmus	Electroencephalogram
Dizziness/Lightheadedness							
Psychogenic	Most common cause of dizziness in children	Recurrent Often persistent Without relation to posture	Many "functional" complaints	Stress reduction	Emotional stress		

Hyperventilation syndrome	More common in adults Anxious	Recurrent	Circumoral or digital paresthesias	Rebreathing in paper bag	Emotional stress	Hyperventilation is not observed often Symptoms may be replicated by having patient hyperventilate voluntarily	
Reactive hypoglycemia		Recurrent Dizziness has temporal periodicity Onset is 2–4 hours after meals	Hypoglycemia-induced paroxysmal tachycardia Trembliness Sweating	Temporary relief from carbohydrates Avoidance of excessive carbohydrate ingestion	Carbohydrate ingestion	Sweating Tachycardia	5-hour glucose tolerance test
Orthostatic hypotension	Elderly Hypertensives Diabetics	Recurrent Giddiness on standing	Occasional syncope	Recumbency	Erect posture Antihypertensive medication	Orthostatic hypotension	
Drugs		Persistent lightheadedness or unsteadiness without true vertigo		Phenytoin Psychotropic drugs Ototoxic drugs			
Sick sinus syndrome	Adults Rare in children	Recurrent dizziness	Syncope Palpitations			Irregular pulse May be normal Bradycardia	EKG Holter monitor His bundle study
Wolff-Parkinson-White syndrome		Recurrent	Palpitations			May be normal between attacks	EKG Holter monitor His bundle studies

younger patients). Older patients with the subclavian steel syndrome feel lightheaded after movement of their arms. These individuals may have a decreased left carotid pulse, a bruit, or a decreased blood pressure in the left arm. Some patients with hemodynamically significant aortic stenosis or idiopathic hypertrophic obstructive myocardiopathy may experience lightheadedness primarily after exertion.

Selected References

Donaldson, J. A.: Differential diagnosis of vertigo. AFP Family Practice Annual, 1982, pp. 5–17.

Drachman, D. A., and Hart, C. W.: An approach to the dizzy patient. Neurology 22:323–334, 1972.

Gantz, B. J.: Differential diagnosis and management of the dizzy patient. Primary Care 9(2):413–427, 1982.

Hinchcliffe, R.: Outpatient problems—Dizziness. Br. J. Hosp. Med. 20:202–203, 1978.

Hybels, R. L.: History-taking in dizziness: the most important diagnostic item. Postgrad. Med. 75(3):41–46, 1984.

Jongkees, L. B. W.: The dizzy, the giddy, and the vertiginous. ORL 40:293–302, 1978.

Singleton, G. T.: Dizziness: an approach to its evaluation. J. Flor. Med. Assoc. 65:712–716, 1978.

Smith, J. D.: Evaluating vertigo. Emerg. Med. 12:45–51, Nov 30 1980.

Torok, N.: When a patient complains "I keep getting dizzy, Doctor!" Med. Times 108:8S–16S, Feb. 1980.

11
EARACHE

Otalgia usually is a sign of an acute or chronic infection of the external auditory canal or mastoid or of an acute infection of the middle ear. These infections can be identified easily with careful examination. **If otologic examination fails to show the source of the pain, referred pain should be considered.** Since the ear is innervated partially by sensory branches of the vagus nerve (Arnold's nerve), glossopharyngeal nerve (Jacobson's nerve), trigeminal nerve (auriculo-temporal nerve), as well as the facial nerve and bunches of C2 and C3, pathologic conditions including infection and malignant disease of the upper aerodigestive tract (carcinoma of the larynx, hypopharynx, oro-pharynx, and base of the tongue) and odontogenic disease also can cause otalgia (Fig. 11–1).

Most earaches are caused by an *acute infection of the middle ear or of the external ear canal.* Usually a careful examination will reveal the cause promptly; occasionally, the differential diagnosis is more difficult. Other common causes of ear pain include *acute serous otitis media, acute otitic barotrauma, mastoiditis, traumatic perforation of the tympanic membrane, foreign bodies,* and *referred pain* (as with temporomandibular joint dysfunction and impacted third molars).

NATURE OF PATIENT

Otitis externa is more frequent in adults, particularly elderly dia-betics. This infectious process also is more common in patients who suffer from seborrheic dermatitis or psoriasis of the scalp. "Swimmer's

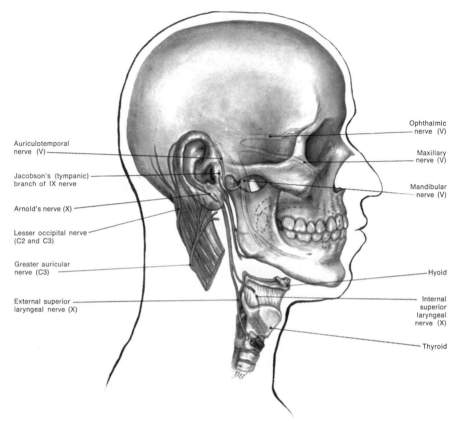

Ophthalmic
nerve (V)

Auriculotemporal
nerve (V)

Maxillary
nerve (V)

Jacobson's (tympanic)
branch of IX nerve

Mandibular
nerve (V)

Arnold's nerve (X)

Lesser occipital nerve
(C2 and C3)

Greater auricular
nerve (C3)

Hyoid

External superior
laryngeal nerve (X)

Internal
superior
laryngeal
nerve (X)

Thyroid

Figure 11–1. Nerve supply to the ear. (From Beddoe, G. M.: Am. Fam. Phys. *11*:108, 1975.)

ear" is common in individuals who swim frequently, but also occurs in those who clean their ears with cotton swabs, paper clips, towel tips, and so forth.

Otitis media is more common in children, particularly those younger than 8 years of age. Various studies suggest that 20 per cent of all children have at least three episodes of otitis media in their first year of life and that two thirds of all children have at least one episode before the age of 2 years. After upper respiratory infection and tonsillopharyngitis, otitis media is the third leading reason for pediatric office visits. Premature children on respirators are at higher risk, as are those with cleft palate and Down's syndrome.

Serous otitis also is more common in children. It usually is not associated with severe pain, except when an acute infection results in an acute otitis media. Serous otitis media often is asymptomatic but frequently is detected on routine audiometric testing of school children, as it is the most common cause of hearing deficiencies in children.

Local causes of ear pain predominate in children, whereas the incidence of referred pain increases with age. One study showed that 60 per cent of patients referred to an ear, nose, and throat (ENT) clinic suffered from referred pain to their ear. The mean age among this group was 36 years. In 80 per cent of the patients, the ear pain was caused by *cervical spine lesions, temporomandibular joint dysfunction,* or *dental pathology. Impacted third molars* are more common in women between the ages of 15 and 25 years and are not an uncommon source of referred ear pain. In the elderly, *malignant lesions* of the oropharynx and larynx can cause referred otalgia. It should be noted, however, that referred pain to the ear does not rule out a local painful process. *Barotrauma* should be considered in patients who have recently traveled by air and in scuba-diving enthusiasts. Pain from direct trauma can result from a blast or a slap on the ear and in ear pickers.

NATURE OF SYMPTOMS

Otitis externa is easily differentiated from otitis media in that patients with otitis externa find movement or pressure on the pinna extremely painful. In addition, they may have tender swelling of the outer ear canal. **Bilateral pain in the ears is more suggestive of otitis externa.** Bilateral pain is unlikely in otitis media and virtually rules out a referred source of the pain. The pain of otitis media has been described as a deep-seated, severe pain that often prevents the patient from sleeping. Children who are too young to talk may present with irritability, restlessness, fever, poor feeding, or rubbing of the affected ear. In addition, there frequently is a history of a recent upper respiratory infection.

Serous otitis usually is painless unless the ear is infected. It generally is not associated with a severe earache, but there usually is some intermittent discomfort. Patients may state that they hear crackling or gurgling sounds. Severe pain in, and especially behind, the ear is experienced in patients with *acute mastoiditis.* Individuals with this condition have exquisite tenderness on pressing over the mastoid process.

The pain of *barotrauma* may be severe and persistent, and a superimposed otitis media occasionally develops. The pain most frequently is experienced during descent in an airplane, especially if the patient has a concurrent upper respiratory infection with eustachian tube dysfunction. The pain may be excruciating.

Patients with *impacted cerumen* also may complain of severe pain in the ear, or they may have only a vague sensation of discomfort that is sometimes associated with impaired hearing. On questioning, the patients may admit to a long-standing problem with cerumen accumulation in their ears, with exacerbation leading to visits to the physician.

The pain of *temporomandibular joint dysfunction* usually is intermittent and often is worse in the morning if associated with night grinding. The pain also may occur toward the end of the day, especially if it is secondary to tension-induced bruxism. For further discussion of temporomandibular joint dysfunction, see chapters on facial pain and headache.

ASSOCIATED SYMPTOMS

The usual sequence of symptoms in *otitis media* is a blocked feeling in the ear, pain, fever, discharge if the tympanic membrane perforates, and some relief of pain and fever with perforation. Patients with *serous otitis* usually are well and afebrile. They frequently present with impaired hearing as their only complaint, although they also may complain of a feeling of fullness in the ear, popping or crackling sounds, or tinnitus. Symptoms commonly associated with *temporomandibular joint dysfunction* include vertigo, tinnitus, headache, and a jaw click. The pain may be worse in the morning if the patient is a night grinder.

PRECIPITATING AND AGGRAVATING FACTORS

Otitic barotrauma is aggravated by upper respiratory infections, hayfever, middle ear effusion, or stuffy nose. It often is precipitated by an increase in atmospheric pressure, as occurs with descent in an airplane. *Acute otitis media* often precedes acute mastoiditis by 10 to 14 days. Pain in the ear that is referred from the second and third spinal nerve may be worse with flexion of the neck.

AMELIORATING FACTORS

Barotrauma may be alleviated somewhat by chewing, Valsalva maneuver, and nasal decongestants. *Temporomandibular pain* may be eased by a dental bite appliance.

PHYSICAL FINDINGS AND DIAGNOSTIC TESTS

The physical findings of otitis externa, otitis media, and serous otitis are well known (see references) and will not be described here. It should be emphasized that the physician must perform an accurate, complete

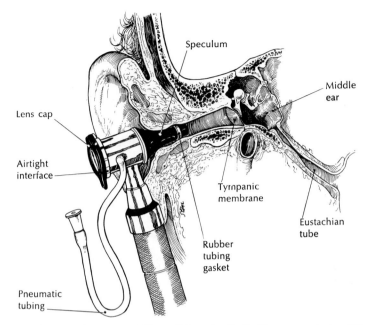

Figure 11–2. Pneumatic otoscopy. (From Schwartz, R. H.: New concepts in otitis media. Am. Fam. Phys. *19(5)*:91–98, 1979.)

examination of the eardrum to rule out otitis media. If an adequate view is obstructed owing to wax accumulation or secondary external ear canal infection, otitis media cannot be ruled out; it can only be excluded if the entire drum is normal and there is no conductive hearing loss. In serous otitis, a serous or glutinous fluid accumulates in the middle ear space. The drum may look abnormal because of the effusion, or it may be injected with noticeable radial vessels. Occasionally, it is retracted and shows decreased mobility on pneumo-otoscopy (Fig. 11–2). Impedance tympanometry (Fig. 11–3) helps one confirm the diagnosis.

When the patient complains of ear pain, has a fever and noticeable swelling behind the ear, or experiences tenderness to palpation over the mastoid process, *acute mastoiditis* is probable. The tympanic membrane often is red, bulging, and immobile because of an associated otitis media. It should be suspected whenever there is a continuous discharge from the middle ear for more than 10 days. Radiographs help one establish the diagnosis.

Whenever a patient complains of pain in the ear and examination of the ear canal and drum is normal, referred pain is most probable. One of the common causes of referred pain to the ear is *temporomandibular joint dysfunction.* This may be either acute, resulting from opening the mouth extremely wide, or chronic, resulting from malocclusion or arthritis of the temporomandibular joint. Malocclusion

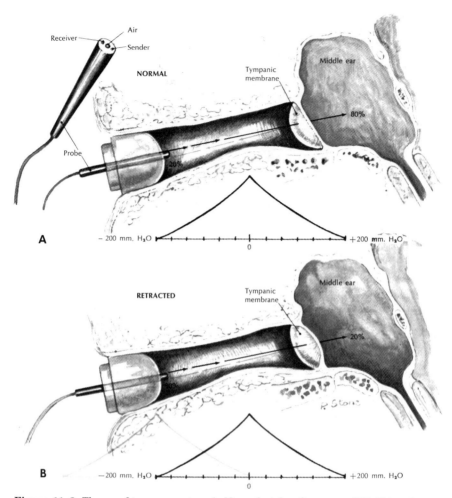

Figure 11–3. Theory of tympanometry. *A,* Normal. A low-frequency (220 Hz) probe tone is emitted from a tiny aperture in the probe tip of the instrument and is directed to the tympanic membrane. When the tympanic membrane is stiffened by positive or negative pressure, a greater amount of sound energy is reflected off the membrane and is directed back down the ear canal. A small microphone housed in the probe assembly reads the amount of reflected sound energy. When the tympanic membrane is in a neutral position, the pressure in the middle ear is equal to that of atmospheric pressure and is thus in its most mobile position. Here, most of the sound energy from the probe tone is absorbed by the tympanic membrane into the middle ear and the least amount is reflected back down the ear canal. *B,* Retracted. The retracted tympanic membrane reflects negative pressure in the middle ear relative to atmospheric pressure. The most compliant position of the membrane (peak of tympanogram) is found when artificially induced negative pressure is introduced from the manometer of the instrument (see blue peak at —200 mm, H_2O). Thus, the pressure point at which the peak of the tympanogram occurs represents an indirect measure of middle ear pressure. Note that greater sound energy is reflected off the tympanic membrane until the pressure introduced down the ear canal is equal to the pressure in the middle ear (in this case, —200 mm. H_2O). (From Schwartz, R. H.: New concepts in otitis media. Am. Fam. Phys. *19(5)*:91–98, 1979.)

DIFFERENTIAL DIAGNOSIS OF EARACHE

CONDITION	NATURE OF PATIENT	NATURE OF SYMPTOMS	ASSOCIATED SYMPTOMS	PRECIPITATING AND AGGRAVATING FACTORS	PHYSICAL FINDINGS AND DIAGNOSTIC STUDIES
Otitis media	Children, especially <8 years	Pain is unilateral, deep, and severe	Irritability Restlessness Fever Poor feeding Ear feels full	Upper respiratory infection	Tympanic membrane inflamed and bulging Decreased light reflex
Serous otitis media	Children Some adults	Not usually painful Unilateral	Decreased hearing Crackling and gurgling sounds		Fluid behind tympanic membrane Tympanic membrane shows decreased mobility Decreased conductive hearing Impedance tympanometry
Otitis externa	Adults Diabetics Patients with seborrhea Ear pickers Swimmers	Often bilateral			Pain on manipulation of pinna

Table continued on following page

DIFFERENTIAL DIAGNOSIS OF EARACHE *Continued*

CONDITION	NATURE OF PATIENT	NATURE OF SYMPTOMS	ASSOCIATED SYMPTOMS	PRECIPITATING AND AGGRAVATING FACTORS	PHYSICAL FINDINGS AND DIAGNOSTIC STUDIES
Otitic barotrauma		Pain may be severe	URI, nasal stuffiness	Worse on airplane descent	
Mastoiditis		Pain in and behind ear	Fever Drainage from middle ear for more than 10 days	Otitis media 10–14 days previously	Exquisite pain with pressure on mastoid process Swelling behind ear Radiograph of mastoid
Foreign body Cerumen	Children Adults	Pain or vague discomfort	May impair hearing Recurrent problem		
Referred otalgia as with TMJ dysfunction, dental problems, and tumors	Adults (increases with age)	Rarely bilateral TMJ dysfunction is intermittent and often worse in morning	Resemble those of TMJ dysfunction: vertigo, tinnitus, jaw click Pain referred from infected tooth may be worse with hot or cold foods	TMJ arthritis Malocclusion or bruxism Impacted molar	Normal ear examination

or enlarged masseter muscles caused by bruxism may be apparent on physical examination. In addition, there often is tenderness to palpation over the temporomandibular joint. Occasionally, the examiner may hear clicking or palpate crepitus over the temporomandibular joint. Patients with *impacted third molars* may have trismus and pain when pressure is applied above and behind the angle of the mandible. The diagnosis can be confirmed by dental radiographs.

LESS COMMON DIAGNOSTIC CONSIDERATIONS

Pain in the ear can be caused by infections such as impetigo, insect bites, chondrodermatitis chronicus helicis (an exquisitely tender nodule of the helix seen in older adults), perichondritis of the pinna, or gouty tophi (which usually are not painful). Rarely, tumors of the middle ear and meatus can produce nonremitting pain. In herpes zoster oticus (Ramsey-Hunt syndrome), there is severe pain in one ear for several days, after which vesicles appear on the auricle or in the meatus. These vesicles also may appear on the tympanic membrane and occasionally on the palate. Concurrent with the vesicles there usually is a complete lower motor neuron lesion of the seventh cranial nerve associated with pyrexia, constitutional disturbances, deafness, tinnitus, vertigo, and nystagmus.

Pain referred to the ear can occur from lesions of the fifth cranial nerve, dental caries, abscesses of lower molars, trigeminal neuralgia, sinusitis, and parotid pathology. Ear pain can be referred from the ninth and tenth cranial nerves with lesions of the vallecula, posterior third of the tongue, tonsils, larynx, migraine, glossopharyngeal neuralgia, and carotidynia (persistent sore throat with normal pharynx, ear pain aggravated by swallowing, and a tenderness over the carotid bulb).

Selected References

Al-Sherkhli, A. R. J.: Pain in the ear—with special reference to referred pain. J. Laryngol. Otol. *94*:1433–1440, 1980.

Clark, J. L.: Otalgia: identifying the source. Postgrad. Med. *70(4)*:99–103, 1981.

Ingvarsson, L.: Acute otalgia in children: findings and diagnosis. Acta Paediatr. Scand. *71(5)*:705–710, 1982.

Fletcher, M. M.: The Painful Ear. Resident and Staff Physician 1980, July, pp. 45–51.

Ludman, H.: Pain in the ear. Br. Med. J. *281*:1538–1541, 1980.

Schwartz, R. H.: New concepts in otitis media. Am. Fam. Phys. *19*(5):91–98, 1979.

Thomas, J. R., and Allard, J. G.: Diagnosis and Treatment of Serous Otitis Media. Miss. Med. *76(9)*:479–488, 1979.

12

FACIAL PAIN

Since the practitioner usually can differentiate headache from other causes of facial pain, the differential diagnosis of headache is discussed separately elsewhere in this book (see Chapter 15). Commonly, by the time a patient consults a physician for facial pain, he already has visited a dentist several times. This illustrates the diagnostic difficulty.

The common causes of facial pain are diseases of local structures such as *eye disease* (glaucoma), *nose* or *sinus disease* (sinusitis), and *dental disease* (dental abscess or temporomandibular joint dysfunction); vascular pain such as *migraine* and *temporal arteritis;* neurologic pain such as *trigeminal neuralgia* and *sphenopalatine ganglion neuralgia;* referred pain, rarely from *angina pectoris* and occasionally due to *muscle contraction headaches;* and psychogenic pain, as seen with *atypical facial pain, hysteria,* and *depression.* Because pain is a symptom and cannot be seen or easily measured, the evaluation and diagnosis must depend on the patient's description; therefore, details that the clinician elicits are important. A patient's reaction to pain can be seen and may indicate the severity of the pain. In cases of chronic pain, the initial symptoms may have been psychologically based, further complicating the diagnostic process. Despite the fact that depressed, anxious, or neurotic individuals may seek help for organic causes of facial pain more frequently than other individuals, chronic or recurrent episodes of facial pain can lead to depression and anxiety.

NATURE OF PATIENT

Trigeminal neuralgia is more common in patients over the age of 50 years. If facial pain occurs in a younger patient (less than 40 years), trigeminal neuralgia is less likely, and other conditions that can mimic tic douloureux should be considered. These include *multiple sclerosis, acoustic neuroma,* and *trigeminal neuroma,* especially if the upper division (pain in the forehead or eye) is involved or if the symptoms are unilateral. Likewise, *glaucoma* is more common in the elderly; it affects 2 per cent of those over 40 years of age. It is more common in individuals who are farsighted than in those who are nearsighted.

Atypical facial pain is most common in women between the ages of 30 and 50 years; 60 per cent of these patients have a similar family history. It tends to occur in individuals presenting with a history of high stress, drug addiction, low self-esteem, impotence or frigidity, marital or family conflicts, or prior episodes of anxiety or depression. The typical patient is an edentulous, haggard-looking, middle-aged woman. She may have a history of concomitant psychiatric illness as well.

Facial pain from sinusitis can occur at any age but is less common in children and teenagers. *Temporomandibular joint (TMJ) dysfunction* is more common after age 40 years, but it can accompany severe malocclusion or mandibular trauma at any age. There appears to be a higher incidence of TMJ dysfunction in patients with rheumatoid arthritis.

NATURE OF SYMPTOMS

Excruciating, lancinating, stabbing, paroxysmal pain is characteristic of the *trigeminal, sphenopalatine,* and *glossopharyngeal* neuralgias. The pain of *glaucoma* generally is described as dull and frontally located. The pain of *acute narrow angle glaucoma,* however, can cause severe pain of abrupt onset.

Pain is relatively uncommon in patients with chronic or subacute sinusitis; it commonly is seen with episodes of *acute sinusitis* (which may be superimosed on subacute sinusitis). Sinusitis pain usually is dull and relatively constant; occasionally, it may be described as throbbing. This pain usually is located over the affected sinus or behind the orbit. With sphenoid sinusitis, however, pain may present at the vertex of the head and radiate to the neck and orbit. Sinusitis pain usually is unilateral but can be bilateral.

The neuralgia pains usually have a sudden onset. A typical attack may consist of two to three stabbing pains over a 1-minute period. Episodes may become more frequent with time, and there may be several attacks in a single day wih spontaneous remission for weeks or months. Although the pain may be recurrent, it usually is paroxysmal and instantaneous. Although the actual pain may last only a few seconds and then disappear, some patients experience a gradual transition from lancinating pain to a vague ache or burning. Trigeminal neuralgia pains usually occur during the day, whereas glossopharyngeal pains often develop at night. Over time, the episodes of trigeminal neuralgia may become more frequent and occur one or more times daily. These pains rarely awaken patients from their sleep.

The pain of *glaucoma* may be worse in dark rooms. It usually is gradual in onset, although the pain of acute narrow angle glaucoma can begin suddenly and present as a dramatic emergency. The pain of sinusitis usually develops gradually and can last days to weeks if not adequately treated.

Most causes of facial pain (including trigeminal neuralgia, sinusitis, glaucoma and temporomandibular joint dysfunction) present with unilateral pain; occasionally, all can be bilateral or alternating. The pain of *trigeminal neuralgia* is located over the course of one of the three divisions of the fifth cranial nerve. It usually is unilateral but can be bilateral in 5 to 10 per cent of patients. These bilateral attacks tend to be more common in certain families and possibly more common in women. Trigeminal neuralgia most commonly occurs along the distribution of the second (maxillary branch) or third (mandibular branch) division and rarely over the first division (ophthalmic branch). The patient generally feels that the pain is on the surface in contrast to being deep inside the head, which is more common with sphenopalatine ganglion neuralgia. **Both the lancinating nature of neuralgia pain and the fact that it tends to be remittent and possibly associated with trigger areas distinguish it from the more chronic pain of sinus infection, dental abscesses, and glaucoma.** The anatomic distribution of the pain helps differentiate neuralgia from *atypical facial pain*, which is not confined to an anatomic distribution of any cranial or cervical nerve. In cases of atypical facial pain, the entire side of the head as well as the face, neck, or throat may be involved.

The pain of *subacute glaucoma* usually causes frontal headaches, whereas the pain of *acute glaucoma* often is described as pain in the eye or just behind the eye radiating to the head, ears, or teeth. The pain of *sinusitis* generally corresponds in location to the sinus involved. Patients with maxillary sinusitis usually complain of pain over the cheek or under the eye; the pain of frontal sinusitis is above the eyes or in the forehead; the pain of ethmoid sinusitis is most often supraorbital and may occasionally radiate to the vertex of the head. Sphenoid and ethmoid sinusitis rarely occur as isolated phenomena; they generally are associated with other forms of sinusitis.

Pain of *temporomandibular arthritis* or *temporomandibular joint dysfunction* generally is located in the TMJ area, although it may be referred to the ear or temples, thus simulating the pain of a tension headache. **Any time a patient complains of pain in the ear and physical examination of the ear is negative, the physician should palpate over the TMJ, question the patient for other signs and**

symptoms of TMJ joint dysfunction, and also consider other causes of referred otalgia. The pain of temporomandibular joint dysfunction may radiate to either the teeth or the ear.

ASSOCIATED SYMPTOMS

Involuntary facial contractions may occur with the severe pain of *trigeminal neuralgia.* Results of suffering from a chronic painful syndrome include sleeplessness, weight loss, anxiety, depression, and, rarely, a suicidal tendency. Patients with *sinusitis* often have—or recently have had—symptoms of an upper respiratory infection. Patients with *atypical facial pain* commonly are depressed and emotional, and they have a large affectual component to their illness. Patients with cluster headaches *(Horton's cephalgia)* may have ipsilateral lacrimation or rhinorrhea.

When patients see halos or rainbows around lights, have temporary obscuring of vision and experience pain in and around the eye, *glaucoma* should be suspected. Occasionally, these patients also will complain of nausea and vomiting. This latter finding sometimes leads to the erroneous diagnosis of migraine headaches. The associated symptoms of *TMJ dysfunction* include clicking, popping, crepitation, tinnitus, vertigo (rarely), pain in the ear, jaw clenching, bruxism, neckache, and headache. Patients may report that it is difficult to open their mouths widely because this action elicits the aforementioned symptoms.

PRECIPITATING AND AGGRAVATING FACTORS

Neuralgia pains often are induced by touching of "trigger points" or by temperature extremes. *Sphenopalatine neuralgia* may be precipitated by sinusitis or a postnasal drip. Coughing and sneezing may exacerbate sinus pain. Erect posture may worsen pain that is due to *maxillary sinusitis,* whereas recumbency exacerbates *frontal sinus* pain. Darkness and drugs, which cause pupillary dilatation, often precipitate the pain of *glaucoma. TMJ pain* may be aggravated by bruxism and by opening the mouth widely. Mastication and temperature extremes may exacerbate dental pain.

AMELIORATING FACTORS

Sinus pain often is relieved by postural changes: Some sinuses drain better when the patient is erect, whereas others drain more effectively when the patient is recumbent. Since frontal sinuses drain better when the patient is erect, the pain of *frontal sinusitis* lessens as the day progresses. In contrast, the pain of *maxillary sinusitis* improves with recumbency, as the maxillary sinuses drain better when the patient is in this position.

Effective relief of pain with carbamazepine (Tegretol) suggests that the pain is due to *neuralgia.* Phenytoin also will relieve neuralgic pain, but it is rarely effective in patients wih migraine headaches. Patients with *atypical facial pain* rarely obtain relief from anything other than psychotherapy or antidepressants. The pain of TMJ dysfunction occasionally is relieved by tranquilizers, anti-inflammatory agents, and muscle relaxants. Depending on what is causing the TMJ pain, bite plates or correction of a malocclusion may be helpful. One should note that correction of the malocclusion may correct the malalignment of the TMJ but not necessarily correct arthritic changes that have occurred in the joint, either primarily or secondarily to the malocclusion. Therefore, even extensive dental work does not always completely relieve TMJ pain.

PHYSICAL FINDINGS

The physician must conduct a meticulous examination of eyes, ears, nose, nasopharynx, mouth, and hypopharynx to determine the source of facial pain. The physical examination usually is normal in patients with atypical facial pain and the various neuralgias. Rarely, patients with trigeminal neuralgia may have a sensory deficit over the division involved and, possibly, pupillary inequality. If the trigemial neuralgia is atypical or bilateral or occurs in patients under age 50 years, the physical examination should focus particularly on findings that could be caused by a basilar artery aneurysm, multiple sclerosis, or cerebellar dysfunction. Patients who have suffered with long-standing undiagnosed *neuralgia* may be partially or completely toothless; extractions may have been performed to relieve pain thought to be of dental origin.

The physical findings of *glaucoma* include increased intraocular pressure, as determined by tonometry, dilated pupil, and conjunctival injection. In the early stages of simple glaucoma, the patient usually does not notice any pain, obscuring of vision, halos, or visual field cuts. Patients with subacute glaucoma may have their vision temporarily obscured and see halos or rainbows around lights. Patients with acute glaucoma may have marked conjunctival injection; acute glaucoma, therefore, is part of the differential diagnosis of the patient with a "red eye." In patients with acute glaucoma, other physical findings include edema of the eyelids, a hazy and "steamy" cornea, decreased corneal sensation, an injected discolored iris, and a pupil that is mildly dilated and occasionally vertically oval. The intraocular tension is raised, and the eye is hard to the touch and tender to gentle palpation. Acute glaucoma can be differentiated from iritis (which may be painful) and conjunctivitis by the appearance of the cornea and the pupil. In conjunctivitis and iritis, the cornea is clear and sensitive (Table 12–1). In conjunctivitis the pupil is active, whereas in iritis it is small and fixed. In both conjunctivitis and iritis, intraocular tension is normal.

Patients with *acute sinusitis* have ipsilateral nasal fullness and pain over the affected sinus that is exacerbated by palpation or percussion. Transillumination over the affected sinus is impaired. Patients may complain of toothaches or tenderness on percussion of the upper teeth because the roots of these teeth are close to the floor of the maxillary sinus. Because maxillary sinusitis is very common, it occasionally is misdiagnosed as hay fever or chronic allergic rhinitis, and vice versa.

There are fewer physical findings and symptoms associated with *subacute or chronic sinusitis.* Patients with subacute sinusitis may complain of headache, postnasal drip, or purulent discharge from the nose or posterior pharynx when the sinus ostea permit drainage in this subacute phase. Patients with chronic sinusitis may have a mucopurulent discharge that is unresponsive to medical management. They may complain of vague ear pain or hearing loss that is secondary to a serous otitis. Often they have a sore throat secondary to a postnasal drip.

Patients with *TMJ dysfunction* may experience pain with palpation of the joint when they open and close the mouth. The masseter muscles may be prominent in patients who grind the teeth. Auscultation over the joint may reveal a clicking sound with opening and closing of the mouth.

DIAGNOSTIC STUDIES

All patients with *unexplained* facial pain should be evaluated with dental, sinus, and skull radiographs or CT scans, tonometry, studies of erythrocyte sedimentation rate, and a very thorough examination of the nose, nasopharynx, larynx, oropharynx, and hypopharynx.

The radiograph in *chronic sinusitis* may be negative or show haziness of the sinus cavity or thickening of the sinus mucosa. Likewise, in *acute sinusitis,* radiographs can be negative in the very early stage and become positive later. In other words, positive radiographic findings are confirmatory, although negative findings do not absolutely rule out the presence of acute or chronic sinusitis. The absence of radiographic changes, however, significantly decreases the likelihood of chronic recurrent sinusitis. Radiographic findings of *temporomandibular joint dysfunction* include the loss of the TMJ space, thinning or loss of lamina over the condylar head or glenoid fossa, flattening of the condylar head,

Table 12–1. A Summary of the Points of Distinction Between Conjunctivitis, Iritis, and Acute Glaucoma

Condition	Conjunctivitis	Iritis	Acute Glaucoma
Conjunctiva	Conjunctival vessels bright red and injected; movable over subjacent sclera; injection most marked away from corneoscleral margin; color fades on pressure	Ciliary vessels injected, deep red or bluish-red; most marked at corneoscleral margin; color does not fade on pressure	Both conjunctival and ciliary vessels injected
Cornea	Clear, sensitive	Clear, sensitive	Steamy, hazy, insensitive
Anterior chamber	Clear; normal depth	Aqueous turbid; anterior chamber slightly shallow	Very shallow
Iris	Normal color	Injected, swollen, adherent to lens, and muddy-colored	Injected
Pupil	Black, active	May be filled with exudate Small, fixed	Dilated, fixed, oval
Intraocular tension	Normal	Normal	Raised

(From Hart, F. D. [Ed.]: French's Index of Differential Diagnosis. 10th ed. © 1973, The Williams & Wilkins Co., Baltimore.)

and spur formation. Often, routine mandibular radiographs may be negative, but tomographic studies may show arthritic changes in the TMJ.

LESS COMMON DIAGNOSTIC CONSIDERATIONS

Vague facial pains, neuralgias and headaches, or aching or sharp stabbing pains on swallowing, head movements, yawning, or coughing suggest the possibility of *Eagle's syndrome*. This may be related to an elongated styloid process that is present in 4 per cent of the population. It should be noted that only 4 per cent of those with elongated styloid process have symptoms. The diagnosis may be confirmed radiographically.

Symptoms of burning, constant, and persistent pain affecting the upper division or any other division of the trigeminal nerve that begins after a recognized bout of herpes may be a postherpetic neuralgia. This is most common in older patients who, after a bout of trigeminal neuralgia, continue to have local neuralgic pain with intermittent exacerbations.

Pain that usually occurs at night (in contrast to trigeminal neuralgia, which usually occurs during the day) should suggest the possibility of a glossopharyngeal neuralgia. Patients (usually older) describe the pain as stabbing, jolting, burning, or continuous. The pain may last seconds to minutes, and attacks tend to occur in clusters, lasting from days to months. The pain often is localized to the posterior half of the tongue, the tonsils, and the pharynx, although it may radiate to the ear, the neck, and the jaw. This diagnosis should be suspected when the pain begins at night or if it is triggered by swallowing, talking, yawning, or eating spicy, salty, or bitter foods. Its incidence is quite rare as compared with that of trigeminal neuralgia.

When a patient complains of constant unilateral burning or aching in the region of the mandible, maxilla, or frontotemporal area, and if the pain is described as "deep" instead of "on the surface," the problem may be sphenopalatine neuralgia (Sluder's syndrome). It can be differentiated from trigeminal and glossopharyngeal neuralgia in that it usually is a constant pain. It will last hours to days, and there may be inflamed nasal mucosa ipsilaterally. It often develops in patients who have sinusitis or postnasal drip. A diagnosis often may be made by anesthetization of the sphenopalatine ganglion. Cocaine or other topical anesthetics can be used on the tip of a nasal swab that is inserted straight back through the nares after the nasal mucosa is shrunk.

The presentation and differential diagnosis of temporal arteritis are described in Chapter 15. If a patient complains of dull, aching pain in

DIFFERENTIAL DIAGNOSIS OF FACIAL PAIN

CONDITION	NATURE OF PATIENT	NATURE OF PAIN	ASSOCIATED SYMPTOMS	PRECIPITATING AND AGGRAVATING FACTORS	AMELIORATING FACTORS	PHYSICAL FINDINGS	DIAGNOSTIC STUDIES
Neuralgia trigeminal	>50 years	Lancinating Stabbing Sudden onset Usually occurs in daytime "On surface" Usually unilateral Maxillary or mandibular division more common		Touching of trigger points Extremes of temperature	Carbamazepine Phenytoin	Tenderness at trigger points	
glosso-pharyngeal		Paroxysmal Recurrent Pain often nocturnal					
spheno-palatine		Constant Pain "in deep"	Postnasal drip				
Sinusitis		Dull Constant Over affected sinus or behind orbit Recurrent or chronic Gradual onset or chronic	Nasal stuffiness Mucopurulent nasal discharge Upper respiratory infection	Upper respiratory infections Coughing and sneezing Frontal sinusitis pain worsens with recumbency Maxillary sinusitis pain may worsen when erect	Maxillary pain eases when recumbent Frontal pain lessens when erect	Tender to palpation or percussion Decreased transillumination Nasal congestion	Sinus radiographs

Table continued on following page

DIFFERENTIAL DIAGNOSIS OF FACIAL PAIN *Continued*

CONDITION	NATURE OF PATIENT	NATURE OF PAIN	ASSOCIATED SYMPTOMS	PRECIPITATING AND AGGRAVATING FACTORS	AMELIORATING FACTORS	PHYSICAL FINDINGS	DIAGNOSTIC STUDIES
Glaucoma	>40 years Farsighted	Dull Severe with acute narrow angle Usually unilateral	Nausea and vomiting			Increased ocular tension Pupil dilated	Tonometry
acute		Orbital Severe Sudden onset		Halos or rainbows around light Temporary visual obscuration	Darkness Drugs that dilate pupils (e.g., sympathomimetics, some psychotropics, and anticholinergics)	Conjunctival injection with acute glaucoma Steamy cornea	
subacute		Frontal Dull Gradual onset					
Temporomandibular joint dysfunction	>40 years Those with rheumatic arthritis	Recurrent or chronic Usually unilateral over TMJ Pain may be in ear, temple, or teeth Worse in morning in night grinders	Tinnitus Clicking Crepitation of TMJ Bruxism	Bruxism Opening mouth widely	Bite plates Correction of malocclusion	Tender to palpation over TMJ Malocclusion Prominent masseter muscles	Radiographs and tomograms of TMJ

Condition	Symptoms	Precipitating/Associated factors	Population	Treatment	Signs	Tests
Cluster headache (Horton's cephalgia) (see Chapter 15)	Eye pain Frontal headaches	Ipsilateral lacrimentation and rhinorrhea				
Temporal arteritis (see Chapter 15)	Headache Transient blindness				Temporal artery tender to palpation	Elevated ESR
Tumors of nasopharynx	Constant pain in nose, ethmoid, midface		Elderly			Skull radiographs and CT scans
Atypical facial pain	Pain does not follow any cranial or cervical nerve "Hemicrania"	Large affectual component	Adult women Anxious Similar family history Often depressed	Psychotherapy Antidepressants	Normal	
Dental abscess	Chronic pain in teeth, jaw, or maxillary region	Temperature extremes Mastication	Any age		Sensitive to hot or cold Tender to percussion over teeth	Dental radiographs

the lower jaw (either unilaterally or bilaterally) that occurs with physical exertion, it may be atypical referred anginal pain. The diagnosis is confirmed if the jaw pain is relieved by administration of sublingual nitroglycerin. Pain that is located in the nasal cavity, in the ethmoid region, or deep in the midface and that is not due to one of the more common causes of facial pain should suggest the possibility of nasal neoplasm, particularly if the patient is elderly.

Pain in the eye most commonly is due to trigeminal neuralgia, postherpetic neuralgia, sinus disease, or cluster headaches. Less common causes of referred pain to the eye can be observed in patients with hypertension, cranial arteritis, orbital tumors, and ophthalmoplegic migraine (pain with a third nerve palsy), which may be due to an intracranial aneurysm. Direct causes of pain in the orbit include herpetic keratitis, herpes zoster of the ophthalmic branch, narrow angle glaucoma, acute iritis, and keratoconjunctivitis sicca.

Obstruction of a salivary duct may be present if the patient complains of submandibular or parotid pain that is worse on chewing or swallowing and particularly if there is tenderness or swelling in the salivary glands. Exacerbation of the pain and swelling following instillation of lemon juice into the oropharynx or ingestion of lemon juice confirms the diagnosis.

Selected References

Birt, D.: Headaches and head pains associated with disease of the ear, nose, and throat. Med. Clin. North Am. *62*:523–531, 1978.

Drinnan, A. J.: Differential diagnosis of orofacial pain. Dent. Clin. North Am. *22*:73–87, 1978.

Gerschman, J., Burrows, G. D., and Reade, R. D.: Orofacial pain. Aust. Fam. Phys. *6*:1219–1225, 1977.

Goodman, B. W.: Temporal arteritis. Am. J. Med. *67*:839–852, 1979.

Gray, G.: Sinusitis—or is it? Aust. Fam. Phys. 7:121–131, 1978.

Schramm, V. L.: A guide to diagnosing and treating facial pain and headache. Geriatrics *35*:78–90, 1980.

Stohoe, N. L.: Ocular pain in the elderly: simple symptom or hidden danger. Geriatrics *35*:41–70, 1980.

Sluder, G.: The role of the sphenopalatine ganglion in nasal headaches. N. Y. Med. J. *87*:989, 1908.

13
FATIGUE

Fatigue can be the presenting symptom of virtually any disease. A thorough history and physical examination will establish a diagnosis in approximately 85 per cent of patients. If in addition to experiencing fatigue the patient complains of localizing symptoms such as abdominal pain or hemoptysis, the diagnosis is easier. Specific attention then can be focused on abdominal or chest causes, respectively. If the patient's only complaint is fatigue, however, the diagnosis is more difficult.

Fatigue can be categorized as acute, chronic, or physiologic. *Acute fatigue* is most often a prodrome or sequela of an acute viral or bacterial infectious process. Heart failure and anemia also may present with a sudden onset of fatigue.

Chronic fatigue (of weeks' to months' duration) can be caused by *depression; chronic anxiety* or *stress; chronic infection,* especially *infectious mononucleosis, hepatitis,* or *tuberculosis; cancer; rheumatoid arthritis* and other rheumatologic disorders; *heart failure; serum electrolyte abnormalities* (hyponatremia, hypokalemia, and hypercalcemia); *chronic lung disease;* or *anemia. Drugs* (both prescribed and over-the-counter) are frequent, often unrecognized, causes of chronic fatigue. These drugs include antihistamines, tranquilizers, psychotropics, hypnotics, and antihypertensives (particularly reserpine, methyldopa, clonidine, and beta blockers).

Patients with *physiologic fatigue* usually recognize the cause of their fatigue and usually do not consult a physician about this problem. Physiologic fatigue can result from overwork (either physical or mental) and insufficient or poor-quality sleep (which may be due to depression, caffeine, drugs, alcohol, or chronic pain).

In approximately 50 per cent of patients presenting with fatigue, the cause is functional (*depression, anxiety* or *stress*) and 50 per cent have an organic cause. It is important for the physician to consider that multiple causes of fatigue may be present. For instance, a patient complaining of fatigue may demonstrate signs and symptoms of depression and have hepatitis, infectious mononucleosis, or bronchogenic carcinoma.

It must be emphasized that depression as a cause of fatigue is NOT a diagnosis of exclusion. Innumerable diagnostic tests to rule out all possible organic causes should not be performed before the diagnosis of depression is made. Rather, if a thorough history and physical examination do not reveal clues to an organic etiology yet do uncover symptoms of depression, depression is the probable cause of fatigue.

NATURE OF PATIENT

Fatigue is an uncommon complaint in children and young adults. When it is the presenting symptom, it usually is due to a prodrome or a sequela of an *acute infectious process*. Chronic fatigue in a young person most often is related to *infectious mononucleosis, hepatitis, drug abuse, depression,* or *chronic anxiety*.

Infants and children rarely manifest depression by lowered mood or fatigue; rather they present with somatic complaints such as headache or acting out. Often, depression is manifested in children and infants by hyperactivity, withdrawal, eating problems, school troubles, sleep disturbances, or vague physical complaints. In adolescents, when fatigue is associated with "acting out" behavior (such as drug abuse or sexual misconduct), depression may be the underlying culprit. Illnesses such as cancer, chronic lung disease, heart disease, and leukemias are quite uncommon in children and adolescents.

As in younger patients, the most common cause of *acute* fatigue in adults is *infection*. The next most frequent causes of fatigue are *depression* and *anxiety*.

In adult patients, particularly the elderly, serious *organic illnesses* such as anemia, cancer, and endocrine abnormalities are more likely to present with fatigue. In the elderly, *masked hyperthyroidism* may present with a chief complaint of fatigue. Patients with this condition do not necessarily show the tachycardia, tremor, and other classic signs of hyperthyroidism.

Because fatigue is such a common symptom of depression in adults, it is important for the physician to recognize that the signs and symptoms of depression vary not only with age but also with sex and socioeconomic status (Table 13–1). Males more commonly manifest depression by guilt,

Table 13–1. **Discriminators of Depression by Socioeconomic Class**

Low	Middle	High
Affective		
Hopelessness	Loneliness	Decreased social life
Self-accusation	Helplessness	Pessimism
Crying	Guilt	Dissatisfaction
Dissatisfaction	Crying	Anxiety–tension
Guilt	Anxiety–tension	
Depressed mood	Depressed mood	
Somatic		
Palpitation	Decreased sex drive	Fatigue
Headache	Urinary complaints	Insomnia
Anorexia	Trouble falling asleep	
Waking early	Headache	
	Anorexia	
	Waking early	

(From Rockwell, D. A., and Burr, B. D.: The tired patient. J. Fam. Pract. *5(5)*:853–857, 1977, and Schwab, J., Bralow, M., and Brown, J.: Diagnosing depression in medical patients. Ann. Int. Med. *67*:695, 1967.)

feelings of helplessness, pessimism, and depressed moods. Early signs of depression in women include headache, insomnia, and withdrawal from social activities. Depressed patients of lower socioeconomic class are likely to have depressed moods, feelings of guilt, hopelessness, dissatisfaction, and crying spells, and they may complain of palpitations, loss of appetite, early-morning waking, and headaches. Depressed middle class patients will state that they feel sad or blue, guilty, helpless, lonely, or anxious. They may complain of crying spells, initial insomnia, early waking, loss of appetite, headache, and decreased libido. Patients of upper socioeconomic class more often complain of fatigue, insomnia, anxiety and tension, dissatisfaction, and decreased interest in work and social life.

NATURE OF SYMPTOMS

The following historical clues suggest fatigue of *organic* origin: Fatigue is of shorter duration, related to exertion, *not* present in the morning but increasingly evident as the day goes on, relieved by rest, and progressive rather than fluctuating over time. Other obvious organic symptoms or signs may be present. The fatigue may be related to a specific muscle group (e.g., weakened arms or drooping eyelids as in myasthenia gravis). Fatigue that increases over several months suggests a progressively deteriorating condition such as anemia or cancer.

Fatigue of *functional* origin usually is of longer duration than that of organic origin; it often is present—and may be worse—in the morning, but it improves gradually as the day progresses; and it usually is not related to exertion. The cause of functional fatigue may become apparent during the history, especially if the onset of symptoms correlates with emotional stresses, including doubts about job security, major life changes, and significant loss (e.g., death of a spouse, loss of a job, or amputation of a limb). Fatigue that tends to be worse in the morning, even while the patient is in bed, and improves as the day progresses suggests a *depressive* etiology. Fatigue that is constant over weeks or months, is not aggravated by effort, is associated with numerous somatic complaints, and shows no diurnal variation is probably due to *chronic anxiety.*

Physiologic fatigue that does not represent a pathologic process should be expected in the following situations: prolonged physical activity without adequate rest; insufficient or poor-quality sleep; dieting; sedentary lifestyle; pregnancy and the postpartum period; and prolonged mental stress.

ASSOCIATED SYMPTOMS

Fatigue associated with dyspnea on exertion or shortness of breath suggests *chronic cardiorespiratory disease.* Fatigue associated with a low-grade fever suggests *infectious processes* such as hepatitis, tuberculosis, or subacute bacterial endocarditis. *Inflammatory diseases* also may present with fatigue and a low-grade fever. Patients with these conditions also may present only with fatigue and no fever

In adults complaining of fatigue who also have vague gastrointestinal symptoms (e.g., constipation, bloating, or indigestion), skin disorders, and chronic pain syndromes, *depression* may be the cause. Fatigue associated with restlessness, irritability, sweating, palpitations, and paresthesias probably is due to *chronic anxiety,* stress, or, rarely, hyperthyroidism.

When fatigue is associated with breathlessness, anorexia, weight loss, and pallor, *anemia* should be suspected. If these symptoms are accompanied by numbness in the legs or arms, pernicious anemia should be considered. If fatigue is associated with shortness of breath, swelling of ankles, or paroxysmal nocturnal dyspnea, *congestive heart failure* should be suspected.

PRECIPITATING AND EXACERBATING FACTORS

Identifying a precipitating factor is often a major clue in diagnosis. Initiation of medications, increased work load, insomnia, loss of job, and family problems all can be precipitating factors. If the onset of fatigue is associated with psychosocial problems, the cause may be chronic anxiety or stress. It is important for the physician to note that in someone subjected to chronic anxiety or stress, a minimal additional stress may exacerbate anxiety and result in a new complaint of fatigue. It is as important to note, however, that patients with organic disease may erroneously attribute their fatigue to a psychosocial problem.

AMELIORATING FACTORS

Fatigue reduced by rest is probably *physiologic*. If fatigue is improved on weekends and vacations, then *chronic stress* related to employment may be underlying the fatigue. *Drugs* are causal if fatigue disappears after they are stopped. If fatigue abates after a viral illness, the *viral infection* caused the fatigue.

PHYSICAL FINDINGS

The most critical component in examining a patient complaining of fatigue is a thorough history that focuses on the onset of symptoms, relationship to exertion, family and social history, a full systemic review, and questions about abuse of drugs or other substances.

Physical findings may provide clues about the etiology of fatigue. Coarse hair, loss of the outer third of the eyebrows, hoarse voice, a doughy consistency to the skin, and myoclonic reflexes (particularly the "hung-up" ankle jerk) all suggest *hypothyroidism*. Tachycardia, tremor, and fine hair as well as warm, moist palms suggest *hyperthyroidism*. Conjunctival or skin pallor suggests *anemia*. Signs of avitaminosis such as a smooth, glossy tongue and cheilosis suggest a *nutritional deficiency*. Distended neck veins, rales at the lung bases, tachycardia, gallop, and edema suggest that *congestive heart failure* is the cause of fatigue. Auscultation of a midsystolic click or a late systolic murmur suggests *mitral valve prolapse*. This is a fairly common condition in which patients often complain of fatigue that is most often a manifestation of *anxiety*.

When associated with splenomegaly or hepatomegaly, adenopathy (particularly posterior cervical adenopathy) suggests *infectious mononucleosis*. Hepatomegaly (with or without jaundice) and pruritis suggest *hepatitis;* diffuse adenopathy suggests a *lymphoma*, such as *Hodgkin's disease*. An enlarged liver with ascites and spider angiomata suggest *cirrhosis*. Increased bruising sometimes associated with pallor suggests a platelet deficiency, which may be part of some other *hematologic problem*.

Fever suggests an *infectious process*. Rales at the lung apices suggest *pulmonary tuberculosis*. Low blood pressure associated with increased

Text continued on page 148

DIFFERENTIAL DIAGNOSIS OF FATIGUE

TYPE	NATURE OF PATIENT	NATURE OF SYMPTOMS	ASSOCIATED SYMPTOMS	AMELIORATING FACTORS	PHYSICAL EXAMINATION	DIAGNOSTIC STUDIES
Physiologic Prolonged physical activity Overwork Inadequate sleep Dieting Pregnancy and postpartum period Sedentary lifestyle	Usually recognizes cause of fatigue and does not complain to physician about it			Rest Increased physical activity		Within normal limits
Functional	May appear depressed	Fatigue on arising Onset may correspond to emotional stress (e.g., job insecurity, major life changes, or significant loss)	Insomnia Vague gastrointestinal symptoms Chronic pain			
Depression				Improvement in life situations	Flattened affect	
Anxiety			Numerous somatic complaints Irritability Breathlessness	Removal of stress	No physical abnormalities	
Emotional stress		Of longer duration than that of organic origin Often present or worse in morning Improves during the day Unrelated to exertion	Irritability Breathlessness	Removal of stress	No physical abnormalities	

Organic	Of shorter duration than that of functional origin Related to exertion Not present in morning but gets worse as day progresses	Symptoms of the disease causing the fatigue: dyspnea on exertion (cardiorespiratory disease), fever (infections), muscle weakness (myasthenia), cold intolerance (hypothyroidism)	Signs of organic pathology causing fatigue: pallor (anemia), rales (pulmonary congestion), weight loss (cancer), tachycardia (hyperthyroidism)	If diagnosis is not clinically apparent: CBC with differential urinalysis, blood sugar, SMA-22, ESR, chest radiograph, PPD, Monospot test, thyroid function tests, serum electrolytes
Acute Viral or bacterial infections	Most common cause of acute fatigue in all age groups Fatigue usually subsides in 2 weeks	Fever	Signs of particular infection	CBC with differential Cultures
Depression	Common cause of fatigue in adults	Sleep disturbances	No physical abnormalities	
Anxiety	Tense, nervous	Somatic complaints	May be signs of mitral valve prolapse	
Drugs and medication		Bizarre behavior Drowsiness	Bradycardia from methyldopa and beta-blockers	
Organic illnesses Anemia	May have acute onset but increases progressively over time	Breathlessness Anorexia and weight loss Pallor Numbness of extremities (with pernicious anemia)	Conjunctival or skin pallor	
Hypothyroidism		Weight gain	Coarse hair Loss of outer third of eyebrow Hoarse voice "Doughy" skin Myoclonic reflexes (especially "hung-up" ankle jerk)	Thyroid function tests

Table continued on following page

DIFFERENTIAL DIAGNOSIS OF FATIGUE *Continued*

TYPE	NATURE OF PATIENT	NATURE OF SYMPTOMS	ASSOCIATED SYMPTOMS	AMELIORATING FACTORS	PHYSICAL EXAMINATION	DIAGNOSTIC STUDIES
Acute *Continued* Serious organic illnesses (e.g., cancer, endocrine disorders)	Rare in children Most common in elderly		Depends on organic illness			
Chronic Depression (not a diagnosis of exclusion)	Does not present with fatigue in children Often overlooked in elderly Adolescents may present with somatic complaints and "acting out" behavior (e.g., abuse or sexual misconduct) Most common cause of chronic fatigue in adults	In adults, worse in the morning, improves as day progresses Signs and symptoms may vary with age, sex, and socioeconomic status	In children: somatic complaints "acting out" hyperactivity school, eating and sleeping problems withdrawal In adults: feelings of guilt, helplessness, pessimism, sadness, loneliness, decreased libido, anxiety, dissatisfaction insomnia early morning awakening weight loss and decreased appetite social withdrawal crying spells headache vague GI symptoms skin disorders chronic pain syndromes		Patient has "flat" affect	Should not perform innumerable diagnostic studies to rule out all possible organic causes before diagnosing depression

Cause	Population	Onset/Characteristics	Symptoms	Physical findings	Tests/Treatment
Medications	Users of antihistamines, psychotropics, tranquilizers, antihypertensives (reserpine, methyldopa, clonidine, beta-blockers)	Onset correlates with beginning of drug ingestion			Cessation of drugs
Chronic anxiety or stress		Constant over weeks or months; Shows no diurnal variation; Is not aggravated by effort; May be precipitated by psychosocial factors	Somatic complaints; Restlessness; Irritability; Sweating; Palpitations; Paresthesias	With mitral valve prolapse, there may be midsystolic click or late systolic murmur	
Organic illnesses Congestive heart failure Cancer Chronic infection	Adults		Varies with illness	Varies with illness	
Mononucleosis	Most common in adolescents and young adults			Posterior cervical adenopathy; Hepatomegaly; Splenomegaly	Monospot test
Hepatitis	Most common in alcoholics and IV drug users			Hepatomegaly with or without jaundice	Abnormal liver function tests and hepatitis antigens

skin pigmentation suggests *adrenal insufficiency.* Polyarticular arthritis suggests *rheumatoid arthritis,* whereas migratory arthritis suggests a *connective tissue disorder.*

DIAGNOSTIC STUDIES

In cases of fatigue in which the diagnosis is not readily apparent, the following routine laboratory tests should be performed: complete blood count with differential, urinalysis, blood sugar, SMA-22, erythrocyte sedimentation rate, and chest radiograph. When the patient has a normal sedimentation rate, it is not likely that serious organic disease is present. Depending on the diagnostic considerations, other laboratory tests may be indicated, such as a tuberculin test, a Monospot test, thyroid function tests, or serum electrolyte evaluation.

LESS COMMON DIAGNOSTIC CONSIDERATIONS

The less common causes of fatigue include neoplasia, connective tissue diseases (e.g., disseminated lupus erythematosus, polymyalgia rheumatica and temporal arteritis); metabolic states (e.g., uremia, hypokalemia, and hyponatremia), endocrine disorders (e.g., hypothyroidism, hyperthyroidism, hypoglycemia, Addison's disease, and diabetes); malnutrition with or without malabsorption; chronic pain; chronic neurologic disorders (e.g., myasthenia gravis and Parkinson's disease); and chronic infections (e.g., brucellosis, subacute bacterial endocarditis, and chronic Epstein-Barr virus infection).

Selected References

Berris, B., and Rachlis, A.: Investigation of fatigue. Can. Fam. Phys. *23*(465):75–76, 1977.
Miller, P. M., Ingham, J. G., and Davidson, S.: Life counts, symptoms and social support. J. Psychosom. Res. *20*(6):515–522, 1976.
Rockwell, D. A., and Burr, B. D.: The tired patient. J. Fam. Pract. *5*(5):853–857, 1977.

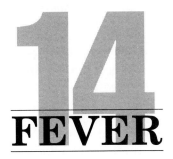

FEVER

This chapter emphasizes fever as the presenting problem rather than fevers of unknown origin (FUO). Only a brief description of FUO will be given here, as excellent, detailed discussions of FUO may be found elsewhere. **Classically, FUO is defined as an oral temperature greater than 100°F occurring on several occasions during a 3-week period in an ambulatory patient or during a 1-week period in a hospitalized patient.** Some authors have suggested that the fever need persist only 10 to 14 days in an outpatient. The fever's etiology should not be apparent, even after a complete history, physical examination, CBC with differential, urinalysis, SMA-22, cardiogram, chest radiograph, Monospot test, and intermediate-strength PPD.

In most febrile patients, a diagnosis is readily apparent or becomes evident within a few days. **Unexplained fever usually is due to a common disorder displaying atypical manifestations or a benign, self-limited illness for which no specific cause is found.** Despite this, it is still important for the physician to search for occult sources of infection, especially if a response to antibiotics is possible.

Normal oral temperature is 37°C or 98.6°F, plus or minus approximately 1°. Body temperature shows a normal diurnal variation: The lowest point is registered in the early morning hours, and the highest is reached in the late afternoon.

Acute fevers most commonly are due to *upper respiratory infections, tonsillitis, viral syndromes* such as influenza and gastroenteritis, *drug reactions,* and *genitourinary tract infections* (e.g., cystitis, pyelonephritis, and prostatitis). Less commonly, acute fevers accompany meningitis, intra-abdominal abscess, and other forms of sepsis.

Chronic low-grade fevers most commonly are due to *hepatitis, tuberculosis, infectious mononucleosis* (especially in children and young adults), *lymphomas,* and *occult neoplasms* (especially in the elderly). If the source of a fever is not readily apparent on the basis of history, symptoms, or physical examination, the possibility of *drug fever* (particularly that due to sulfa drugs, streptomycin, isonicotinic hydrazide, methyldopa, and barbiturates), *sinusitis, dental abscess, prostatitis, tuberculosis, infectious mononucleosis* (especially if there is associated fatigue), and *hepatitis* (both anicteric and icteric) should be considered.

Less common causes of fever whose etiology is not readily apparent by presenting symptomatology include diverticulitis, subacute bacterial endocarditis, osteomyelitis, thrombophlebitis, and Crohn's disease.

NATURE OF PATIENT

The most common cause of fever in children is a viral upper respiratory tract infection. Young children usually have signs or symptoms of a respiratory infection but may show only fever. Common causes of fever in children who have no localizing signs or symptoms at time of examination include *upper respiratory infections, gastroenteritis, tonsillitis, otitis media, urinary tract infections, measles,* and *roseola.* A true FUO in a child has serious implications: In one study, 41 per cent of children with true FUO were found to have a chronic or fatal disease.

Prior history of urinary tract infection, sinusitis, prostatitis, and recurrent pneumonia on the same side increase the likelihood that the current febrile episode may be similar to those in the past.

In the absence of physical signs or symptoms suggesting the etiology of fever, the physician should question specifically about occupational history (particularly exposure or contact with animals or chemicals), drug ingestion, and travel away from the patient's usual residence. In febrile, elderly patients who lack signs or symptoms that suggest an etiology, *tuberculosis, occult neoplasm, cranial arteritis,* and *recurrent pulmonary emboli* must be considered.

NATURE OF SYMPTOMS

Contrary to common belief, studies have shown that the fever pattern is not likely to be helpful diagnostically, although the magnitude may. Temperatures above 105°F suggest *intracranial pathology, factitious fever, pancreatitis,* or *urinary tract infection,* especially if there are shaking chills as well. A mild fever suggests *upper respiratory infection* or *flu-like syndrome.* Low-grade fever (especially when associated with fatigue) may be the initial manifestation of *tuberculosis, infectious mononucleosis,* or *hepatitis.* The fever range may also be helpful. A narrow range of fever, without spikes or chills, may be seen in lymphomas such as *Hodgkin's disease, lymphatic leukemia,* and *hypernephroma.* A fever in an emotionally disturbed patient who is otherwise in good health, is frequently associated with the medical profession, has no weight loss, and demonstrates no related or proportional increase in pulse rate should make the physician suspect a factitious etiology. Some investigators report that this is more likely in female patients. If a factitious etiology is suspected, a simultaneous measurement of urine and rectal temperature should be obtained. **The temperature of the urine normally approximates rectal temperature, and a factitious etiology should be suspected if the rectal temperature is significantly (usually more than 2.7°C) higher than the urine temperature.** Other clues to a factitious etiology include failure of temperature to follow a diurnal pattern, rapid defervescence without sweating, high temperature without prostration, and high temperature without weight loss or night sweats.

ASSOCIATED SYMPTOMS

The following clues may help the physician differentiate viral from bacterial infections. **If the fever is high and there appears to be a sparsity of systemic symptoms (e.g., aches, pains, malaise, backache, fatigue), with the more specific findings limited to either the pharynx, abdomen, or chest, a *bacterial infection* is more likely. However, if there is a relatively low-grade fever of less than 101.5°F associated with systemic complaints (e.g., aches, pains, backache, fatigue, and headache) and the localizing findings are sparse, a *viral infection* is more likely.** For example, the combined findings of a temperature of 103°F, a red, sore throat, hoarseness, and possible dysphagia suggest a bacterial pharyngitis. A viral etiology is more likely if the temperature is less than 101°F, the pharynx is injected and edematous but little evidence of follicular tonsillitis is present, and the patient complains of aches, pains, myalgia, and headache.

Shaking chills suggest a bacteremia frequently due to *pyelonephritis.* When fatigue is associated with a low-grade fever, *infectious mononucleosis* or *tuberculosis* is likely. Persistent fever after an upper respiratory infection, occasionally associated with a frontal headache, should suggest the possibility of *sinusitis.*

PRECIPITATING AND AGGRAVATING FACTORS

Contact with people with an upper respiratory infection or influenza or a local endemic increases the likelihood of *upper respiratory infection* or *influenza*. These two conditions are particularly common in the winter and late summer.

In women, a marked increase in sexual activity may precipitate *cystitis* or *urethritis*, referred to as "honeymoon cystitis." In men, a sudden decrease in sexual activity, particularly following an increase in sexual relations, (e.g., during a vacation) may precipitate *prostatitis*.

The pain of *sinusitis* may be exacerbated by bending foward, coughing, sneezing or blowing the nose.

PHYSICAL FINDINGS

In addition to conducting a careful, thorough physical examination, the physician should pay special attention to certain areas when evaluating a patient whose chief complaint is fever. The sinuses should be percussed and transilluminated for evidence of *sinusitis*. The throat should be examined for signs of *bacterial* or *viral infection* as well as the enanthems of *measles* or *infectious mononucleosis*. Carious teeth should be tapped for signs of *periapical abscess*. All lymph nodes should be palpated. Rectal examination must be performed for evidence of a *perirectal abscess* or *prostatitis*.

If an obvious source of fever is not made apparent by history or physical examination, attention should be focused on sources of fever that initially present without any clue other than fever. This is particularly true in children. Because significant physical findings and symptoms other than fever may be absent in young children, the physician may use the following clues to assess the severity of the illness: decreased playfulness, decreased alertness, reduced motor ability, respiratory distress, and dehydration. It is not uncommon to see fever as an early manifestation of many illnesses, ranging from *teething* to *roseola*. If the source of the fever in a child is not apparent, a urinalysis should be performed; pyuria and albuminuria may be the only manifestations of a urinary tract infection. In teenagers and young adults, *infectious mononucleosis* should be suspected if the fever is associated with any one or more of the following: pharyngitis (either exudative or nonexudative), an enanthem on the soft palate, posterior cervical or generalized adenopathy, hepatosplenomegaly, or exanthema. If these patients are given ampicillin, a rash similar to that seen after administration of penicillin may develop. If this occurs in patients with proven infectious mononucleosis, the likelihood of a true penicillin sensitivity is small.

DIAGNOSTIC STUDIES

Laboratory tests useful in determining the etiology of a fever include complete blood count with differential (particular attention should be given to monocytes and atypical lymphocytes), urinalysis, Monospot test, erythrocyte sedimentation rate, SMA-22, antistreptolysin titers, tuberculin test, antinuclear antibodies, febrile agglutinins, and cultures of blood, urine, pharynx, and stools. In certain instances, CT scans, sonograms, technetium and gallium scans, and special radiographic studies may be helpful.

LESS COMMON DIAGNOSTIC CONSIDERATIONS

Uncommon illnesses that cause fever are legion and include subacute bacterial endocarditis, acute bacterial endocarditis, bacteremia, disseminated fungal infection, myocarditis, lung abscess, osteomyelitis, encephalitis, neoplasms in any location, retroperitoneal lesions, lymphomas, connective tissue disorders, inflammatory bowel disease, diverticulitis, periodic fever, malaria, rat-bite fever, and pulmonary emboli (Table 14–1).

Table 14–1. **Causes of Fever of Unknown Origin in Adults***

Category	Authors				
	Petersdorf and Beeson	Sheon and Van Ommen	Howard et al.	Gleckman et al.	Esposito and Gleckman
Infection	36	21	37	18	36
Tuberculosis	11	5	4	6	8
Abdominal abscess	4	3	9	6	11
Hepatobiliary	7	0	7	0	6
Endocarditis	5	8	9	0	8
Pyelonephritis	3	0	4	0	0
Other	6	5	4	6	3
Neoplasm	19	17	31	9	24
Lymphoma	6	7	22	9	14
Carcinoma					
Renal	1	0	2	0	4
Pancreatic	2	0	0	0	1
Hepatobiliary	0	2	0	0	3
Unknown primary	2	2	2	0	2
Other	8	6	5	0	0
Connective tissue disorder	15	13	19	9	25
Giant cell arteritis	2	0	4	3	17
Systemic vasculitis	0	6	5	3	6
Lupus erythematosus	5	5	3	0	0
Still's disease	0	0	1	3	0
Rheumatic fever	6	2	0	0	1
Other	2	0	6	0	1
Miscellaneous	23	10	8	29	10
Pulmonary emboli	3	0	0	9	5
Factitious fever	3	0	0	0	0
Periodic disease	5	0	0	3	3
Drugs	1	0	2	0	2
Inflammatory bowel disease	0	4	4	3	0
Other	11	6	2	14	0
Undiagnosed	7	39	5	35	5

*All values are expressed as per cent of total cases.

(From Esposito, A. L., and Gleckman, R. A.: A diagnostic approach to the adult with fever of unknown origin. Arch. Int. Med. *139*:575, 1979. Copyright 1979, American Medical Association.)

DIFFERENTIAL DIAGNOSIS OF FEVER

TYPE	NATURE OF PATIENT	NATURE OF SYMPTOMS	ASSOCIATED SYMPTOMS	PRECIPITATING AND AGGRAVATING FACTORS	PHYSICAL FINDINGS	DIAGNOSTIC STUDIES
Acute						
Upper respiratory infections						
viral	Any age	Oral temperature usually <101.5°F	Signs of URI May be systemic symptoms	Contact with people with URI Local endemic	Cough Oropharynx injected but not beefy red	
bacterial	More common in children	Often high fever, >101°F	Marked signs of URI Sparsity of systemic symptoms Children are restless		Pharyngotonsillar exudate Pulmonary findings	Positive culture
Other viral syndromes						
influenza	Any age	Usually mild fever	Muscle aches Nausea Vomiting Cramps Diarrhea		Minimal	
gastroenteritis	Any age					
Drug reactions	Taking prescription or over-the-counter drug	Often high fever	Occasional rash		Fever abates when patient stops taking drug	
Urinary tract infection	More common in adults	Often high fever with chills	Backache Urinary frequency and urgency	Obstructive uropathy	CVA tenderness	Urinalysis Urine culture
Prostatitis			Dysuria Backache	Marked change in sexual frequency	Prostate tenderness	Culture of prostate secretions
Bacterial sepsis		Often high fever with chills				Blood culture

Condition	History	Fever	Symptoms	Physical findings	Tests
Chronic Hepatitis	More common in IV drug users	Usually low-grade fever	Fatigue, Jaundice, Anorexia	Hepatomegaly; Liver is tender to percussion; Jaundice	Liver function tests; Hepatitis antigens
Tuberculosis	More common in diabetics	Usually low-grade fever		Chest findings	Chest radiograph; Tuberculin test
Infectious mononucleosis	Teenagers; Young adults	Usually low-grade fever	Fatigue	Enanthema; Pharyngitis; Adenopathy (especially postcervical); Splenomegaly	Monospot test
Neoplasm	Adults and elderly	Usually narrow fever range	Weight loss		
Occult infection (e.g., sinusitis, dental abscess, prostatitis, diverticulitis, SBE, osteomyelitis, inflammatory bowel disease)		Usually low-grade fever	Depends on cause	Depends on cause	Many
Drug reaction	Taking prescription or over-the-counter drug				CBC may show hematologic abnormality
Factitious fever	May be emotionally disturbed; Associated with health care	Usually >105°F; Can be low-grade	No weight loss; Pulse rate not proportional to fever	Emotional stress; Disparity between rectal/oral temperature and urine temperature	

Selected References

Esposito, A. L., and Glechman, R. A.: A diagnostic approach of the adult with fever of
   unknown origin. Arch. Int. Med. *139*:575–579, 1979.
Everett, M. T.: Definition of FUO in general practice. Practitioner *218*:388–393, 1977.
McCarthy, P. L., et al.: History and observation variables in assessing febrile children.
   Pediatrics *65*:1090–1095, 1980.
Musher, D. M.: Fever of unknown origin: diagnostic principles. Hosp. Pract. *17*:89–95,
   1982.
Rezmik, L.: Diagnosis of fever of unknown origin. J. Am. Osteopath. Assoc. *79*:714–725,
   1980.
Vickery, D. M., and Quinnell, R. K.: Fever of unknown origin—an algorithmic approach.
   J.A.M.A. *238*:2183–2188, 1977.

15

HEADACHE

It has been estimated that 80 per cent of Americans experience some form of headache each year. Fifty per cent of these patients have severe headaches, and 10 to 20 per cent of them consult a physician with headache as the chief complaint. The most common type of headache is the *muscle-contraction,* or *tension,* headache. About 10 per cent of the population have *vascular* headaches. Headaches caused by acute *sinusitis* also are fairly common. Less common causes of headaches include glaucoma, temporal arteritis (more common in the elderly), *cervical arthritis, temporomandibular joint* (TMJ) *dysfunction,* and *trigeminal neuralgia.* **Eye strain and hypertension are not common causes of headaches. Most patients with hypertension do not have headaches; most patients with headaches do not have hypertension. When headaches and hypertension coexist, the headaches usually are not related to the hypertension.**

In order to establish a correct diagnosis, the physician must first differentiate acute headaches from recurrent or chronic headaches. Most common headaches are recurrent; a few are chronic. Therefore, the physician should first elicit the "temporal profile" of the particular headache and history of prior headaches. It is very important for the examiner to ask any patient complaining of headaches about the number and types of headaches; age and circumstances at the time the headaches began; any family history of headaches; the character of pain (including location of pain, frequency of attacks, duration of headache, and the time of onset of attack); any prodromal symptoms; associated symptoms; precipitating factors; emotional factors; previous medical history (especially past illnesses, concurrent disease, recent trauma or surgery); allergies; and responses to medication.

NATURE OF PATIENT

Tension headaches, *vascular* headaches (including migraine), and headaches due to *temporal arteritis* are significantly more common in women, whereas *cluster* headaches are much more common in men (ratio of men to women, 9:1).

Muscle-contraction, or *tension,* headaches are the most common type of headaches in children and adults. These headaches usually are of psychogenic origin and often are induced by situational (home, family, school, or work) problems. Although most children with tension headaches may be suffering from simple anxiety or stress, the headache also may be a manifestation of depression, particularly if it is associated with mood change, withdrawal disturbances, aggressive behavior, loss of energy, self-deprecation, or weight loss. **If a headache has been present continuously for 4 weeks in the absence of neurologic signs, it is most likely psychogenic in origin.**

Studies of young children with *chronic* headaches have revealed that only a small fraction had an organic etiology. In children, headaches may be the presenting symptom of a *febrile illness* such as pharyngitis, particularly with otitis media. A child with a sore throat or otitis media therefore may present complaining of headache.

Studies have shown that among children up to the age of 7 years, there is a 1.4 per cent incidence of *migraine;* among patients who are 17 years of age, the incidence is 5 per cent. Population studies indicate a 12 per cent incidence of migraine in postpubescent males and up to a 20 per cent incidence in postpubescent females. Despite these studies, it is important for one to realize that 20 per cent of all adults who experience migraine headaches have onset of symptoms before the age of 5 years, and 50 per cent have onset of migraine symptoms prior to the age of 20 years. **Although combination headaches (i.e., tension and migraine) are common in adults, they are rare in children and their frequency increases with adolescence.**

Sinus headaches are uncommon in children, but they may occur in young patients, particularly in association with persistent rhinorrhea, cough, otitis media, or allergies. The maxillary sinus is most frequently involved in children. Likewise, headaches of ocular origin are uncommon in children; the possibility of *astigmatism, strabismus* or *refractive error* must be considered, however. This is particularly true if the headaches appear to be related to reading or school work or if they occur late in the afternoon or evening.

Increased intracranial pressure should be suspected if a child who complains of headache has other signs of neurologic dysfunction or projectile vomiting without nausea or if the headache is precipitated or exacerbated by coughing or straining. Causes of increased intracranial pressure in children include tumors (the headache usually is progressive and chronic), *pseudotumor cerebri, hydrocephalus* (detected by serial head measurements), *subdural hematoma* (more common in battered children or after trauma), and *brain abscess* (which may be a complication of otitis media). *Malingering* can be the cause of headaches in children as well as in adult.

In *classic migraine,* the aura and prodrome are prominent, and the headaches are throbbing and unilateral. The patient often goes to sleep and, on awakening, frequently finds that the headache has disappeared. *Common migraine* occurs more frequently than classic migraine. In common migraine, the aura may be vague or not present. The prodrome may be vague and manifested only by personality change or malaise, nausea, and vomiting. Common migraine headaches are less often unilateral than classic migraine. It should be noted that cluster headaches are extremely rare in children, although they may occur in teenagers. Cluster headaches have their highest frequency in the fourth to sixth decades of life. A family history of "vascular," "sinus," or "sick" headaches is present in the majority of patients with migraine. A positive family history, however, is not usually present in patients with cluster headaches. Most patients with vascular headaches have a history of headaches caused either by tension or by vascular problems. Prior diagnoses may be incorrect because of an inadequate or an incomplete history.

Because the incidence of significant disease causing the headaches increases with age, the onset of headaches in patients after the age of 50 years requires careful evaluation and differential diagnosis. **It should be noted that fewer than 2 per cent of patients over the age of 55 years experience new, severe headaches. If patients over 55 have an acute onset of an unrelenting headache that lasts for hours or days, significant disease such as tumor, meningitis, encephalitis, or temporal arteritis should be suspected.** Headache may precede the onset of neurologic deficit. Sudden new onset of headaches in the elderly occasionally strongly suggests *cerebral ischemia* and *impending stroke* as well as *arteritis.*

In patients over 50 years of age, there are only a few conditions that cause chronic severe headaches. They include *temporal arteritis, cluster headaches, mass lesions, posttraumatic headaches, cervical arthritis,* and *depression.* **Depression is a common cause of chronic headache in patients over 50 years, but these patients usually experienced chronic headaches prior to age 50 as well.** Temporal arteritis, although uncommon, occurs more frequently in elderly women; it should be suspected in elderly patients over age 60 years who have unilateral chronic head pain, unexplained low-grade fever, proximal myalgia, markedly elevated erythrocyte sedimentation rate, or an unexplained decrease in visual acuity. Other less common causes of headache in the elderly include congestive heart failure, glaucoma, trigeminal neuralgia, and TMJ dysfunction. Iritis, cerebral vascular insufficiency, cerebral hemorrhage, subdural hematoma, and meningitis are even less common but are more serious causes of chronic headache.

NATURE OF PAIN

The type, severity, and location of pain are important in the differentiation of the cause of headaches (Tables 15–1 to 15–3). *Tension, or muscle-contraction,* headaches usually are dull, not throbbing, steady, and of low, but persistent, intensity. If a patient suffering from chronic tension headaches awakens with a headache, its severity may increase as the day progresses and then decrease toward evening. The pain of

Table 15–1. **Causes of Headaches (by Location)**

Area of Pain	Possible Cause
Generalized	Muscle tension
	Hypertension
	Arteriosclerosis or anemia
	Central nervous system tumor
	Head trauma or chronic subdural hematoma
	Systemic: uremia, thyrotoxicosis
Frontal	
upper	Muscle tension
	Frontal ethmoid sinusitis
	Rhinitis
midfacial	Dental disease, maxillary sinusitis, nasal disease
	Ocular or vascular disease, tumor
	Neurologic (cranial nerve) or vascular degenerative disease
Lateral	
temporal	Muscle tension
	Temporomandibular joint disorders, myofascial disease
	Vascular: arteritis, migraine, cluster headache
facial or ear	Pharyngeal disease (referred pain)
	Otologic or dental disease; Ramsay Hunt syndrome
	Myofascial disease
Vertex	Sphenoid or ethmoid disease
	Hypertension
	Muscle tension
	Central nervous system, nasopharyngeal neoplasm
Occipital	Uremia
	Fibromyositis
	Subarachnoid hemorrhage
	Hypertension
	Muscular tension

(From Schram, V. L.: A guide to diagnosing and treating facial pain. Geriatrics *35*:78–90, 1980.)

Table 15–2. **Diagnosis of Tension Headache Versus Migraine by History**

| Characteristics | Tension Headache (Muscle-Contraction) | | | Migraine* Type of Vascular Headache | |
	Description	Percentages of Patients 1970s†	1950	Description	Percentages of Patients 1950
Laterality	Bilateral	86	90	Unilateral	80
Locus	Occipital	25	—	Supraorbital frontal region	55
	Occipital and suboccipital	26	—		
	Frontal and occipital/ frontal	61	<50		
Quality of head pain	Nonthrobbing	73	70	Throbbing or pulsating	80
Onset of head pain	Severity increases gradually	81	—	Severity increases rapidly in classic, steadily in common	
Frequency	≤8/months	54	—	<1 week	60
	Constant or daily	—	50		
Duration	≤7 hours	50	—	<12 hours	50
	1–12 hours	—	33		
	1–3 hours	—	10		
Prodromes	None	88	90	Present	75
Autonomic symptoms	None	75	90	Present	50
Age at onset	15–24 years	52	—		
	Before 20 years	—	30	Before 20 years	55
Family history	No	54	60	Yes	65

*Percentages for both common and classic combined.
†Percentages calculate from data of 1,420 tension-headache patients in three multicenter studies.
(From Friedman, A. P.: Characteristics of tension headache. Psychosomaties 20(7):451–457, 1979.)

migraine headaches is severe, initially throbbing, and later boring. The severity of this pain increases rapidly and steadily. The pain of *cluster* headaches is much more severe, stabbing, and burning in quality than the usual vascular or tension headaches. Acute sinus headache pain usually is described as severe, throbbing, and pressure-like.

Common migraine headaches are usually unilateral, but may be bilateral. Most often they are located in the frontotemporal or supraorbital region. *Classic migraine* headaches are unilateral. *Cluster* headaches are unilateral and periorbital in any given cluster; the pain is described as in the eye and radiating to the front of the face or the temporal regions. *Tension* headaches are most often occipital, suboccipital, and bilateral, and patients describe the pain as similar to that caused by a constrictive band around the head or as tightness of the scalp. These headaches may radiate down the back of the head and neck. The pain of *sinus* headaches is usually over the involved sinus or sinuses: maxillary, ethmoid, or frontal. Patients with *ethmoid sinusitis* occasionally present complaining of pain behind the eye that intensifies with coughing or sneezing.

Classic migraine headaches usually last approximately 2 to 8 days. Common migraine lasts 12 hours to several days. The onset of most

Table 15–3. Factors in Neuralgia and Vascular Pain

Factor	Typical Neuralgia	Atypical Neuralgia	Migraine	Cluster Headache	Temporal Arteritis
Age	50–70 years	30–50 years	15–30 years	30–50 years	50–70 years
Sex	Equal	Predominantly female	About equal	Predominantly female	Predominantly male
Family history	Not significant	60%	Frequent	20%	Not significant
Pain location	Usually limited to one cranial nerve	Deep, diffuse, crosses sensory boundaries	Unilateral head and face	Unilateral face or orbit	Distribution of cranial artery, but may be multiple locations
Pain duration	Short, paroxysmal, seconds to minutes	Fluctuating, hours to days	Minutes to hours	Minutes to hours	Fluctuating, persistent
Pain character	Sharp, localized	Aching, drawing, pulling	Progressive, dull, boring; then throbbing	Repetitive burning or intense throbbing	Intense, deep boring, or throbbing
Precipitating factors	Touch, wind, and others	Variable	None	None	None
Trigger zone	Usual	No	No	No	Artery tenderness only
Autonomic nervous system or other signs or symptoms	Unusual	Occasional lacrimation, flushing	Nausea, photophobia scotomata, hemianopsia, paresthesia	Common: lacrimation, rhinorrhea, flushing, congested nose, and conjunctiva; nose, and conjunctiva; occasionally Horner's sign	Fever, malaise, anorexia, progressive decreased visual acuity
Effect of drugs					
vasoconstrictors	None	Occasional relief	Relief	Relief	None
analgesics	Inadequate	Relief with narcotic	Not adequate	Not adequate	Variable
local anesthetics	Relief	Occasional relief	None	None	None
steroids	None	None	None	None	Gradual relief
Effect of surgery					
cranial nerve	Generally effective	Not effective	None	None	None
biopsy	None	None	None	None	Diagnostic

(From Schram, V. L.: A guide to diagnosing and treating facial pain. Geriatrics 35:78–90, 1980.)

migraine headaches is gradual. *Tension* headaches usually persist all day for several days. Some patients state that these headaches are constant. *Cluster* headaches have a much shorter duration than tension headaches or migraines do; most cluster headaches last from 20 to 60 minutes. Patients with *trigeminal neuralgia* usually complain of facial pain, but occasionally their presenting symptom is headache. This pain is usually short, sharp, severe, and stabbing. Each episode lasts less than 90 seconds, but repeated pains persist for 2 to 3 minutes. Headaches caused by mass lesions are persistent but intermittent, whereas headaches due to intracranial infections are usually constant.

Headache Patterns

The common varieties of headaches have a typical pattern for each patient. A change in the pattern should suggest the development of a new problem. If a patient who usually has tension headaches in the occipital region or in a bandlike region around the head develops unilateral headaches associated with nausea and vomiting, migraine headaches may have developed as an additional problem. *Migraine* headaches recur at irregular intervals and have no specific pattern; they may recur once or twice weekly or once a year. They often occur around the menstrual period.

The pattern of *tension* headaches varies with the cause of tension. They most often occur daily but may also occur several times a week. **It is not uncommon for a patient with chronic tension headaches to awaken in the morning with a headache, but it is rare for one to be awakened at night by it.** A specific form of muscle-contraction headaches is due to *bruxism* (grinding of the teeth). Patients may present with a constant headache on awakening if they are night grinders. Typically, *hypertensive* headaches also occur in the morning after nighttime recumbency. They are usually throbbing in nature.

The frequency patterns of *cluster* headaches are diagnostic because these types of headaches usually occur in close succession. They often occur at appoximately the same time of day for 3 to 8 weeks and may recur one to three times a day. They may have an inexplicable remission for months or years and an equally inexplicable recurrence. Although early morning onset (1:00 A.M. to 5:00 A.M) is typical of cluster headaches, some attacks occur during the day. If they happen at night, which is rare, they possibly are related to rapid eye movement during sleep. *Sinus* headaches also often begin in the morning, get progressively worse, but tend to get better towards evening.

Migraine headaches have prodromes, which are uncommon in *cluster* headaches; occasionally, some patients experience a burning sensation on the forehead before the onset of pain. The classic migraine prodrome occurs 15 to 30 minutes before the headache. It is abrupt in onset, lasts for 10 to 15 minutes, and is often contralateral to the headache. Visual auras include a variety of scotomata, transient blindness, blurred vision, and hemianopsia. Nonvisual auras may include weakness, aphasia, mood disturbances, and photophobia. In contrast to classic migraine, common migraine usually has no specific aura. When prodromes are present, they vary widely and may present as psychic disturbances, fatigue, gastrointestinal symptoms, or mood changes.

ASSOCIATED SYMPTOMS

With *classic migraine* the most common associated symptoms include anorexia, nausea and vomiting, sonophobia, photophobia, and irritability. Less common are dizziness, fluid retention, abdominal pain, and sleepiness. Symptoms associated with the *common migraine* include all those associated with classic migraine as well as fatigue, chills, diarrhea, and urticaria. Cyclic abdominal pain or vomiting in children and motion sickness in adults are commonly seen in patients with migraine headaches.

Pain in the posterior cervical region that is exacerbated by neck extension often is seen in patients with *tension* headaches. The patients frequently are tense, anxious, significantly depressed, and fatigued. Patients with chronic tension headaches seem to be more emotionally involved in their headache symptoms; they seem to focus on their symptoms more than patients with migraines do. In addition, the intensity of the affective disturbance is more marked in those with tension headaches than in those with migraine.

Patients with acute *sinus* headaches may complain of toothaches; this indicates a maxillary infection. If they complain of pain in the eye, this indicates an ethmoid sinusitis. There frequently are nasal discharge, percussion tenderness over the sinus area, and symptoms of an upper respiratory infection. A *nasal* or *sinus neoplasm* may be present if the physician suspects a sinus headache which does not improve after approximately 2 weeks of appropriate therapy (including antibiotics and nasal decongestants) and if there is blood-tinged rhinorrhea. These symptoms recur despite therapy, and sinus radiographs may show evidence of bone destruction.

The symptoms associated with *cluster* headaches are significantly different and help the physician establish this diagnosis. Patients may complain of injection of the involved eye, a blocked nose with rhinorrhea, and marked ipsilateral lacrimation. There may be an ipsilateral Horner's syndrome. About 25 per cent of patients with cluster headaches have peptic ulcer disease.

Organic brain disease should be suspected if one or more of the following signs or symptoms are noted:

1. Intermittent or continuous headache that progressively increases in frequency and severity.

2. Headache that is exacerbated by coughing or straining at stool.

3. Headache that is worse in the morning (note that sinus and hypertensive headaches also may be worse in the morning).

4. Vomiting.

5. Headache that disturbs sleep.

6. Inequality of pupils.

7. Fever.

8. Seizures.

9. Confusion.

10. Recent onset of neurologic deficit.

11. Papilledema.

12. Onset of severe headaches after 50 years of age.

PRECIPITATING AND AGGRAVATING FACTORS

Although migraine headaches may be precipitated by *menstruation,* their frequency increases as estrogen levels fall. Migraine headaches frequently are precipitated by emotional stress. Less frequently, they are precipitated by fatigue, bright lights, fasting, hypoglycemia, odors, exercise, weather changes, and high altitude.

Patients may have a history of headaches that are caused by ingestion of certain *foods* and *beverages* (e.g., aged cheese, chocolate, yogurt, buttermilk, and red wine). Headaches may be precipitated by foods that contain nitrites ("hot dog headache") or monosodium glutamate ("Chinese restaurant syndrome"). *Alcohol* and *caffeine* also are frequent offenders, as is *caffeine withdrawal. Drugs* such as reserpine, vasodilators, and contraceptives also may cause headaches. Some patients who have been heavy users of ergot drugs to control migraine may experience migraine headaches when these therapeutic agents are stopped.

Muscle-contraction, or *tension,* headaches can be precipitated by emotional or physical stress, extended periods of mental concentration, and prolonged, somewhat abnormal positions of the neck. Some tension headaches may ocur with cessation of analgesics or tranquilizers used in their treatment. Dental malocclusion may stimulate contraction of the muscles of mastication, thus causing spasm of the muscles and headache. Ill-fitting dentures, particularly if they have been worn for 10 or more years, also may lead to muscle-contraction headaches.

Cluster headaches may be precipitated by short naps, alcohol ingestion, nitroglycerin, tyramine, and emotional stress. *Sinus* headaches may be aggravated by coughing or sneezing, but this is also true of other types of headaches, especially vascular. Eye pain due to *glaucoma* often is precipitated by darkness or sympathomimetic drugs, which cause pupillary dilatation.

AMELIORATING FACTORS

If the patient states that ergot-containing drugs improved the acute headaches, a vascular etiology is probable. Likewise, relief with nasal decongestants and antibiotics suggests a sinus etiology. A headache that is severe; associated with nausea, vomiting, scotomata, or aura; and relieved by sleep is probably migraine.

PHYSICAL FINDINGS

In patients with *tension* or *migraine* headaches the physical findings rarely contribute to the differential diagnosis. Patients with *trigeminal neuralgia* may have a trigger point. During an attack of *cluster* headache there may be ipsilateral lacrimation and rhinorrhea. Patients with acute *sinus* headaches may have a mucopurulent or blood-tinged nasal discharge. In addition, there may be tenderness to percussion or palpation over the involved sinus, which also may demonstrate impaired transillumination. The presence of fever suggests an *infectious process* as the etiology of the headache. Severe *hypertension* may suggest that the headaches are of hypertensive origin, although most patients with hypertension do not have headaches. Tenderness to palpation over the temporal artery suggests *temporal arteritis* as an etiology.

When nuchal rigidity is found, *meningitis* or a *subarachnoid bleed* should be suspected. Nuchal rigidity must be differentiated from the stiff neck of patients with cervical arthritis (more common in elderly patients). In patients with true nuchal rigidity, the neck is stiff throughout the arc as the examiner flexes it but not in extension or lateral rotation. In contrast, with *cervical arthritis,* the early phase of flexion of the neck is supple; this is followed by a sudden, boardlike rigidity with resistance in other directions of movement as well.

Patients with *psychogenic* or *conversion* headaches may describe the pain in very vivid terms with much affect; the patient does not really appear to be in great pain.

Pain localized to one or both eyes with increased intraocular pressure indicates *glaucoma*. The presence of a jaw click or point tenderness to palpation over the temporomandibular joint suggests that the headache may be due to TMJ dysfunction.

Most patients with headaches do not exhibit any abnormalities on neurologic examination. However, a transient ipsilateral Horner's syndrome may be seen with some migraine headaches.

DIAGNOSTIC STUDIES

There are only a few laboratory tests that help in the differential diagnosis of headaches. Radiographs may confirm *acute sinusitis* if there is a typical fluid level in one or more of the sinuses. Patients may experience sinus headaches and still have normal sinus radiographs. The erythrocyte sedimentation rate is markedly elevated with *temporal arteritis*. A biopsy of the arterial wall showing giant cell infiltration is pathognomonic of arteritis.

If there is sudden onset of headache in patients over 50 years of age, the physician must make a difficult decision regarding whether to perform lumbar puncture. It is indicated in suspected instances of *cerebral hemorrhage* or *bacterial encephalitis,* but it is dangerous in patients with mass lesions or increased intracranial pressure. Noninvasive tests such as a CT scan or nuclear magnetic resonance (NMR) should be done first if intracranial disease is suspected. Arteriograms may show vascular abnormalities and mass lesions.

LESS COMMON DIAGNOSTIC
CONSIDERATIONS

Glaucoma, eye strain, and systemic problems are less common conditions that also may present with headaches.

Patients with glaucoma may complain of pain in one or both eyes; they describe a visual halo around objects; headaches often come on in a darkened environment; and there is increased intraocular pressure and occasionally tenderness to palpation over the globe.

Eye strain is a diagnosis that often is applied incorrectly. Headache from eye strain is unusual. It tends to occur in people who do work that requires close vision. In addition, the headaches tend to occur after a prolonged period of using the eyes.

Systemic causes include uremia, thyrotoxicosis, severe anemia, brain tumors, chronic subdural hematoma, subarachnoid hemorrhage, and ocular disease. Tumors of the eye, ear, nose, or throat also may present with headaches.

The key to diagnosing headaches consists of a careful, detailed clinical history and neurologic examination. There is usually time to

Text continued on page 172

DIFFERENTIAL DIAGNOSIS OF HEADACHE

TYPE	NATURE OF PATIENT	NATURE OF SYMPTOMS	ASSOCIATED SYMPTOMS	PRECIPITATING AND AGGRAVATING FACTORS	AMELIORATING FACTORS	PHYSICAL EXAMINATION	DIAGNOSTIC STUDIES
Tension headaches (muscle-contraction headache)	Most common cause of headache at any age More common in females	Usually of psychogenic origin In children: may be manifestation of stress, anxiety, or depression In adults: usually dull, non-throbbing, with persistent, low intensity may last a few days severity may increase as day progresses and then decrease toward evening usually occipital, suboccipital, and bilateral described as constrictive band around head or tightness of scalp rarely wakes patient from sleep	Fatigue	Emotional or physical stress Abnormal neck positions (especially neck extension) Prolonged mental concentration Withdrawal of analgesics or tranquilizers Dental malocclusion or ill-fitting dentures Bruxism (nightgrinding of teeth)	Stress reduction		
Vascular headaches	Affect 10% of U.S. population More common in women Family history of headaches			Coughing Sneezing	Ergot-containing drugs Beta-blockers		

Common migraine	More frequent in children	Vague or absent aura and prodrome Gradual onset Lasts 12 hours to several days Not always unilateral Usually in frontotemporal or supraorbital region	Those of classic migraine General malaise Fatigue Chills Diarrhea Urticaria Motion sickness		Sleep
Classic migraine	More common in women Incidence: 1.4% in children (under age 7 years) 5% in children at age 17 years 17% in postpubescent males 20% in postpubescent females 50% of adults with migraines have symptoms before age 20 years	Prominent aura The prodrome: has abrupt onset lasts 10–15 min. precedes headache by 15–30 minutes Headache: severe throbbing unilateral gradual onset intensity increases steadily and rapidly lasts 2–8 days	Visual auras (scotomata, transient blindness, blurred vision, hemianopsia) Nonvisual auras (weakness, aphasia, mood disturbances, photophobia) Nausea and vomiting Anorexia Sonophobia Photophobia Irritability Dizziness Fluid retention Abdominal pain Sleepiness	Menstruation Emotional stress Fatigue Bright lights High altitude Weather changes Exercise Certain foods Fasting Hypoglycemia	Sleep
Cluster headaches	Highest incidence in fourth to sixth headache Rare in children Much more common in men than in women (9:1) Family history of cluster headaches uncommon	Pain is more severe, stabbing, and burning than in vascular or tension headache Unilateral and periorbital in any given cluster May radiate to front of face or to temporal regions Duration ranges from 20–60 minutes	25% of patients have peptic ulcer disease Injection of involved eye Rhinorrhea Marked ipsilateral lacrimation May be ipsilateral Horner's syndrome	Short naps Alcohol Nitroglycerine Tyramine Emotional stress	

Table continued on following page

DIFFERENTIAL DIAGNOSIS OF HEADACHE *Continued*

TYPE	NATURE OF PATIENT	NATURE OF SYMPTOMS	ASSOCIATED SYMPTOMS	PRECIPITATING AND AGGRAVATING FACTORS	AMELIORATING FACTORS	PHYSICAL EXAMINATION	DIAGNOSTIC STUDIES
Cluster headaches *Continued*	Recur at same time of day for 3–8 weeks, 1–3 times per day Typical early morning onset						
Headaches due to febrile illnesses	Common cause of headache in children	Headache may be only presenting symptom in children	Fever	Pharyngitis, especially with otitis media		Fever	
Sinusitis (see Chap. 12)	Uncommon in children	Pain: severe, throbbing, and intense pressure usually over involved sinus begins in morning, gets progressively worse during the day, improves toward evening Maxillary sinus is most often involved in children	Persistent rhinorrhea Otitis media Allergies Symptoms of URI Toothache, with maxillary involvement Eye pain with ethmoid involvement	Coughing Sneezing		Mucopurulent or blood-tinged nasal discharge Percussion tenderness over involved sinuses	Transillumination of sinuses Sinus radiographs
Depression	Common cause of headache in patients > 50 years	Constant, chronic headache	Those of depression		Treat depression		

Condition						
Temporomandibular joint (TMJ) dysfunction (see Chap. 12)	Adults	Usually pain in TMJ or ear, but may present with headache (temporoparietal)	Bruxism	Opening mouth too wide	Jaw clicks Point tenderness to palpation over TMJ Prominent masseter muscle	Radiograph of TMJ
Temporal arteritis	Most common in elderly women	Unilateral, chronic headache	Unexplained low-grade fever Proximal myalgia Decreased visual acuity		Tenderness to palpation over the temporal artery	Erythrocyte sedimentation rate (ESR) is markedly elevated
Cervical arthritis	Most common in elderly	Occipital or nuchal headache			Stiff neck Early phase of flexion is supple but followed by sudden, board-like rigidity with resistance in other directions	Radiograph of cervical spine
Trigeminal neuralgia (see Chap. 12)	Adult	Pain is short, episodic, sharp, severe, and stabbing Each episode lasts < 90 seconds but recurs for 2 to 3 minutes	Pain in face along distribution of one division of nerve	Trigger point Extremes of temperature	Patient may have a trigger point	
Increased intracranial pressure		Progressive, chronic headache	In children; neurologic dysfunction and projectile vomiting without nausea	Coughing Straining	Papilledema	CT scan Increased cerebrospinal fluid pressure
Glaucoma (see Chap. 12)		Frontal headache	Patient sees halos Pain in eye	Darkened areas Drugs that dilate pupils	Increased intraocular pressure	Tonometry

observe patients and to evaluate the whole patient in relation to the family and environment, which is helpful in determining the underlying cause of headache. The physician should try to avoid the use of habituating drugs in the treatment of patients with chronic headaches.

Selected References

Appenzeller, O., Feldman, R. G., and Friedman, A. P.: Migraine, headache, and related conditions—Panel 7. Arch. Neurol. *36*:784–804, 1979.

Caviness, V. S., and O'Brien, P.: Current concepts—headache. N. Engl. J. Med. *302*(8):446–450, 1980.

Kunkel, R. S.: Evaluating the headache patient: history and workup. Headache *19*:122–126, 1979.

Schramm, V. L.: A guide to diagnosing and treating facial pain and headache. Geriatrics *35*:78–90, 1980.

Thompson, J. A.: Diagnosis and treatment of headache in the pediatric patient. Curr. Probl. Pediatr. *10*:1–52, 1980.

16

HEARTBURN AND INDIGESTION

Heartburn and indigestion are common presenting complaints. Because these symptoms are often vague, it is difficult for the physician to determine a precise etiology, and therefore treatment is frequently ineffective. For purposes of this discussion, heartburn is described as a sensation of burning, warmth, or heat in the retrosternal region between the xiphoid and manubrium that occasionally radiates toward the jaw or, rarely, the arms. Water brash may be present. Indigestion is described as a separate entity. A patient with indigestion may complain of one or more of the following symptoms: a vague feeling of abdominal discomfort, belching, bloating, borborygmi, dysphagia, and abdominal burning.

The most common causes of heartburn and indigestion include *reflux esophagitis* (with or without hiatal hernia), *gastritis,* excessive consumption of *food* or *alcohol, gallbladder disease, pregnancy, aerophagia,* and *functional gastrointestinal disorder.* Although patients with tumors of the gastrointestinal tract may complain of heartburn or indigestion, neoplasms are not a common cause of these symptoms. This chapter focuses on indigestion and heartburn unassociated with abdominal pain. Conditions associated with abdominal pain are discussed in the chapters on abdominal pain.

NATURE OF THE PATIENT

Children rarely complain of indigestion or heartburn, although vague abdominal discomfort may affect children who experience *malabsorption* or *food intolerance.* In these conditions, certain foods may

173

cause crampy abdominal pain or diarrhea. Weight loss may be noted if there is significant malabsorption. When children complain of distention or awareness of peristalsis and gurgling, they often have *functional gastrointestinal disease*. If these complaints are intermittent and not disabling, if the patient is otherwise healthy, and if the results of the physical examination are normal, an emotional etiology should be suspected. Questioning the child may reveal depression or other emotional problems. These problems frequently occur with external environmental stress, such as divorce, birth of a sibling, illness in a family starting school, and problems with boyfriend or girlfriend.

In adults, heartburn is almost always due to *reflux esophagitis*. This is more common in pregnant women, particularly during the later months. Patients with esophagitis may complain of severe heartburn that is relieved by alkali and aggravated by recumbency. Although *hiatal hernia* is three times more common in multiparous patients than in primigravid women, it should be remembered that the *symptoms of heartburn are due to esophageal reflux and not to the hiatal hernia*. Pregnant patients have delayed gastric emptying, increased intra-abdominal pressure, and increased estrogen levels, all of which facilitate esophageal reflux. It has been reported that 30 to 50 per cent of adults demonstrate hiatal hernias on radiographs; only 5 per cent of this population report symptoms of heartburn.

Indigestion due to gastritis occurs frequently in patients who ingest large quantities of *alcohol* or *drugs* such as salicylates, corticosteroids, nonsteroidal anti-inflammatory agents, theophylline, quinidine, and some antibiotics.

Elderly patients are more likely to complain of vague feelings of indigestion, possibly related to bloating. Many of the symptoms of indigestion and abdominal bloating are due to excessive amounts of *intestinal gas*. Virtually all intestinal gas is the result of bacterial fermentation, although the amount of discomfort is not necessarily proportional to the amount of gas in the intestines. The complaints of indigestion and bloating are more common in the elderly because of relative gastric and intestinal stasis, hypomotility of the gut, altered intestinal bacteria, increased incidence of constipation, and lack of exercise, all of which tend to facilitate the production of intestinal gas.

Tense and *anxious patients* are more likely to be aware of normal intestinal movement and are also more likely to complain about these feelings. Patients with *gallbladder disease* and *ulcers* frequently complain of vague abdominal discomfort and occasional distention.

NATURE OF SYMPTOMS

Heartburn is a burning sensation that occurs in the xiphisternal region with occasional proximal radiation. It may vary in intensity from a mild feeling of warmth to extreme pain. Occasionally, the pain may be indistinguishable from that of severe angina pectoris; it is therefore important for the physician to note that heartburn has *no relation to physical activity*. The pain is usually caused by esophageal spasm, is intermittent over several minutes, and recurs over long periods of time. Pain may radiate into the neck and occasionally into the arms, back, or jaw. According to one study, the pain radiated to the back in 40 per cent of patients with proven *esophageal reflux* but radiated to the arms or neck in only 5 per cent.

Initially, the pain of heartburn may be felt only after heavy meals or while the patient is lying down or bending over. In more advanced cases, the pain is more easily provoked, lasts longer, and is accompanied by dysphagia.

Patients with *gastritis* may have abdominal pain, vague indigestion, or heartburn as a presenting complaint. Epigastric discomfort that is worse after eating, loss of appetite, a sense of fullness, nausea, and occasional vomiting are also common complaints in patients with gastritis. Heartburn is also a common complaint in patients with *bile gastritis,* which often occurs after gastric resection or pyloroplasty. In these cases bile refluxes into the stomach and subsequently into the distal esophagus, causing heartburn. Some patients who have *peptic ulcer* do not complain of the classic symptoms but only of vague indigestion that is sometimes relieved by vomiting.

Gastrointestinal symptoms in patients with *functional gastrointestinal disorders* are often vague and nonspecific. Patients do not get consistent relief with any medication or therapeutic regimen. Other neurotic symptoms are often present, and there is no evidence of systemic disease or weight loss despite a long history of vague symptoms. Because various patients who present with an organic pathology (e.g., peptic ulcer, gallbladder disease, or colonic tumors) may also have vague symptoms, a specific work-up will be required in some cases. When these vague symptoms occur in young adults, it is unlikely that a malignant process in present. Likewise, if the symptoms have been present for many years without any significant progression or evidence of systemic disease, a major disease process is also unlikely.

There are other distinguishing characteristics that often help the physician differentiate functional from organic pain. With functional illness, patients may present with severe and continuous pain but will not experience significant weight loss. The patients often give exaggerated descriptions of their pain and have a significant emotional investment; they may come into the office with a list of their symptoms written on a piece of paper—"Le malade avec le petit morceau de papier." With organic disease, the pain, although severe, is often periodic and not uncommonly associated with weight loss.

ASSOCIATED SYMPTOMS

Patients with *peptic esophagitis* frequently have chest pain. They may complain of heartburn or chest pain when there is esophageal spasm. In some instances, the patients will complain only of substernal pain, which may radiate into the neck, jaw, or upper arms.

Belching secondary to *aerophagia* is often seen in patients with reflux esophagitis and in patients with functional gastrointestinal disease. If indigestion is associated with nausea, right upper quadrant pain, or pain in the right shoulder (particularly the inferior angle of the right scapula), duodenal *loop distention* or *cholelithiasis* should be considered. Hematemesis suggests *peptic ulcer disease* or *variceal bleeding,* regardless of how vague the other symptoms are.

PRECIPITATING AND AGGRAVATING FACTORS

In many patients whose symptoms are due to *reflux esophagitis,* coronary artery disease or hysteria has been previously diagnosed. **Clues to the correct diagnosis of esophagitis are that the pain is not usually brought on by exercise, frequently occurs in the recumbent position, and is often relieved by antacids.** Anything that distends the lower third of the esophagus, irritates its mucosa, or reduces lower esophageal pressure can precipitate *reflux esophagitis*. This includes recumbency, acidic foods, gastric stasis, large meals, and fatty foods (which delay gastric emptying). Several studies show that in addition to gastric juices, bile and other duodenal juices may play a role in the pain of reflux esophagitis. Conditions that increase intra-abdominal pressure (e.g., pregnancy and marked ascites) can facilitate regurgitation of gastric or duodenal contents into the distal esophagus. Caffeine frequently causes heartburn in susceptible individuals. Certain spices, carminatives (e.g., oil of spearmint and peppermint), garlic, onions, chocolate, fatty foods, alcohol, and carbonated beverages may reduce lower esophageal pressure and thus facilitate reflux. Cigarette smoking also reduces lower esophageal pressure and stimulates gastric acidity. It is important for the physician to remember that certain drugs (particularly theophylline derivatives, isoproterenol, and anticholinergics) lower esophageal pressure and may precipitate reflux and heartburn. Other precipitating factors include straining, recumbency, lifting, and ingestion of orange juice, tomato juice, and spicy foods and drinks.

In some patients who swallow air, chew gum, or eat rapidly, heartburn develops as a result of belching and subsequent regurgitation of gastric juices into the distal esophagus. Although there are some instances in which patients with hiatal hernia have heartburn or chest pain, the presence of a hiatal hernia does not establish the presence of esophagitis.

AMELIORATING FACTORS

In general, avoidance of the aforementioned precipitating factors reduces and may eliminate the discomfort. In addition, raising the head of the bed (by tilting the entire bed, not by merely using another pillow), retiring with an empty stomach, sucking on antacid tablets, eating small frequent meals, following a low-fat diet, and avoiding tight garments may help.

The pain of peptic esophagitis is frequently relieved by antacids. These substances reduce gastric acidity and re-establish more normal lower esophageal sphincter pressure, thus reducing reflux. It is particularly important for the physician to remember that the pain of peptic esophagitis may be relieved by nitrates, ordinarily thought to relieve only the pain of angina pectoris. **Relief of substernal pain by nitroglycerin does not necessarily establish the diagnosis of angina pectoris, as this drug can also relieve the pain of lower esophageal spasm.** In fact, patients with peptic esophagitis who obtain inadequate relief from the usual therapeutic measures (antacids, bethanechol, cimetidine, and metoclopramide) may receive additional relief from nitroglycerin. **If the pain is relieved by ingesting viscous Xylocaine or lidocaine, it is probably due to peptic esophagitis.** Some authors suggest using viscous Xylocaine or lidocaine as a diagnostic tool because studies have shown that when chest pain was relieved by ingestion of viscous Xylocaine or lidocaine, it usually was due to peptic esophagitis. There were a few false-positives, however, among patients who had chest pain of coronary origin. Therefore, this test is useful but will not rule out coronary artery disease with absolute certainty.

Once the diagnosis of serious disease is excluded, patients with vague symptoms of indigestion and functional gastrointestinal complaints should be treated with reassurance and, occasionally, tranquilizers. In some instances, antispasmodics and digestants may be helpful.

PHYSICAL FINDINGS

Most patients who complain of indigestion or heartburn demonstrate no abnormal physical findings, despite a careful examination. Auscultation of peristalsis in the chest should suggest a large diaphragmatic hernia. Mild, diffuse, abdominal tenderness associated with abdominal distention sometimes is observed with *pancreatitis* or *excessive swallowed air* in the intestinal tract. A succussion splash can often be elicited in

DIFFERENTIAL DIAGNOSIS OF HEARTBURN AND INDIGESTION

CAUSE	NATURE OF PATIENT	NATURE OF SYMPTOMS	ASSOCIATED SYMPTOMS	PRECIPITATING AND AGGRAVATING FACTORS	AMELIORATING FACTORS	PHYSICAL FINDINGS	DIAGNOSTIC STUDIES
Reflux esophagitis	Adults More common in pregnant women in later months	Severe heartburn Water brash often occurs with recumbency Recurrent pain radiates to back (40%), arms, or neck (5%) Not induced by exercise	Chest pain Dysphagia Belching (due to aerophagia)	Recumbency Straining or lifting Drinking alcoholic, caffeinated, or carbonated beverages Eating heavy meals or fatty, spicy, or acidic foods Smoking Pregnancy	Raising head of bed Antacids Nitrates Small, frequent, low-fat meals Avoidance of tight garments		Pain often relieved by ingestion of viscous Xylocaine or lidocaine Esophagoscopy Bernstein test Upper GI radiograph
Gastritis	Alcoholics	Abdominal pain Vague indigestion Heartburn	Decreased appetite Sense of "fullness" Nausea and vomiting	Alcohol Meals Drugs (aspirin, nonsteroidal anti-inflammatory agents, corticosteroids)	Bile gastritis may be relieved by vomiting	Tenderness to abdominal palpation or epigastric percussion	Endoscopy Upper GI radiograph
"Functional" gastrointestinal disorder	Children and adults	Abdominal distention Awareness of peristalsis and "gurgling" Intermittent symptoms Vague, nonspecific symptoms No weight loss Continuous pain	Significant emotional investment Other neutoric symptoms Belching (secondary to aerophagia)	Social/environmental stresses		No signs of systemic disease	Studies normal

Excessive intestinal gas	Common in elderly	Vague feelings of indigestion	Abdominal bloating, Belching, Passing flatus	GI stasis, Hypomotility of gut, Changed intestinal bacteria, Constipation, Lack of exercise	Belching, Passing flatus		
Gas entrapment (hepatic or splenic flexure syndrome)		Abdominal discomfort, Pain often referred to chest	Chest pain	Bending over, Wearing a tight garment	Passing flatus	Flexion of thigh on abdomen replicates symptoms	Abdominal radiograph shows "trapped" gas in hepatic or splenic flexure
Gallbladder disease		Vague abdominal discomfort, Occasional distention, Indigestion	Nausea, Pain in right shoulder	Fatty foods			Cholecystograms, Sonograms

patients with *gastric dilatation,* whether due to reflex or secondary to pyloric obstruction. Some patients with *gastritis* will have tenderness on abdominal palpation, whereas others may have no physical findings other than midepigastric tenderness to percussion. The same is true for patients with *peptic ulcer disease.* Patients with *cholelithiasis* may have no symptoms, although there occasionally may be right upper quadrant tenderness to palpation or percussion. In some patients with *hydrops of the gallbladder,* a dilated gallbladder is palpable or ballotable.

DIAGNOSTIC STUDIES

Esophageal reflux can be observed on upper gastrointestinal radiographs. Esophagitis can be detected by esophagoscopy, and its symptoms can be produced by instillation of dilute hydrochloric acid in the distal esophagus (Bernstein test).

Gastritis can be diagnosed by radiographic studies or gastroscopy.

Gallbladder disease can be diagnosed by sonography, cholecystography, and isotopic studies.

LESS COMMON DIAGNOSTIC CONSIDERATIONS

When the patient finds that abdominal discomfort is intensified by bending over or wearing a tight garment, gas entrapment (e.g., hepatic or splenic flexure syndrome) should be suspected. Sometimes, this discomfort is relieved by passage of flatus. Gas entrapment can be confirmed if flexion of the right or left thigh on the abdomen replicates the pain or if an abdominal radiograph shows a large bubble of "trapped" gas in the hepatic or splenic flexure. The pain of gas entrapment in the hepatic or splenic flexure is often referred to the chest, and the patient may present with a complaint of chest pain.

Heartburn may be caused by viral esophagitis and moniliasis of the esophagus. Disseminated sclerosis that invades the esophagus may also cause severe heartburn. Indigestion may be the presenting symptom in uremia, pulmonary tuberculosis, migraine, gastric dilatation, glaucoma, hypercalcemia, diabetes, and coronary artery disease.

Selected References

Hunt, T.: Indigestion in Harvey's time. Am. J. Med. *85*:891–893, 1978.
Long, W. B., and Cohen, S.: The digestive tract as a cause of chest pain. Am. Heart J. *100*:567–572, 1980.
Reed, P. I.: Oesophageal reflux. Practitioner *224*:357–363, 1980.
Thompson, W. Grant, and Heaton, K. W.: Functional bowel disorders in apparently healthy people. Gastroenterology *79*:283–288, 1980.
Volpicelli, N. A., Yardley, J. H., and Hendrix, T. R.: The association of heartburn with gastritis. Dig. Dis. *22*:333–339, 1977.

17
INSOMNIA

Of all the sleep disorders, insomnia is the most common. Studies have shown that hypnotics are used on a regular basis by approximately 20 per cent of the adult population. Insomnia includes the following problems: delay in falling asleep, poor quality of sleep (deficiency of deep and REM sleep), frequent awakening, and early morning wakefulness. Insomnia can be caused by *physical disorders* (e.g., congestive heart failure, pregnancy, hyperthyroidism, nocturnal asthma, or nocturnal seizures); *painful* or *uncomfortable syndromes* (e.g., toothache, arthritis, or restless legs syndrome), *psychiatric illnesses* (e.g., depression, anxiety, or mania); and the use or withdrawal of *drugs* (e.g., caffeine, alcohol, antidepressants, beta blockers, or hypnotics).

NATURE OF PATIENT

Nocturnal enuresis (bedwetting), *sleep-walking, talking while asleep,* and *night terrors* are thought to be arousal disorders because they usually occur with emergence from deep non–REM sleep. Children who experience nocturnal enuresis and sleep-walking often have difficulty sleeping. Bedwetting is the most common sleep-arousal disorder in children between the ages of 3 and 15 years. It is more frequent in males than in females. When there is no obvious organic or psychologic cause, bedwetting generally occurs in the first part of the night as the child emerges from delta sleep and before the first REM sleep. The change of sleep state often is accompanied by body movements and increased muscle tone; urination occurs during this period. Although these problems usually have a psychologic etiology, many investigators believe that such disorders stem from a basis that is psychophysiologic rather than from one that is strictly psychologic.

Nightmares and night terrors often disturb sleep. Nightmares, in both children and adults, occur during REM sleep. Night terrors, characterized by sudden screams and arousal, occur during deep sleep. **Insomnia in children is most often due to psychologic stress, although occasionally it can be due to organic disease (e.g., a disorder of the hip).**

Some patients who *snore* have *sleep-induced apnea,* which causes wakefulness. These patients are often obese males. Typically, their sleep companions complain that they snore very loudly. These loud snorers may have as many as 100 episodes of sleep apnea each night; many episodes lead to brief arousal.

Sleep patterns often change with aging; elderly people frequently require less sleep than they needed in their younger years. Elderly patients often complain of both delay in falling asleep and poor sleep quality.

Patients who ingest products that contain *caffeine* (e.g., coffee, tea, and cola) frequently complain of insomnia. Even those patients who previously tolerated caffeine well often develop sleeping problems. Because the half-life of caffeine may range from 2 to more than 6 hours in different people, the ingestion of caffeine, especially after 6 P.M., may contribute significantly to insomnia. Patients may or may not be aware that caffeine is the cause of their insomnia. People who drink *alcohol,* even in moderate amounts (i.e., two drinks at night), as well as cured alcoholics, often experience poor sleep quality with frequent awakening.

Often, poor sleep at night may be related to napping or dozing during the day. Elderly patients with *dementia* are often restless and wakeful at night. *Depression,* a common cause of sleep disturbances, is frequently undiagnosed in the elderly.

Depressed (unipolar affective disorder) patients of all ages frequently experience insomnia characterized by delayed sleep onset (prolonged latency), frequent awakening, and, classically, early morning wakefulness. Patients with *manic depression (bipolar affective disorder),* may experience marked insomnia, especially just prior to and during the manic phase. Patients suffering from *anxiety* may have trouble falling asleep but rarely experience early morning wakefulness.

NATURE OF SYMPTOMS

Patients usually describe insomnia rather loosely as "trouble sleeping." A patient may have one or more types of insomnia. Therefore, the physician must question specifically for each type of insomnia to diagnose the cause correctly and to provide effective, specific therapy. It is very helpful to ask patients what they are thinking about before they fall asleep and what they are thinking about on awakening. This often provides significant clues to the etiology of their insomnia.

Prolonged sleep latency (the time from turning the lights out until stage-one sleep) is most common in anxious patients, caffeine and alcohol users, and elderly patients, especially those who sleep during the day. It should be noted that the latency period is generally overestimated by the patient. Some patients complain of a poor quality of sleep when they do not feel rested despite an adequate amount of sleep; this is usually due to a deficiency of deep-REM sleep and is particularly common in patients with painful syndromes, pregnant women, people who consume alcohol, and cured alcoholics. Some patients, particularly alcoholics, complain of frequent awakening; this is usually from stage-two sleep. **Early morning awakening from which a patient cannot return to sleep is most common and particularly characteristic of depressed patients.** Some studies show depressed patients to have prolonged sleep latency, decreased total sleep, increased intermittent awakening, and less deep sleep than other patients.

ASSOCIATED SYMPTOMS

Painful and *uncomfortable conditions* such as pleurisy, peptic esophagitis, toothaches, pregnancy, and even severe itching can interfere with normal sleep. Paroxysmal nocturnal dyspnea, nocturnal asthma, hyperthyroidism, alcoholism, use of caffeine or other drugs, recent cessation of hypnotics or antidepressants, and severe snoring may also contribute to sleeping problems. **The most common causes of insomnia are ingestion of caffeine, alcohol consumption, anxiety, and depression.**

Although anxiety and depression often cause insomnia, patients with these conditions usually have additional symptoms. *Anxious patients* often have somatic complaints such as headaches, chest pain, palpitations, dizziness, gastrointestinal distress, nervousness, and feelings of foreboding. *Depressed patients* frequently complain of decreased appetite, weight loss, lack of energy, lack of interest in activities, decreased libido, constipation, and vague aches and pains. Patients with fibrositis and insomnia (which some investigators attribute to depression) may obtain excellent relief of their aches, pains, and insomnia with antidepressant medication.

PRECIPITATING AND AGGRAVATING FACTORS

Patients who complain of insomnia should be questioned about whether certain situations (e.g., death in the family, financial concerns,

DIFFERENTIAL DIAGNOSIS OF INSOMNIA

CAUSE	NATURE OF PATIENT	NATURE OF SYMPTOMS	ASSOCIATED SYMPTOMS	PRECIPITATING AND AGGRAVATING FACTORS
Bedwetting (nocturnal enuresis)	Children (especially 3–15 years) More common in males	Arousal after deep sleep	Sleep-walking	Environmental or psychologic stresses and fears
Nightmares and night terrors	More common in children	Arousal during REM sleep		
Painful or uncomfortable conditions Physical disorders	Any age	Delayed latency Poor sleep quality	Symptoms related to physical disorder or painful or uncomfortable condition	Toothache Pleurisy Arthritis Pregnancy Esophagitis Nocturnal asthma or seizures Congenital hip lesions Hyperthyroidism Nocturia
Change in sleep habits	Elderly	Delayed sleep latency Poor sleep quality	Daytime naps or dozing	
Unipolar depression	Depressed	Delayed sleep latency Early morning wakefulness	Anorexia Fatigue Lack of interest in activities Decreased libido Constipation Vague aches and pains	Conditions, medications, and situations that produce depression
Bipolar depression	Manic Manic-depressive	May not sleep at all during manic phases	Agitation Hyperactivity Flight of ideas	Worse just before and during manic phase

Table continued on opposite page

DIFFERENTIAL DIAGNOSIS OF INSOMNIA *Continued*

CAUSE	NATURE OF PATIENT	NATURE OF SYMPTOMS	ASSOCIATED SYMPTOMS	PRECIPITATING AND AGGRAVATING FACTORS
Anxiety	Any age	Delayed sleep latency	Somatic complaints Headaches Chest pain Palpitations Dizziness GI symptoms Nervousness Feelings of foreboding	Situations that produce anxiety
Snoring	Adults Often obese males	Frequent awakening Poor sleep quality	Snoring	Sleep apnea Obstruction Central apnea
Caffeine	Any age	Delayed sleep latency Poor quality sleep	May have previously tolerated caffeine well	Use of caffeine (especially after 6 P.M.)
Alcohol	Teenagers Adults Elderly	Delayed latency Frequent awakening	Nervousness Signs of alcoholism	Alcohol Alcoholic withdrawal "Cured" alcoholics
Withdrawal of antide-pressants or hypnotics	Any age	Similar to prior symptoms	May redevelop symptoms of anxiety, depression	
Medications	Any age	Poor sleep quality Prolonged sleep latency	Depends on drug responsible	Psychotropics Beta blockers Diuretics Hypnotics Appetite suppressants Amphetamines

family crises, school examinations, changes in life patterns, alterations in work schedules, or changes in drug habits) coincided with the onset of insomnia. The patient should also be questioned about prior episodes of insomnia and what may have precipitated them. Transient insomnia may also occur in anticipation of a joyous event or during periods of excitement.

According to one study of patients referred to a sleep center, the most common cause of insomnia is ingestion of caffeine in any form. Many of these patients previously tolerated caffeine well. The second most common cause is alcohol. Although small amounts of alcohol may facilitate sleep onset for some patients, it may also cause early awakening or nightmares, contrary to common belief. These patients often note poor quality of sleep and frequent awakening.

In evaluating sleep disturbances, physicians should have patients keep a sleep diary for 1 week. Patients should note the time they retire; their latency period; number of awakenings; time of last awakening; any sleep events such as dreams, nightmares, and the need to urinate; and any comments made by the sleep partner. It is particularly important for patients to note their thoughts during latency and on awakening, as these may help establish the cause of their insomnia.

Other precipitating and aggravating factors in insomnia include fear of illness and even pruritus. Although these factors may be tolerated during the day when the patient is active, they may be distracting enough to cause insomnia when the patient is at rest.

AMELIORATING FACTORS

Hypnotics, including over-the-counter preparations, are occasionally helpful for short periods of insomnia. However, their continued use (for more than 1 week) may exacerbate insomnia, particularly if REM sleep has been suppressed. Hypnotics are *rarely* indicated to treat the symptom "insomnia." **One must treat insomnia by dealing with its cause.** Daytime naps or pain can be identified as the probable cause of insomnia if cessation of the former or relief of the latter results in improved sleep. If avoidance of caffeine (in all forms) after noon permits the return of normal sleep patterns, caffeine was probably responsible for the insomnia. When changes in work shifts are associated with insomnia, patients should be advised to try to return to their original sleep schedule to determine whether this eliminates their insomnia. Avoidance of noisy or extremely warm environments and strenuous exercise at night also may facilitate a return to normal sleep patterns.

PHYSICAL FINDINGS

The physical examination is usually not helpful in determining the etiology of insomnia. Occasionally, medical conditions that contribute to insomnia may yield abnormal physical findings; this occurs in hyperthyroidism, congestive heart failure, peptic esophagitis, pulmonary disease, ulcer disease, seizure disorders, and prostatism. It should be noted that any condition that causes frequent nocturia may interfere with normal sleep patterns.

DIAGNOSTIC STUDIES

When the etiology for insomnia cannot be determined and the patient cannot be relieved of this symptom, he should be referred to a sleep center for sleep studies. Centers are located in many regions and are discussed by several other authors (Reynolds et al., 1979).

LESS COMMON DIAGNOSTIC CONSIDERATIONS

Conditions that occur less frequently include nocturnal myoclonus, painful erections, central sleep apnea, and "restless legs" syndrome. These last two conditions are more common in the elderly. Sleep apnea often is exacerbated by hypnotics and alcohol.

Selected References

Gillen, J. C., et al.: Successful separation of depressed, normal, and insomniac patients by EEG sleep data. Arch. Gen. Psych. *36*:85–90, 1979.

Kales, A., et al.: Insomnia and other sleep disorders. Med. Clin. North Am. *66*:5, 1982.

Kogeorgos, J., and Scott, D. F.: Sleep and sleep disorders. Practitioner *224*:717–721, 1980.

Mathis, J. L.: Insomnia. J. Fam. Pract. *6*:873–876, 1978.

Pagel, J. F.: Sleep disorders and insomnia. Am. Fam. Phys. *17*:165–169, 1978.

Reynolds, C. F., et al.: Sleep and its disorders. Symposium on psychological issues in primary care. Primary Care *6*:417–438, 1979.

18
MENSTRUAL IRREGULARITIES

ABNORMAL BLEEDING

Bleeding from the vagina is considered abnormal whenever it occurs at an unexpected time of life (before menarche or after menopause) or when it varies from the norm in amount or pattern. *Spontaneous abortions, pregnancy complications,* and *bleeding from polyps* or other pathologic processes account for approximately 25 per cent of the cases of abnormal vaginal bleeding.

Dysfunctional uterine bleeding is a somewhat confusing nonspecific diagnostic term. It has been defined as abnormal uterine bleeding not due to organic gynecologic disease. Therefore, this diagnosis may be reached only by a process of exclusion. With advances in the understanding of the neuroendocrinologic basis of the menstrual cycle, diagnosis and therapy have become more specific. The reader can find detailed reviews of these developments in several excellent articles (see references). In order to understand and diagnose the various causes of menstrual irregularities, one must have a thorough knowledge of normal physiology (Fig. 18–1). Although the history is very important, it is rarely diagnostic and serves only as a guide to the origin of the bleeding. In most instances, hormonal or cytologic studies are necessary to establish the correct diagnosis.

Anovulatory Bleeding

Hormonal mechanisms of endometrial bleeding include *estrogen-withdrawal bleeding, estrogen-breakthrough bleeding, progesterone-with-*

189

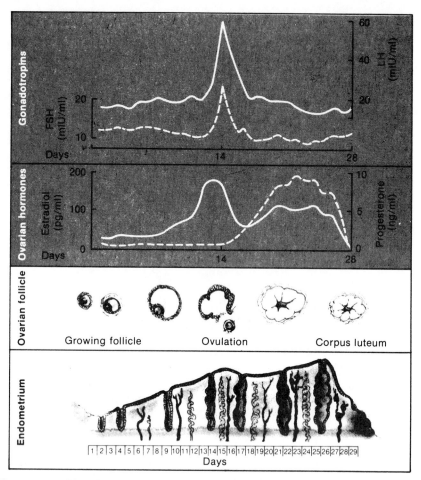

Figure 18–1. Physiology of the normal ovulatory menstrual cycle. (From Lopez, R. I.: Menstrual irregularities in teenage girls. Drug Therapy, April, 1981, p. 47.)

drawal bleeding, and *progesterone-breakthrough bleeding.* **Anovulatory, hormone-related bleeding is most common.** This form of dysfunctional uterine bleeding is due to estrogen-withdrawal or estrogen-breakthrough bleeding.

Estrogen-Withdrawal Bleeding. In instances of estrogen-withdrawal bleeding, the endometrium proliferates and remains stable as long as the estrogen level remains above the threshold. When the estrogen falls below the threshold, there is bleeding. When this occurs in the absence of progesterone, the endometrium is not in the secretory phase, and bleeding is often prolonged and profuse. This type of bleeding often occurs during adolescence and the climacteric.

Estrogen-Breakthrough Bleeding. This type of bleeding has been divided into two categories. The first is associated with low but constant levels of estrogen (near the threshold). This causes portions of the endometrium to degenerate and results in spotting. **This type of threshold-breakthrough bleeding occurs with the use of low-dose oral contraceptives.** The second type of estrogen-breakthrough bleeding occurs when estrogen levels are initially well above the threshold. This causes the endometrium to proliferate and become hyperplastic; areas of endometrium outgrow their blood-borne hormone supply, with degeneration and irregular, prolonged bleeding resulting.

Progesterone-Withdrawal Bleeding. This type of bleeding occurs only with an estrogen-primed endometrium. When estrogen therapy is continued as progesterone is withdrawn, progesterone-withdrawal bleeding occurs. This type of bleeding is observed when intramuscular progesterone or oral medroxyprogesterone acetate (Provera) is administered as a test for the presence of endogenous estrogen.

Progesterone-Breakthrough Bleeding. This is a form of estrogen-breakthrough bleeding that occurs when a high dose of a progestational drug is given.

Ovulatory Dysfunctional Bleeding

Ovulatory dysfunctional bleeding may be suspected by history and confirmed with simple investigations (Table 18–1). Ovulatory bleeding is usually associated with a regular cycle length, occasional ovulation pain (mittelschmerz); premenstrual symptoms (e.g., breast soreness, bloating, weight gain, and mood changes), and a biphasic basal body temperature. *Anovulatory bleeding* causes an irregular cycle in which bleeding is not preceded by or associated with, subjective symptoms. In such cases, there is a monophasic basal body temperature pattern.

Bleeding Patterns

Recognition of particular bleeding patterns is another way of considering cases of abnormal vaginal bleeding (Table 18–2). *Menorrhagia,* or *hypermenorrhea* (excessive menstrual bleeding), is often due to local gynecologic disease (e.g., polyps, malignancy, salpingitis, and uterine fibroids). It also commonly occurs in association with intrauterine devices. *Metrorrhagia* (intermenstrual spotting between otherwise normal periods) is also often caused by local disease. It frequently is associated with exogenous estrogen therapy. *Menometrorrhagia* is bleeding that is unpredictable with regard to amount and frequency; it can be caused by local lesions, complications of early gestation, or endocrine dysfunction (e.g., dysfunctional bleeding). *Polymenorrhagia* is excessive cyclic hemorrhage occurring at intervals of 21 days or less. This type of bleeding is most commonly the result of anovulatory cycles.

Table 18–1. **Differentiation of Ovulatory and Anovulatory Bleeding**

Criteria	Ovulatory Bleeding	Anovulatory Bleeding
History	Regular cycle length, ovulation pain (mittelschmerz), premenstrual molimina (breast soreness, bloating, weight gain, mood change), dysmenorrhea (cramps up to 12 hours before flow and/or for first 2 days of flow)	Irregular cycles in which bleeding is not preceded by or associated with subjective symptoms
Basal body temperature record	Biphasic pattern	Monophasic pattern
Cervical mucus	Preovulatory: Thin, clear, watery mucus with stretchability (spinnbarkeit) and ferning Postovulatory: Thick, cloudy, cellular mucus that lacks stretchability and ferning	Always dominated by estrogen
Maturation index	Preovulatory: Dominated by superficial cells Postovulatory: Shift to high percentage of intermediate cells	Always a marked right shift due to high estrogen level
Premenstrual endometrial biopsy	Secretory endometrium	Proliferative and possible hyperplastic changes
Serum progesterone level	Preovulatory: <1 ng/ml Postovulatory: >5 ng/ml	Never exceeds 5 ng/ml; usually preovulatory values

(From Strickler, R. C.: Dysfunctional uterine bleeding—diagnosis and treatment. Postgrad. Med. *66*:135–146, 1979.)

Table 18–2. **Nomenclature to Describe Menstrual Disturbances**

Term	Bleeding Pattern
Menorrhagia	Excessive flow (amount and/or duration) with normal cycle (21–35 days)
Polymenorrhea	Normal flow with cycle less than 21 days
Polymenorrhagia	Excessive flow with cycle less than 21 days
Metrorrhagia	Excessive flow that is acyclic
Metrostaxis	Continuous bleeding
Ovulation bleeding (pseudopolymenorrhea)	Spotting or light flow at time of midcycle estrogen nadir
Premenstrual staining	Spotting or light flow up to 7 days prior to menstruation in ovulatory cycle

(From Strickler, R. C.: Dysfunctional uterine bleeding—diagnosis and treatment. Postgrad. Med. *66*:135–146, 1979.)

Nature of Patient

Prior to menarche, there is a characteristic sequence of events that begins at about 8 years of age (Fig. 18–2): Breast buds develop, pubic hairs appear, breasts enlarge, axillary hairs appear, and finally a height spurt occurs. Menstrual function usually begins after the height spurt. Approximately 6 months before menarche, there is a physiologic leukorrhea. One must remember that in the first year after menarche, 55 per cent of menses are anovulatory, with a sharp decline to approximately 7 per cent by 8 years after menarche. Usually, 15 months are required for completion of the first 10 menstrual cycles. This means that when menses begin, it is unusual for them to occur at regular monthly intervals.

The average age at which girls begin to menstruate is 12 years. The characteristics of normal menstruation are shown in Table 18–3. Bleeding that occurs before 9 to 10 years of age is abnormal, and local pathology as well as adrenal and ovarian tumors must be suspected. Since some teenage girls are reluctant to volunteer information about their menstrual periods, it is absolutely essential that physicians routinely ask a series of questions: (1) When did your menses begin? (2) How often do your menstrual periods occur? (3) On what date did your last period occur? (4) Is there any pain associated with menstruation? (5) Are you sexually active? (6) Are you practicing any form of birth control? These questions must be asked in a nonthreatening way so that the patient feels at ease and understands that the physician is willing to listen. Likewise, when asking questions about sexual activities, it is essential that the physician remain nonjudgmental. The teenager should be reassured that any discussion of this nature will remain a private matter between patient and physician.

The adolescent frequently has cycles of variable length. Anovulation may be associated with both short and long cycles together with short follicular and luteal cycles. Another important point is that menarche may be delayed in underweight adolescents. In some teenage girls who are on strict diets to remain fashionably thin and in athletes with normal body weight but low body fat, menarche may be delayed. Likewise, there is often a familial pattern of menarche: It is common for girls to start menstruating at approximately the same age as their mothers and sisters did.

There are several significant age-associated conditions that can cause abnormal vaginal bleeding. In children, insertion of *foreign bodies* into the vagina may cause bleeding. During the reproductive years, *dysfunctional uterine bleeding* and bleeding from *pregnancy complications, tumors,* and *fibroids* may occur (Table 18–4). In postmenopausal women, bleeding may result from *endometrial* and *cervical cancers.* Anovulatory *estrogen-withdrawal bleeding* is the most common cause of

Stage	Description

Breast development

	Stage	Description
	B1	Preadolescent: elevation of nipple only
	B2	Breast-bud stage: elevation of breast and nipple as a small mound
	B3	Further enlargement of breast and areola with no separation of contours
	B4	Projection of areola so as to form a secondary mound
	B5	Mature stage: nipple projects from general contour of breast

Pubic hair development

	Stage	Description
	PH1	None
	PH2	Sparse growth of long straight hair along labia; no hair on mons pubis
	PH3	Thicker, coarse, curled hair on mons pubis
	PH4	Adult-type hair on mons pubis but not reaching the medial aspect of thighs
	PH5	Hair reaches the medial surface of thighs

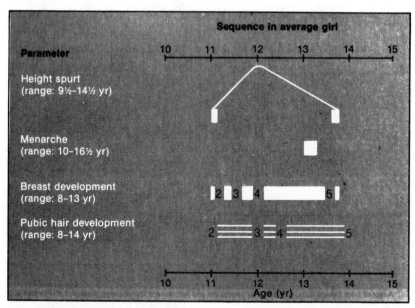

Figure 18–2. Relationship of pubertal events in adolescent girls. (From Lopez, R. I.: Menstrual irregularities in teenage girls. Drug Therapy, April, 1981, p. 49.)

Table 18–3. **Characteristics of Menstruation***

Characteristics	Range	Average
Menarche (age of onset)	9–17 years	12.5 years
Cycle length (interval)	21–35 days	28 days
Duration of flow	1–8 days	3–5 days
Amount of flow	10–80 ml	35 ml
Onset of menopause	45–55 years	47–50 years

*Range and averages for American women.
(From Hamilton, C.: Vaginal bleeding: evaluation and management. Resident and Staff Physician, November, 1981, pp. 62–64.)

irregular menses during the reproductive years and accounts for 40 per cent of menstrual disturbances occurring in the perimenopausal years.

Nature of Symptoms

Prolonged irregular and profuse bleeding may occur with either estrogen-breakthrough or estrogen-withdrawal bleeding. The bleeding may be spotty (threshold-breakthrough bleeding). Anovulatory bleeding is usually unexpected and painless. Anovulatory cycles may result in *polymenorrhagia*. With ovulatory menstrual abnormalities, there may be a short luteal phase, in which case menstrual cycles may be variable but long. Patients with these problems may also complain of premenstrual bleeding or staining. When *menorrhagia* is present, *tumors, fibroids, malignancy, polyps, salpingitis,* or *intrauterine contraceptive devices* may be the cause. *Endometriosis, salpingitis,* and *cancer* may also cause minimal bleeding and should be suspected if there is also a purulent discharge. The sympoms of endometriosis are reviewed in detail in Chapter 19.

During the reproductive years, abnormal vaginal bleeding often represents *pregnancy complications.* There may be a history of sexual activity without adequate contraceptive measures. In addition, symptoms of pregnancy such as missed periods, morning sickness, or breast tenderness may be present. In these cases, the uterine bleeding initially results from endometrial sloughing, and therefore spotting rather than amenorrhea may occur prior to gross hemorrhage.

Gross hemorrhage may be concealed or visible. *Ectopic pregnancy* is strongly suggested by an adnexal or cul-de-sac mass in a pregnant woman who has a normal or only slightly enlarged uterus. Concealed pelvic hemorrhage from a ruptured ectopic pregnancy can occur either with or without vaginal bleeding. This diagnosis should be suspected when there is amenorrhea, pelvic or abdominal fullness, abdominal pain (particularly if the pain is unilateral or referred to the shoulder), tenesmus, urinary frequency, or urinary urgency. Fever, signs of peritoneal irritation, purulent vaginal discharge, or pain can be seen in patients with ectopic pregnancy or salpingitis. **It is axiomatic that copious vaginal bleeding is most often the result of pregnancy complications and less often due to local gynecologic disease or dysfunctional bleeding.** Bright red hemorrhage with clots suggests a brisk nonmenstrual flow. A darker tint of blood implies slower hemorrhage acted upon by cervical or vaginal secretions. Irregular bleeding during pregnancy may be due to separation of the placenta or the embryo from its attachment, but malignant cervical erosions, polyps, and local vaginal lesions must be excluded.

Menorrhagia during puberty is usually due to anovulation. This gradually abates within several months of the onset of the menarche. Menorrhagia during the reproductive years can also be due to anovulation, as can *polymenorrhagia*. Menorrhagia that occurs during the reproductive years may be caused by *fibromyomas*. **The chief characteristic of a uterine fibroid is an asymmetrically enlarged uterus.** There may be more than one fibroid in the uterus, and the shape can be extremely irregular. As a rule, the consistency of the fibroid is hard and unyielding. Usually the cervix and uterine fibroid move together.

In some instances, it is difficult for the physician to distinguish a fibromyoma from an *ovarian cyst*. **A helpful point in the differentiation of fibroids from ovarian cysts is that ovarian cysts almost never cause menorrhagia.** Ovarian tumors usually create no menstrual disturbances. *Adenomyoma* of the uterus usually causes symmetric uterine enlargement, but absolute differentiation must be accomplished by pathologic examination.

Chronic salpingo-oophoritis (hydrosalpinx, tubo-ovarian abscess, or *chronic salpingitis)* as well as *ovarian endometriosis* can cause menorrhagia, and congestive (premenstrual) dysmenorrhea is usually present as a prominent symptom. Menorrhagia can also be caused by IUD's, thrombocytopenia, and other coagulation defects.

Irregular menstrual bleeding may be divided into three groups: (1) irregular bleeding during menstrual life, (2) bleeding before puberty and after menopause, and (3) bleeding during pregnancy.

Irregular Bleeding During Menstrual Life
(Table 18–4)

Metrorrhagia. The lesions of the reproductive organs that cause metrorrhagia include *cervical carcinoma, benign* and *malignant uterine tumors, endometritis* and, rarely, *tuberculous endometritis*. Usually *fibromyomas* cause menorrhagia but occasionally can cause metrorrhagia. Fibroids tend to produce irregular bleeding when they are submucosal or in the process of extrusion. A carcinoma can develop in a patient known to have uterine fibroids, and a fibroid occasionally can undergo sarcomatous degeneration. Rapid enlargement of the uterus associated

Table 18–4. **Etiologies of Vaginal Bleeding in the Reproductive Years**

Menstruation and Variations
  Ovulational spotting (midcycle)
Pregnancy Complications
  Early (< 20 weeks)
    Implantational bleeding
    Abortion
    Ectopic pregnancy
    Trophoblastic disease
  Late (> 20 weeks)
    Placenta previa, vasa previa, other
  Postpartum
    Uterine atony
    Retained products
Normal Delivery
Disorders of the CNS-Hypothalamic-Ovarian-Pituitary Axis
  Dysfunctional uterine bleeding (DUB)
    Anovulatory (80% to 90%)
    Ovulatory
  Functioning ovarian cysts or tumors
  Emotional stress
  Anticholinergic drugs
Exogenous Hormones
  Estrogen
  Estrogen-progestin oral contraceptives
Trauma
Anticoagulant Drugs
Organic Gynecologic Disease
  Pelvic infections
  Neoplastic diseases
    Benign
    Malignant
  Adenomyosis
Systemic Disease
  Generalized bleeding disorders
  Thyroid disease

(From Hamilton, C.: Vaginal bleeding: evaluation and management. Resident and Staff Physician, November, 1981, pp. 62–64.)

with irregular bleeding is very suggestive of a *sarcoma*. However, several fibroids can be present in the same uterus and are a common cause of rapid uterine enlargement. *Choriocarcinoma* is a rare cause of uterine enlargement that follows a *hydatidiform mole* in about 50 per cent of the recorded cases. It should be suspected during early pregnancy in women in whom there is a threat of abortion and in whom the uterus is extremely enlarged.. Choriocarcinoma is also likely in women who have persistent uterine enlargement.

Cervical erosions usually do not bleed. If there is irregular bleeding from the erosion or if the cervix bleeds during an examination, malignancy should be excluded.

Menorrhagia. *Polyps* and *fibroids* are common causes of menorrhagia. *Dysfunctional uterine bleeding* can occur at any age. Fifty per cent of cases occur in women between the ages of 40 and 50 years, approximately 10 per cent develop at puberty, and the remaining 40 per cent occur between puberty and age 40 years. Bleeding related to dysfunctional uterine bleeding—frequently due to an anovulatory cycle—is generally in the form of menorrhagia, although the interval between periods may be shortened.

Women who are using *estrogen preparations* to control menstrual symptoms or to prevent conception may develop menorrhagia while the drugs are being taken or following their withdrawal. The menorrhagia is often related to the dosage of estrogen.

Bleeding associated with *ovulation* is uncommon; when it occurs, it is midway between the periods (approximately at the time of ovulation). Mid–menstrual cycle bleeding accompanied by lower abdominal pain is referred to as *mittelschmerz*.

Bleeding Before Puberty and After Menopause

When vaginal bleeding occurs in newborn infants, it is usually due to a temporarily *high concentration of estrogen* in the *fetal circulation*. Postmenopausal bleeding may be due to *malignant growths, polyps, senile endometritis,* or *cervicitis. Carcinoma of the body of the uterus* rarely causes much uterine enlargement, and any increase in size usually occurs slowly. It should be noted that the post-menopausal uterus decreases considerably in size. Thus, a uterine size that would be regarded as normal in a younger woman indicates abnormal enlargement in a postmenopausal woman.

Bleeding During Pregnancy

It is important for the physician to differentiate the uterine hemorrhage of extrauterine gestation from that due to threatened abortion. Bleeding can be caused by *placenta previa* and by *abruptio placentae*.

Associated Symptoms

Ovulatory irregular bleeding is often associated with midcycle ovulation pain (mittelschmerz), premenstrual symptoms, and dysmenorrhea. Fever, purulent vaginal discharge, and pain may be clues to pregnancy complications, including spontaneous and induced abortions. These same symptoms also may be observed in cases of ectopic pregnancy and salpingitis. Irregular menses associated with galactorrhea suggests a prolactinoma.

Precipitating Factors

Anovulatory irregular menstrual bleeding often occurs during the first 12 to 18 months after menarche. It is seen most frequently in obese patients; in women who have adrenal disease, pituitary tumors, polycystic ovary syndrome, Cushing's disease, diabetes, malnutrition, chronic illness, or hypothyroidism; and in patients who use phenothiazines or opiates.

Physical Findings

Physical examination should be complete and include thorough pelvic and abdominal evaluations. It should be directed at detection of systemic diseases such as *endocrinopathies*, including adult-onset adrenal hyperplasia, Cushing's disease, thyroid dysfunction, polycystic ovaries, and obesity. Vaginal examination must be thorough.

Diagnostic Studies

Diagnostic tests that are useful in the differential diagnosis of patients with abnormal vaginal bleeding include a complete blood count, platelet count, coagulation studies, thyroid function tests, pituitary function tests, blood sugar tests, and urinalysis. Other diagnostic tests that help the physician evaluate the etiology of abnormal vaginal bleeding include uterine curettage, vaginal and cervical biopsies, and Papanicolaou's smear for detection of cancer; Gram stains and cultures for determination of infections; and serum and urine pregnancy tests for confirmation or exclusion of pregnancy.

Pelvic sonography helps the physician diagnose ectopic pregnancies, ovarian cysts, and tumors. Because most patients of reproductive age who have severe uterine bleeding are pregnant, human chorionic gonadotropin (HCG) should be determined. HCG is produced during uterine and ectopic pregnancies, development of hydatidiform moles, and formation of choriocarcinoma. The most sensitive test for detection of early pregnancy is radioimmunoassay for the beta subunit of HCG. This test often will allow the physician to detect pregnancy as early as 1 week after fertilization, whereas less sensitive urine tests may not confirm a normal pregnancy until the seventh week. This test is particularly important since the physician cannot exclude the possibility of an ectopic pregnancy on the basis of a negative urine test. However, a negative serum radioimmunoassay for the beta subunit of HCG will almost always exclude an ectopic pregnancy. Although ectopic pregnancy accounts for only 0.5 per cent of all pregnancies, it is the cause of 10 to 15 per cent of maternal deaths. More than 90 per cent of ectopic pregnancies are due to tubal implants that rupture during the first trimester. Major risk factors for ectopic pregnancy include history of a previous ectopic pregnancy, salpingitis, previous tubal procedure, and pregnancy that occurs when an intrauterine contraceptive device is in place. The physician is unlikely to miss a catastrophic rupture; however, some ectopic pregnancies leak slowly over several days, so they may go unrecognized until the patient's second or third visit. Ultrasonography helps rule out an ectopic pregnancy by confirming the presence of a uterine gestational sac with an intrauterine pregnancy. When there is a positive culdocentesis or a suspicious sonogram, laparoscopy must be performed, followed by surgical exploration if an ectopic pregnancy is seen. A negative radioimmunoassay for the beta subunit of HCG essentially excludes any pregnancy complication.

Less Common Diagnostic Considerations

Patients with endometriosis may have abnormal vaginal bleeding, but usually these women have dull backaches and dyspareunia associated with their congestive dysmenorrhea. Cervical erosions can be detected on physical examination. Bleeding disorders, including idiopathic thrombocytopenic purpura (ITP), may present with menometrorrhagia. Thrombocytopenia is often seen in patients with disseminated lupus.

Because clear cell adenocarcinoma of the vagina or cervix can be fatal, the possibility of this tumor must always be considered. It is most common in daughters of the 2 to 3 million women who took diethylstilbestrol (DES) as a fertility drug. These "DES daughters" also may have congenital abnormalities of the cervix, uterus, and upper vagina. In addition, they demonstrate an increased risk of pregnancy complications (e.g., threatened abortion, spontaneous or induced incomplete abortion, and ectopic gestation). Abnormal vaginal bleeding may also be a symptom of a coagulation defect, especially platelet deficiency, von Willebrand's disease, or leukemia.

AMENORRHEA

Primary amenorrhea refers to the condition in women who fail to menstruate at all. Most of the young patients simply have delayed menarche. Because weight loss and severe malnutrition can result in delayed menarche, it is particularly important for the physician to determine the patient's diet. In addition, medications such as amphetamines and phenothiazines may interfere with the onset of menstruation. Primary amenorrhea is rare; it usually is associated with an endocrine imbalance or congenital abnormalities. In patients with this condition, it is particularly important for the physician to rule out chromosomal aberrations and genital malformations. In all of these cases, a chromatin analysis of a buccal smear should be performed (Table 18–5). Age is a significant factor in the diagnosis. For example, a 16-year-old girl who has not yet menstruated usually has a delayed menarche; whereas an 18-year-old girl who has not begun to menstruate is considered to have primary amenorrhea (Fig. 18–3).

Patients with *secondary amenorrhea* have menstruated but then stop. **During the reproductive years, the most common cause of secondary amenorrhea is pregnancy.** An endocrine imbalance may be an associated factor, but tumors rarely cause secondary amenorrhea. A vaginal smear and evaluation of the cervical mucous will help in determining whether there is ovarian estrogen production. Various endocrinologic tests help determine whether there is normal ovarian progesterone production and whether there are normal or elevated levels of ovarian androgen. If a patient with secondary amenorrhea has galactorrhea, a prolactinoma is probable. The various causes of secondary amenorrhea are shown in Table 18–6.

Diagnostic studies that are useful in the evaluation of amenorrhea include buccal chromatin analysis, blood and urine hormone estimation, chromosome analysis, basal body temperature, vaginal smear, radiographs of the pituitary fossa, CT scans, and a progesterone withdrawal test for determination of whether estrogen is being manufactured.

Less Common Diagnostic Considerations

Less common causes of amenorrhea include nutritional disorders and strict dieting; systemic disorders such as tuberculosis, diabetes, prolactinoma, hypothyroidism, hyperthyroidism, and anorexia nervosa; psychogenic disturbances, including severe stress; and polycystic ovarian disease. This polycystic ovary syndrome should be suspected in obese young women who have normal sexual development, hypertension, and hirsutism. They may have secondary amenorrhea or oligomenorrhea. In early polycystic ovarian disease, there may be severe dysfunctional bleeding, and serum gonadotropins may be elevated. The patient also may have severe acne.

Congenital adrenal hyperplasia (virilizing tumor) is also manifested by hirsutism and severe acne. Secondary amenorrhea has been reported in female marathon runners, a finding that probably is related to the marked decrease in total body fat in these women. It also has been reported in competitive swimmers and ballet dancers for the same reason. Asherman's syndrome is amenorrhea due to destruction of the basal layer of the endometrium and adhesions following "overenthusiastic" uterine curettage.

Table 18–5. **Diagnostic Scheme for Evaluation of Primary Amenorrhea**

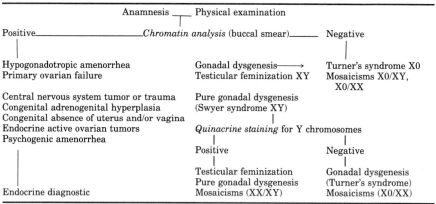

Anamnesis — Physical examination

Positive ———————————— *Chromatin analysis* (buccal smear) ———— Negative

Hypogonadotropic amenorrhea	Gonadal dysgenesis——→	Turner's syndrome X0
Primary ovarian failure	Testicular feminization XY	Mosaicisms X0/XY, X0/XX
Central nervous system tumor or trauma	Pure gonadal dysgenesis	
Congenital adrenogenital hyperplasia	(Swyer syndrome XY)	
Congenital absence of uterus and/or vagina		
Endocrine active ovarian tumors	*Quinacrine staining* for Y chromosomes	
Psychogenic amenorrhea		
	Positive	Negative
	Testicular feminization	Gonadal dysgenesis
	Pure gonadal dysgenesis	(Turner's syndrome)
Endocrine diagnostic	Mosaicisms (XX/XY)	Mosaicisms (X0/XX)

(From Lehmann, F.: Diagnostic approach to ovarian dysfunction. Hormone Res. *9*:319–338, 1978.)

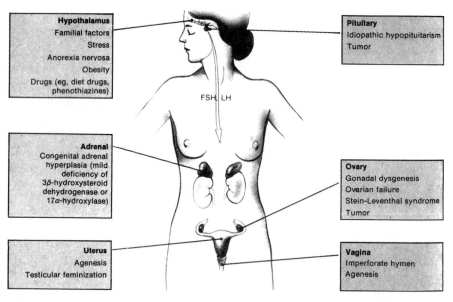

Hypothalamus
Familial factors
Stress
Anorexia nervosa
Obesity
Drugs (eg, diet drugs, phenothiazines)

Pituitary
Idiopathic hypopituitarism
Tumor

FSH LH

Adrenal
Congenital adrenal hyperplasia (mild deficiency of 3β-hydroxysteroid dehydrogenase or 17α-hydroxylase)

Ovary
Gonadal dysgenesis
Ovarian failure
Stein-Leventhal syndrome
Tumor

Uterus
Agenesis
Testicular feminization

Vagina
Imperforate hymen
Agenesis

Figure 18–3. Possible causes of primary amenorrhea and delayed menarche. (From Lopez, R. I.: Menstrual irregularities in young girls. Drug Therapy, April, 1981, p. 42.)

Table 18–6. Possible Causes of Secondary Amenorrhea

	Ovarian Hormone Production	
Normal (Cyclic)	Decreased (Acyclic)	Increased (Acyclic)
Asherman's syndrome	High gonadotropin levels Low or normal gonadotropin levels	Polycystic ovary syndrome
Endometrial destruction		Virilizing ovarian tumors
infective (tuberculosis,	Premature ovarian failure Functional aberrations of the	(arrhenoblastoma, hilus cell
schistosomiasis)	Castration < surgical hypothalamic pituitary axis	tumor)
iatrogenic (curettage,	radiation Psychogenic factors	Feminizing ovarian tumors
irradiation)	Nutritional factors	(granulosa cell tumor, theca
	Nongonadal endocrine disorders	cell tumor)
	(thyroid, adrenals, pancreas)	
	Systemic infections and chronic	
	diseases	
	Pharmacologic factors (psychotropic	
	drugs, postpill oversuppression,	
	drug addiction)	
	Central nervous system disease	
	(tumor or trauma)	

(From Lehmann, F.: Diagnostic approach to ovarian dysfunction. Hormone Res. 9:319–338, 1978.)

DIFFERENTIAL DIAGNOSIS OF MENSTRUAL IRREGULARITIES

CAUSE	NATURE OF PATIENT	NATURE OF SYMPTOMS	ASSOCIATED SYMPTOMS	PRECIPITATING AND AGGRAVATING FACTORS	PHYSICAL FINDINGS	DIAGNOSTIC STUDIES
Dysfunctional Uterine Bleeding (Hormonal Causes)	Can occur at any age; 10% of cases occur at puberty; 50% of cases occur between 40 and 50 years	Usually due to anovulatory cycles; Menorrhagia; Interval between periods may be decreased				Diagnosis may be reached only by a process of exclusion
Anovulatory cycles	Normal occurrence in 55% of girls within first year of menarche	Irregular cycle length; Polymenorrhagia; Bleeding not preceded by or associated with subjective symptoms		Obesity; Adrenal or pituitary disease; Polycystic ovaries; Diabetes; Malnutrition; Chronic illness; Hypothyroidism; Use of phenothiazines or opiates		Monophasic basal body temperature; Serum progesterone never exceeds 5 ng/ml
Estrogen-withdrawal bleeding	Most common cause of irregular menses in reproductive years, especially adolescence and climacteric	Prolonged, irregular, profuse bleeding	Painless			
Estrogen-breakthrough bleeding						
Threshold bleeding		Spotty bleeding		Low-dose oral contraceptives		
With estrogen levels above threshold		Prolonged, irregular, profuse bleeding				

Progesterone-break-through bleeding / Progesterone-withdrawal bleeding				High doses of progestational drugs Intramuscular progesterone or oral medroxyprogesterone acetate (Provera) administered as test for presence of endogenous estrogen
Ovulatory cycles		Cycle length is usually regular / Premenstrual staining/bleeding / Dysmenorrhea	Mittelschmerz / Premenstrual syndrome (PMS)	Biphasic basal body temperature
Complications of Pregnancy	Reproductive age			
Ectopic pregnancy	Increased risk for women with previous ectopic pregnancy, salpingitis, previous tubal procedure or pregnancy that occurs with IUDs	Spotting precedes gross hemorrhage (may be visible or concealed) / Amenorrhea / Pelvic or abdominal fullness / Abdominal pain (usually unilateral) / May refer to shoulder / May or may not be vaginal bleeding / Purulent vaginal discharge	Missed periods / Morning sickness / Breast tenderness Tenesmus / Increased urinary frequency or urgency	Positive HCG / Pelvic sonogram Adnexal or cul-de-sac mass / Normal or slightly enlarged uterus / Peritoneal irritation
During uterine pregnancy		Irregular bleeding due to separation of placenta or embryo from its attachment		

Table continued on following page

DIFFERENTIAL DIAGNOSIS OF MENSTRUAL IRREGULARITIES *Continued*

CAUSE	NATURE OF PATIENT	NATURE OF SYMPTOMS	ASSOCIATED SYMPTOMS	PRECIPITATING AND AGGRAVATING FACTORS	PHYSICAL FINDINGS	DIAGNOSTIC STUDIES
Complications of Pregnancy *Continued* Spontaneous abortion		Hemorrhage (some times with clots)	Fever Purulent vaginal discharge or pain			
Endometriosis (see Chapter 19)		Slight bleeding	Dysmenorrhea Purulent vaginal discharge Dull backache		Implants may be palpable	
Endometrial and Cervical Cancer	Postmenopausal women	Extent of bleeding may vary	Purulent vaginal discharge			
Fibroids	Women of reproductive age	Menorrhagia, occasionally metrorrhagia Irregular bleeding			Uterus is asymmetrically enlarged Fibroids are hard and unyielding Cervix and fibroids usually move together	
IUDs		Menorrhagia	Cervical discharge			
Salpingitis	Usually occurs in reproductive years	Menorrhagia or slight bleeding	Purulent discharge Fever Abdominal pain Dysmenorrhea		Signs of peritoneal irritation	

Insertion of Foreign Bodies into Vagina	Commonest cause of abnormal vaginal bleeding in children		
Amenorrhea Primary	In girls up to age 17 years, delayed menarche is the most common cause Girls 18 years of age or older who have not yet menstruated (rare)	Severe malnutrition Weight loss Amphetamines Phenothiazines Endocrine and congenital abnormalities Chromosomal aberrations	Chromatin analysis of a buccal smear
Secondary	Patients have menstruated and then stop menstruating	Pregnancy Endocrine imbalance Tumors Breastfeeding	Vaginal smear and evaluation of cervical mucus to determine whether there is ovarian estrogen production and to determine other hormone levels
Prolactinoma	Galactorrhea		Serum prolactin

Selected References

Altchek, A.: Dysfunctional uterine bleeding in adolescence. Clin. Obstet. Gynecol. *20*:633–650, 1977.

Dewhurst, J.: Secondary amenorrhea. Pediatr. Ann. *10(12)*:38–42, 1981.

Goldfarb, J. M., and Little, A. B.: Abnormal vaginal bleeding. N. Engl. J. Med. *302*:666–669, 1980.

Hamilton, C.: Vaginal bleeding: evaluation and management. Resident and Staff Physician, November, 1981, pp. 62–74.

Lehmann, F.: Diagnostic approach to ovarian dysfunction. Hormone Res. *9*:319–338, 1978.

Lopez, R. I.: Menstrual irregularities in teenage girls. Drug Therapy, April, 1981, pp. 39–50.

Marul, E. L., and Dawood, M. Y.: Amenorrhea. Clin. Obstet. Gynecol. *26(3)*:749–761, 1983.

Spellacy, W. N.: Abnormal bleeding. Clin. Obstet. Gynecol. *26(3)*:702–709, 1983.

Strickler, R. C.: Dysfunctional uterine bleeding—diagnosis and treatment. Postgrad. Med. *66*:135–146, 1979.

Taber, B.: Manual of Gynecologic and Obstetric Emergencies. 2nd ed. Philadelphia, W. B. Saunders Co., 1984.

MENSTRUAL PAIN

Dysmenorrhea is the term used to describe painful menstruation. Approximately 50 per cent of postpubescent women experience dysmenorrhea; 10 per cent of these women are incapacitated by pain for 1 to 3 days per month. As the greatest single cause of lost working hours and school days among young women, dysmenorrhea has been found to be associated with substantial economic losses to the entire community as well as to the patient. In some instances, anticipatory fear of the next menstrual period can cause anxiety during the intermenstrual period.

In evaluating a patient with pelvic pain at time of menstruation, the physician must first decide whether the patient has *premenstrual syndrome (PMS)* or dysmenorrhea. **Premenstrual syndrome usually begins 2 to 12 days before the menstrual period and subsides at the onset of, or early in the course of, menstruation.** The major symptoms of PMS are a diffuse, dull pelvic ache, mood changes (irritability, nervousness, headaches, and depression), swelling of the breasts and extremities, occasional weight gain, and a sensation of abdominal bloating. The diagnostic process is sometimes more difficult when, as is commonly the case, the symptoms of PMS overlap or are followed by those of dysmenorrhea.

It is helpful to classify dysmenorrhea as primary or secondary. *Primary dysmenorrhea* is the most common menstrual disorder and occurs in 30 to 50 per cent of young women. Dysmenorrhea is classified as primary (intrinsic, essential, or idiopathic) if it occurs in a woman who has no pelvic abnormality. It has been estimated that 95 per cent of female adolescents have primary dysmenorrhea and that this problem is a major cause of school absenteeism. *Secondary dysmenorrhea* (extrinsic or acquired) results from organic pelvic diseases such as fibroids,

209

endometriosis, bacterial infections, and infections caused by intrauterine contraceptive devices. Because effective therapy is now available for secondary dysmenorrhea, it is not sufficient merely to diagnose "dysmenorrhea." The physician must distinguish among premenstrual syndrome, primary dysmenorrhea, and secondary dysmenorrhea.

It must be emphasized that some women will not initiate a discussion of dysmenorrhea with their physician. They may have been taught that it is normal or that relief cannot be obtained. It is therefore essential that the practitioner ask the patient whether dysmenorrhea is a problem.

NATURE OF PATIENT

Severe *primary dysmenorrhea* is common in young women during the first hours of their menstruation. **When dysmenorrhea begins within the first 2 or 3 years of menarche, primary dysmenorrhea is the most likely diagnosis.** Primary dysmenorrhea usually occurs with ovulatory cycles; these generally begin 3 to 12 months after menarche when ovulation occurs regularly. Primary dysmenorrhea usually begins a few months after menarche and becomes progressively more severe. If a patient has gradually increasing monthly pain without menstruation, a *congenital abnormality* obstructing menstrual flow must be considered. These rare abnormalities may lead to hematocolpos, to hematometra, and eventually to intraperitoneal bleeding.

Secondary dysmenorrhea usually begins many years after menarche. Dysmenorrhea that develops after the age of 20 years is usually of the secondary type. Dysmenorrhea often can be caused by an *intrauterine device (IUD)*. If dysmenorrhea develops after cervical conization, cautery, or radiation, *acquired cervical stenosis* or *cervical occlusion* may be the cause. Dysmenorrhea following uterine curettage may be due to *intrauterine synechiae* (Asherman's syndrome). Secondary dysmenorrhea due to *endometriosis* is usually late in onset (beginning when the patient is in her 30s) and worsens with age. Endometriosis is uncommon in teenagers.

NATURE OF SYMPTOMS

Pain that begins with menstrual flow or a few hours before flow commences and that lasts for 6 hours to 2 days is most characteristic of *primary dysmenorrhea*. In teenagers, endometriosis may mimic the pain of primary dysmenorrhea in that the pain may be limited to the first day of menstruation. The pain of primary dysmenorrhea is usually crampy but may be a dull ache. It is usually located in the midline of the lower abdomen just above the symphysis. It occasionally radiates down the anterior aspect of the thighs or to the lower back.

The pain of *secondary dysmenorrhea* often begins several hours or even a few days before menses and is often relieved by the menstrual flow. This pain is usually a dull, continuous, diffuse lower abdominal pain but may be crampy. Like the pain of primary dysmenorrhea, it can radiate down the thighs and into the back.

When *pelvic inflammatory disease (PID)* causes dysmenorrhea, the pain is greatest premenstrually and is relieved with the onset of vaginal bleeding. A common cause of secondary dysmenorrhea that deserves special attention is *endometriosis*. Symptoms in these patients become progressively more severe with each cycle; the pain usually begins (and increases in severity) 2 to 3 days premenstrually and persists for more than 2 days after the onset of flow. It is most severe on the first and second days of bleeding, and the usual drop in basal body temperature (BBT), which normally occurs 24 to 36 hours after menses, is delayed until the second or third menstrual day.

Despite the differences between primary and secondary dysmenorrhea, their symptoms can overlap, can vary greatly in intensity, and do not necessarily occur with every menstrual period. It is important for the physician to recognize that patients with primary dysmenorrhea may develop pelvic pathology and have additional, superimposed symptoms of secondary dysmenorrhea. These patients can have constant, crampy pain beginning 1 or 2 days before menstrual flow and continuing for 2 to 3 days after menstrual flow.

ASSOCIATED SYMPTOMS

Systemic symptoms such as nausea, vomiting, diarrhea, headache, fatigue, nervousness, and dizziness are more characteristic of primary dysmenorrhea than of secondary dysmenorrhea. If menorrhagia and colicky pain are associated with menstruation, *uterine fibroids* should be suspected, although fibroids are rarely responsible for menstrual pain. If a nonpregnant patient with an enlarged, soft uterus complains of menorrhagia and dysmenorrhea, *adenomyosis* should be suspected. Bleeding from glandular tissue located deep within the myometrium has been implicated as the cause of the pain.

The pain of *endometriosis* may continue into the intermenstrual period. Rectal pain on defecation during the menstrual period also suggests endometriosis as a cause of dysmenorrhea. When dysmenorrhea is associated with dyspareunia, rectal pain, tenesmus, backache, and urgent micturition, endometriosis should be suspected.

DIFFERENTIAL DIAGNOSIS OF MENSTRUAL PAIN

CAUSE	NATURE OF PATIENT	NATURE OF SYMPTOMS	ASSOCIATED SYMPTOMS	AMELIO-RATING FACTORS	PRECIPITAT-ING AND AGGRAVATING FACTORS	PHYSICAL FINDINGS	DIAGNOSTIC STUDIES
Premenstrual syndrome		Begins 2–12 days before menses and subsides at onset of, or during first days of period Diffuse, dull, pelvic ache May coexist with dysmenorrhea	Irritability Nervousness Headaches Swelling of breasts and extremities Bloating and weight gain Breast tenderness	Menses	Emotional stress Dysmenorrhea		
Primary dysmenorrhea	30–50% of young women 95% of adolescents	Most common menstrual disorder Begins within 3–12 months of menarche Becomes more severe with age Pain: just precedes or begins with menstrual flow; lasts for 6 hours to 2 days; is crampy or a dull ache; is usually in midline of lower abdomen; may radiate down thighs and to lower back	Nausea and vomiting Diarrhea Headache Fatigue Nervousness Dizziness	Pain may lessen as menstrual cycles become regular Pregnancy	Premenstrual syndrome IUDs Emotional stress	None	

Secondary dysmenorrhea	Over 20 years	Secondary to organic disease; Begins years after menarche; Pain: begins several hours before menses; is a dull, continuous, diffuse, lower abdominal pain; may be crampy; can radiate down thighs and into back		Menses	Cervical stenosis secondary to cervical conization or radiation; IUD	Depends on cause of secondary dysmenorrhea	PAP smear; Gonorrhea culture
Endometriosis	Usually over 30 years; Uncommon in teen-agers	Symptoms worsen with each cycle; Pain: begins 2–3 days before menses and persists for 2 days after; may continue into intermenstrual period	Rectal pain with defecation; Dyspareunia; Tenesmus; Backache; Urgent micturition	Pregnancy; Birth control pills		Pelvic examination best done in late luteal phase; Nodularity felt in uterosacral ligaments or other sites of endometrial implants	Fern test; Basal body temperature
Fibroids		Uncommon cause of dysmenorrhea; Pain is greatest premenstrually	Menorrhagia				
PID			Menorrhagia		Onset at menses	Cervical discharge; Chandelier sign	Gonorrhea culture

PRECIPITATING AND AGGRAVATING FACTORS

Primary dysmenorrhea is aggravated by *premenstrual syndrome.* *Intrauterine devices* may cause secondary dysmenorrhea and, in some instances, may aggravate pre-existing primary dysmenorrhea. *Menstrual flow* that continues longer than 8 days and *emotional stress* also appear to intensify dysmenorrhea. By itself, retroversion does not cause dysmenorrhea; however, there are some conditions that cause retroversion that also cause dysmenorrhea.

AMELIORATING FACTORS

Dysmenorrhea is not consistently alleviated by any known physical measure. Some patients may state that lying on the floor in the knee–chest position gives some relief. Dysmenorrhea that occurs soon after the onset of menarche frequently disappears as the menstrual cycles become more regular. Pregnancy often relieves primary dysmenorrhea and secondary dysmenorrhea due to endometriosis. The pain may be alleviated for several months or, on occasion, permanently. Birth control pills often alleviate the pain of primary dysmenorrhea and endometriosis. Spontaneous alleviation of dysmenorrhea may occur with advancing age, but this is not usually the case.

PHYSICAL FINDINGS

In patients who have primary dysmenorrhea, no physical abnormalities are usually found. In patients who have secondary dysmenorrhea, physical findings depend on the specific cause.

The practitioner must perform a careful physical examination to check for pelvic infection, endometriosis, pelvic mass, uterine enlargement, and other pelvic disease. When evidence of endometriosis is being sought, the pelvic examination should ideally be performed in the late luteal phase, immediately prior to menstruation, when the endometrial implants (often in the uterosacral ligaments) are largest and therefore most palpable. Using a laxative to promote bowel evacuation facilitates pelvic examination for endometrial implants. **Special attention should be paid to genital development, vaginal discharge, stigmata of pelvic infection, appearance of the cervix, and the size, shape, consistency, and position of the uterus.**

DIAGNOSTIC STUDIES

A Papanicolaou smear and a gonorrhea culture should be obtained for all patients with secondary dysmenorrhea. A fern test and basal body temperature may help diagnose endometriosis. Uterine curettage, laparoscopy, and sonography are often useful diagnostic tools.

LESS COMMON DIAGNOSTIC CONSIDERATIONS

Less common causes of dysmenorrhea include congenital malformations; uterine hypoplasia; and true cervical stenosis or obstruction occurring as the result of cauterization, conization, or radiation therapy. Endometrial carcinoma and tuberculosis are rare causes of secondary dysmenorrhea. A foreign body (e.g., an intrauterine contraceptive device or any object inserted into the vagina) can cause dysmenorrhea.

Selected References

Friederich, M. A.: Dysmenorrhea. Women and Health *8(2–3)*:91–106, 1983.

Heinrichs, W. L., and Adamson, G. D.: A practical approach to the patient with dysmenorrhea. J. Reprod. Med. *25*:236–242, 1980.

Renaer, M., and Guzinski, G. M.: Pain in gynecologic practice. Pain *5*:305–331, 1978.

Schwartz, M. B.: Adolescent gynecology for the pediatrician. Pediatrician *8*:113–323, 1979.

Ylikarkala, O., and Dawood, Y. M.: New concepts in dysmenorrhea. Am. J. Obstet. Gynecol. *130*:833–847, 1978.

20
NAUSEA AND/OR VOMITING WITHOUT ABDOMINAL PAIN

Nausea is a vague, unpleasant sensation; it may herald the onset of vomiting or occur without vomiting. *Vomiting* is the forceful expulsion of gastric contents through the mouth and must be differentiated from *regurgitation*. The latter is an effortless backflow of small amounts of ingested food or liquid during or between meals or feedings. Dribbling of milk from a child's mouth is an example of regurgitation. When a patient complains of vomiting it is helpful for the physician to distinguish acute from chronic vomiting.

The most common cause of acute nausea and vomiting in adults and children is *gastroenteritis*. Other common causes of acute nausea and vomiting include *gastritis, excessive alcohol ingestion,* certain *drugs,* and, in children *otitis media.* Common causes of chronic nausea and vomiting include *gastritis, drugs* (especially codeine, digitalis glycosides, quinidine, salicylates, theophylline, chemotherapeutic agents, and antibiotics), *uremia,* and *hepatic failure.* Recurrent nausea that occurs without vomiting is often a reaction to *environmental* or *emotional stresses.* This form of nausea is temporally related to the stressful period and usually disappears when the stress is removed.

NATURE OF PATIENT

In newborns, vomiting with the first feeding is suggestive of *esophageal atresia.* The most common causes of vomiting in the first year are *feeding problems, gastrointestinal* and *urinary tract infections,* and *septicemia.* When projectile vomiting occurs in infants less than 3 months old (usually 2 to 3 weeks of age), *pyloric stenosis* must be considered. Although uncommon, recurrent vomiting of bile-stained material in neonates may indicate *intestinal obstruction* due to atresia, stenosis, or volvulus of the small bowel.

The most common causes of vomiting in children are *viral* and *bacterial infections, high fevers* of any cause, and *otitis media.* Otitis media has its highest incidence in young children and may present with unexplained vomiting and fever.

In adults, the common causes of acute nausea or vomiting are *gastritis* (alcohol- or drug-induced), *viral gastroenteritis, psychogenic conditions,* and occasionally *labyrinthine disorders.* Nausea and vomiting can also be the presenting symptoms in patients with *hepatitis, myocardial infarction,* and *diabetic ketoacidosis.* Chronic vomiting in adults is usually due to *gastritis, mechanical obstruction, gut motility disorders, achalasia, drugs, labyrinthine disorders,* and *uremia.* Both *food contamination* and *chemical poisoning* must be considered as causes of vomiting, particularly if several people are affected at the same time; in cases of food poisoning, there is usually more than one person experiencing symptoms. Nausea and vomiting of *pregnancy* must be considered in women of reproductive age; some pregnant women experience morning sickness in the first trimester of pregnancy, often before they are aware of their condition.

Self-induced vomiting should be suspected in neurotic individuals. If these patients are questioned carefully, they may admit to a feeling of nausea, which they attempt to relieve by gagging themselves to produce vomiting. If an elderly patient presents with persistent vomiting, gastric or intestinal obstruction secondary to *neoplasm* should be suspected.

NATURE OF SYMPTOMS

When vomiting is painless or has preceded abdominal pain by a considerable amount of time, a surgical lesion is unlikely. Repeated episodes of unexplained vomiting and nausea may indicate *pancreatitis,* which is not always associated with abdominal pain. Persistent vomiting without any bile staining is an indication of *pyloric obstruction.* In children this may be due to *pyloric stenosis;* in adults pyloric obstruction may be secondary to ulcer scarring or tumor. Vomiting or regurgitation of undigested food indicates *esophageal obstruction.* Vomiting secondary to *increased intracranial pressure* is often projectile and not preceded by nausea. Nausea and vomiting are frequent manifestations of *digitalis toxicity.* These symptoms are not necessarily due to high serum levels of the digitalis glycoside; there may be a gastrointestinal side effect of the drug occurring at normal serum levels. Although patients with *gastritis* often have abdominal pain, it is not uncommon for these patients to present with unexplained nausea or vomiting without pain. *Substance abuse* (alcohol, caffeine, and recreational drugs) also may be associated with unexplained nausea or vomiting.

The timing of vomiting may be of diagnostic importance. Patients with *uremia, pregnant* women, and *chronic alcoholics* often experience early morning nausea and vomiting. Vomiting immediately before food is ingested may be a manifestation of *neurosis,* whereas vomiting shortly after eating may be a consequence of *gastric outlet obstruction* caused by a pyloric channel ulcer, adenocarcinoma, or other infiltrative lesions.

Postprandial vomiting may also be of *functional origin,* although organic gastric disease should be suspected. Vomiting soon after eating occurs frequently in patients with *gastritis* and in those with *digitalis toxicity.* Vomiting beginning 20 to 40 minutes after meals suggests *gastric atony* associated with diabetes, prior gastric surgery, or peritonitis. If vomiting begins 1 to 2 hours after a meal, disease of the biliary tract or pancreas may be the cause. In these latter instances, pain usually is not relieved by vomiting. Recurrent vomiting occurring 1 to 4 hours after eating may be due to gastric or duodenal lesions causing *gastric outlet obstruction.* Vomiting that follows and relieves an episode of epigastric pain is usually due to an *intragastric lesion* or *pyloric spasm.*

The odor of vomitus may also provide a clue to the etiology. If the vomitus lacks the pungent odor of gastric acid, a *dilated esophagus* (possibly due to a stricture or achalasia) may be the cause. Patients frequently vomit in the morning and not uncommonly will vomit or regurgitate undigested food. If vomitus has a fecal odor, *intestinal obstruction* or *gastrocolic fistula* should be suspected.

ASSOCIATED SYMPTOMS

If headache (especially a unilateral one) is associated with nausea or vomiting, *migraine* should be suspected. If vertigo and tinnitus are associated with nausea and vomiting, *Meniere's disease* or other middle ear disturbances should be considered. If symptoms of depression are present and there is little or no weight loss despite a history of long-standing emesis, psychogenic vomiting is probable. As in *anorexia nervosa,* women experience psychogenic vomiting more often than men.

If chest pain or other signs of myocardial infarction are associated with vomiting, the vomiting is probably due to myocardial infarction. Nausea and vomiting often precede the development of chest pain. Rarely, chest pain and vomiting are caused by a strangulated diaphragmatic hernia. In these instances, electrocardiographic abnormalities may be erroneously suggestive of a posterior infarction.

Acute nausea and vomiting associated with diarrhea and occasionally with abdominal pain are most frequently due to *gastroenteritis*. When vertigo accompanies vomiting, *labyrinthine disorders* should be suspected. When vomiting, without vertigo, is induced by a recumbent posture, a *posterior fossa lesion* should be suspected. Vomiting may be the initial manifestation of *diabetic ketoacidosis*. It is a particularly common presentation in juvenile (insulin-dependent) diabetics.

PRECIPITATING AND AGGRAVATING FACTORS

Nausea and vomiting are frequently precipitated by medications such as digitalis, theophylline, quinidine, potassium preparations, chemotherapeutic agents, antibiotics, and antihypertensives. Iron preparations, salicylates, and nonsteroidal anti-inflammatory agents also cause nausea and occasional vomiting. Nicotine poisoning and excessive use of "Nicorette" gum may cause vomiting. Radiation therapy may also cause nausea and vomiting.

AMELIORATING FACTORS

Vomiting usually relieves the symptoms of fullness and pain caused by pyloric obstruction. Vomiting relieves nausea if it is being caused by nauseating substances in the stomach. It does not usually alleviate nausea caused by gastroenteritis, gastritis, uremia, or drugs that cause nausea through a central effect.

PHYSICAL FINDINGS

The presence of fever in a vomiting patient suggests that *infection* is etiologic. In children, physical findings of *otitis media* suggest that this is the probable cause of the vomiting. A walnut-size mass may be palpable in the epigastrium of infants with hypertrophic pyloric stenosis. A cloudy sensorium or papilledema suggests an *intracranial lesion,* whereas nystagmus suggests a labyrinthine cause. Jaundice or hepatomegaly suggests *hepatitis* or *cirrhosis* as the cause. A distended abdomen accompanying nausea and vomiting may indicate paralytic ileus or mechanical obstruction of the intestine. Abdominal tenderness, distention, and occasionally visible peristalsis suggest *gastrointestinal obstruction*. The location of abdominal pain may provide clues about which organ is responsible for the symptoms.

Chronic vomiting results in weight loss. If a patient's weight is maintained despite a history of chronic nausea and vomiting, the origin of symptoms is probably psychogenic. Decreased skin turgor suggests that the vomiting has caused significant fluid loss. Physical findings consistent with congestive heart failure (e.g., tachycardia, gallop, and peripheral edema) suggest that nausea may be from hepatic capsule distention and mesenteric congestion.

DIAGNOSTIC STUDIES

Studies to confirm a visceral origin of nausea and vomiting include survey films of the abdomen, upper gastrointestinal series, cholecystography, and endoscopy. Detailed neurologic studies including spinal tap and CT scan should be performed only if an intracranial process is suspected. A metabolic etiology may be suspected if laboratory tests indicate abnormal levels of substances such as blood urea nitrogen, creatinine, blood sugar, bilirubin, and calcium. An elevated amylase suggests pancreatitis. Digitalis excess may be diagnosed on the basis of elevated serum digitalis levels. Toxicology screening may detect toxins and drugs that cause vomiting.

More sophisticated tests include radioisotope studies of liquid and solid gastric emptying, esophageal and gastrointestinal manometry, and electrogastrography (Table 20–1). Psychiatric assessment, including the Minnesota Multiphasic Personality Inventory test, may also be helpful.

LESS COMMON DIAGNOSTIC CONSIDERATIONS

Several authors have categorized the causes of vomiting as follows: allergies, cerebromedullary factors, toxins, visceral problems, deficiency states, and motion sickness. Gastrointestinal allergies should be considered if sudden nausea or vomiting consistently follow ingestion of specific food. The less common cerebromedullary causes include increased intracranial pressure such as that caused by cerebral tumors, abscesses,

Table 20–1. Tests That May Be Necessary in Diagnosis of Unexplained Vomiting

History, including psychiatric assessment and family history
Physical examination, with particular attention paid to
    Orthostatic hypotension
    Succussion splash, skin rash, Raynaud's phenomenon
    Neurologic assessment, especially cranial nerves, vestibular and pupillary function,
       peripheral neuropathy, extrapyramidal signs
Laboratory tests
    Routine hematologic and biochemical screening
    Amylase
    Drug screening, such as digoxin levels
    Hormonal levels: thyroxine, thyroid-stimulating hormones; plasma cortisol
       (0900 h, 2400 h), orthostatic catecholamines
    Serum (and urine) protein electrophoresis
    Immunologic tests: rheumatoid factor, DNA-binding titer, autoantibody screening
    Gastric intubation for residual volume after overnight fast
Radiologic tests
    Plain abdominal radiograph
    Gastrointestinal tract contrast series
    Intravenous urogram
    Computed tomographic scan of abdomen and head
Upper gastrointestinal tract endoscopy
Gastric emptying tests
    ^{99m}Tc chicken liver (absorbable solid)
    ^{131}I-fiber (nondigestible solid)
    ^{111}In-pentetic acid (aqueous phase)
Conventional esophageal and anorectal manometry
Gastrointestinal manometry and electrogastrography
    Manometry: low compliance perfusion system (peroral or intraoperative)
    Electrogastrography: internal, external, intraoperative
Formal psychiatric assessment, such as Minnesota Multiphasic Personality Inventory
    and inpatient evaluation
Laparotomy and full-thickness biopsy of small bowel, including electrophysiologic study
    of muscle

(From Malagelada, J. R., and Camilleri, M.: Unexplained vomiting: A diagnostic challenge. Ann. Int. Med. *101*:211–218, 1984.)

hydrocephalus, and intracranial hemorrhage. Hepatic coma and Addison's disease are less common causes of nausea and vomiting. Disorders of the gastrointestinal tract such as ulcers, obstructive tumors (particularly those of the stomach and proximal small bowel), adhesive bands, volvulus, and gastritis may also cause nausea and vomiting. Blood in the gastrointestinal tract also causes nausea and vomiting. Patients with pyelonephritis and pelvic inflammatory disease may present with a chief complaint of vomiting, particularly if they also have reflex ileus. Patients with anorexia nervosa, particularly in the early stages, may practice vomiting. Because anorectic patients rarely complain of this symptom, however, it may be difficult for the physician to diagnose the condition before pronounced weight loss has occurred. Vomiting may also be caused by conditions that alter neural control of gut motility.

DIFFERENTIAL DIAGNOSIS OF NAUSEA AND/OR VOMITING WITHOUT ABDOMINAL PAIN

CAUSE	NATURE OF PATIENT	NATURE OF SYMPTOMS	ASSOCIATED SYMPTOMS	PRECIPITATING AND AGGRAVATING FACTORS	PHYSICAL FINDINGS	DIAGNOSTIC STUDIES
Gastroenteritis	Most common cause at any age	Acute nausea and vomiting	Diarrhea Fever Abdominal pain		Hyperactive peristalsis	
Gastritis		Acute or chronic nausea and vomiting occur postprandially	Abdominal pain	Viral infection Alcohol- or drug-induced		Endoscopy
Viral or bacterial infection	Common cause of vomiting in children	Acute nausea and vomiting	Fever		High temperature	
Drugs		Acute or chronic nausea and vomiting Postprandial vomiting		Codeine Digitalis glycosides Quinidine Salicylates Theophylline Antihypertensives Antibiotics Iron preparations Nonsteroidal anti-inflammatory agents Nicotine and "Nicorette" gum		Serum drug levels
Otitis media	Children	Acute nausea and vomiting	Fever Earache			
Excessive alcohol ingestion	Alcoholics Social drinkers	Early morning vomiting				

Table continued on following page

DIFFERENTIAL DIAGNOSIS OF NAUSEA AND/OR VOMITING WITHOUT ABDOMINAL PAIN *Continued*

CAUSE	NATURE OF PATIENT	NATURE OF SYMPTOMS	ASSOCIATED SYMPTOMS	PRECIPITATING AND AGGRAVATING FACTORS	PHYSICAL FINDINGS	DIAGNOSTIC STUDIES
Uremia		Chronic nausea and vomiting Usually in early morning				Elevated BUN and creatinine
"Morning sickness"	Pregnant females	Early morning nausea and vomiting Usually in first trimester				Serum HCG
Environmental or emotional stresses		Episodic nausea usually without vomiting				
Pyloric obstruction	In infants <3 months old may be due to pyloric stenosis In adults may be secondary to ulcer scarring or tumor	Projectile vomiting	Abdominal pain		Palpable mass Succussion splash	
Esophageal obstruction and achalasia		Vomiting or regurgitation of undigested food Odorless vomitus Usually occurs in early morning or after large meals				Esophageal radiograph Endoscopy
Increased intracranial pressure		Projectile vomiting not preceded by nausea			Papilledema	Neurologic examination Spinal tap CT scan
Pancreatitis	Alcoholics	Repeated episodes of unexplained nausea and vomiting	Abdominal pain	Excessive alcohol intake		Elevated serum amylase CT of pancreas

Selected References

Bockus, H.: Gastroenterology. 4th ed. Philadelphia, W.B. Saunders Co., 1985.

Bramble, M. G., and Record, C. O.: Drug-induced gastrointestinal disease. Drugs *15*:451–463, 1978.

Greenberg, A., et al.: Severe theophylline toxicity. Am. J. Med. *76*:854–860, 1984.

Ingram, D. A., et al.: Vomiting as a diagnostic aid in acute ischemic cardiac pain. Br. Med. J. *281*:636–637, 1980.

Malagelada, J. R., and Camilleri, M.: Unexplained vomiting: a diagnostic challenge. Ann. Int. Med. *101*:211–218, 1984.

Rosenthal, R. H., et al.: Diagnoses and management of persistent psychogenic vomiting. Psychosomatics *218*:722–730, 1980.

Toccalino, H.: Vomiting and regurgitation. Clin. Gastroenterol. *6*:267–282, 1977.

Valman, H. B.: The first year of life—vomiting. Br. Med. J. *280*:620–623, 1980.

21

PAIN IN THE FOOT

Foot pain is usually due to local disease or abnormality but occasionally results from referred pain. Therefore, examination of the foot should begin with the spine and proceed distally. Foot pain is most frequently due to *muscular* or *ligamentous strain* associated with *trauma,* unaccustomed or strenuous *physical activity,* and *sport.* New shoes or change in heel size also may cause foot pain. Other common causes include *gout, plantar warts, callosities,* and *metatarsal fracture (march fracture).* Isolated pain in the heel can result from a *calcaneal spur, arterial insufficiency, Achilles tendonitis* or *bursitis,* and *jogger's trauma.* In adolescents, pain in the heel may be caused by *calcaneal apophysitis.*

NATURE OF PATIENT

Because foot pain is usually due to *muscular* or *ligamentous strain,* it is more likely to occur in people who are physically active, particularly those who are unaccustomed to physical exercise and muscular strain in their feet, such as unconditioned athletes and weekend sportsmen. *Gout* is more common in males over the age of 40 years but does occur in women, especially those who are postmenopausal. The patient may present with a history of previous attacks of painful joints or urolithiasis. Often, a family history of gout may be elicited.

Pain in the heel caused by a *calcaneal spur* and its associated soft-tissue irritation is most frequent in patients over the age of 40 years. When adolescents complain of pain in the heel, it most likely is caused by *calcaneal apophysitis*. *Achilles tendonitis,* which also causes heel pain, is usually due to trauma (e.g., injury from jogging), although the trauma may not be recalled by the patient. It is interesting to note that Achilles tendonitis is more common in patients with Reiter's syndrome and ankylosing spondylitis who are HLA-B27–positive, even without a history of trauma.

NATURE OF SYMPTOMS

As with other types of pain, a careful history of the location and quality of the pain, how it began, and what intensifies it are most helpful in determining its etiology.

If the foot pain is described as a dull ache, it is most likely due to *foot strain*. This is more likely to occur in older adults, overweight individuals, people wearing new shoes, and those who are on their feet for a large part of the day. It is critical that the physician establish the precise location of the ache because this will determine which ligaments, tendons, or fascia are involved (torn or under strain). For example, pain below the ankle on the inner aspect of the heel suggests a tear or strain of the ligamentous fibers attached to the internal malleolus.

Plantar warts and callosities can cause severe pain, particularly with weight-bearing. These commonly are located on the plantar surface of the foot in the metatarsal region. Pain from a *calcaneal spur* or *plantar fasciitis* is usually continuous, although it may worsen with weight-bearing. The spur is usually located in the center of the under-surface of the heel, about 2.25 cm from the back of the foot; the pain, however, may be more toward the back of the heel. The condition called *jogger's foot* may produce complaints of a burning pain in the heel, aching in the arch, or diminished sensation in the sole of the foot behind the large toe.

The pain of *Achilles tendonitis* is usually over the Achilles tendon and may be associated with tenderness to palpation and swelling.

With *gout,* the pain is usually acute, frequently recurrent, and often agonizing, although atypical cases of gout may present with less severe symptoms. The attacks usually have a sudden onset and characteristically start during the early hours of the day, while the patient is still in bed. Before a patient knows that he suffers from gout, he may attribute the bouts of pain to minor trauma such as "stubbing the toe" or "spraining the involved joint." Once the diagnosis of gout has been established, the patient usually recognizes subsequent attacks. Although the metatarsophalangeal joint of the big toe is classically affected, one or more other joints, including the ankle, may also be affected.

PRECIPITATING AND AGGRAVATING FACTORS

Most foot pain is precipitated by *trauma,* unaccustomed or *strenuous physical activity,* and *sport.* Change in occupation or work that involves constant jarring of the foot, walking on concrete floors, or standing may lead to foot strain. Constant vibration or jarring frequently leads to heel pain that may result from calcaneal periostitis. Likewise, new shoes or change in heel size can lead to foot strain. Gouty pain in the foot may have no particular precipitating factors, although several reports have indicated that a gouty diathesis may be caused by minor trauma to the involved joint.

PHYSICAL FINDINGS

In addition to careful examination of the foot for local discoloration, swelling, and areas tender to palpation, patients who complain of foot pain should have a careful examination of the lower back and legs, as foot pain may result from referred pain.

The following are some clues to the etiology of foot pain. When pain is due to *foot strain,* the forefoot may flatten on weightbearing, and calluses under the metatarsal heads may be present. When the pain is due to gout, there is usually a warm, violaceous, tender, swollen joint (commonly the metatarsophalangeal joint of the big toe or the ankle). Tophi may be present in the foot, other joints, or the ear lobe. When the pain is due to a *calcaneal spur* or *plantar fasciitis,* there may be spot tenderness with deep palpation, particularly on the undersurface of the heel. If this is associated with radiographic evidence of calcaneal spur, the diagnosis is obvious. In cases in which there is no radiographic confirmation of a calcaneal spur, this pain may be due to plantar fasciitis.

Although the diagnosis of *ankle sprain* is usually obvious by history, patients may not remember the traumatic incident. Sprained ankles are most commonly due to an inversion injury and have tenderness and swelling over the anterior talofibular ligament. Likewise, *fractures* are usually associated with a history of significant trauma. A radiograph is usually necessary to diagnose small fractures of the ankle. In patients with a history suggesting a sprained ankle, the physician should suspect an associated fracture if the swelling appears disproportionate to the severity of the sprain.

Bunions can also cause foot pain, particularly at the metatarsophalangeal joint. This pain is usually worse with extension of the big toe. *Heel fasciitis,* also called *calcaneal periostitis,* may produce chronic pain

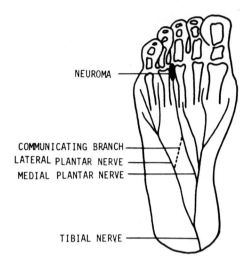

NEUROMA

COMMUNICATING BRANCH
LATERAL PLANTAR NERVE
MEDIAL PLANTAR NERVE

TIBIAL NERVE

Figure 21–1. Anatomy of Morton's neu-roma. (From Morris, M. A.: Morton's metatarsalgia. Clin. Orthop. Rel. Res. *127*:203–207, 1977.)

Table 21–1. **Twenty-three Diagnoses in Ninety-eight Patients with Pain in the Fore Part of the Foot**

Diagnosis	Number
Primary metatarsalgia	
Static disorders	12
Iatrogenic (postoperative)	12
Secondary to hallux valgus	9
Hallux rigidus	3
Morton's foot	3
Congenital	3
Long first ray	2
Freiberg's disease	1
Total	45
Secondary metatarsalgia	
Rheumatoid arthritis	11
Sesamoiditis	10
Posttraumatic	4
Neurogenic	3
Stress fractures	2
Gout	1
Short ipsilateral lower limb	2
Total	33
Pain under the fore part of the foot	
Morton's neuroma	5
Plantar fasciitis	3
Causalgia	2
Tarsal tunnel syndrome	2
Tumors	2
Intermittent claudication	1
Buerger's disease	1
Plantar verrucae (warts)	4
Total	20

(From Scranton, P. E.: Metatarsalgia: diagnoses and treatment. J. Bone Joint Surg. *62*:723–732, 1980.)

in the bottom of the foot. Patients with this condition usually have pain and tenderness localized to the insertion of the long plantar tendon into the base of the calcaneus. When *peripheral ischemia* gives rise to isolated heel pain without other evidence of peripheral vascular disease, there is often cornification of the heel skin and coolness in this area.

DIAGNOSTIC STUDIES

Doppler studies help the physician detect arterial insufficiency. Radiographs may demonstrate calcaneal spurs and fractures, including small stress fractures. Quantitative scintigraphs help the physician identify abnormal weight distribution and its associated fasciitis.

LESS COMMON DIAGNOSTIC CONSIDERATIONS

Metatarsalgia is not a cause but a symptom of pain in the forefoot (Table 21–1). Primary metatarsalgia is pain in the forefoot due to a chronic disorder of weight distribution across the metatarsophalangeal joints. Pain in the metatarsal region can be due to other local processes (e.g., plantar warts, tarsal tunnel syndrome, and plantar fasciitis) or systemic disease (e.g., rheumatoid arthritis, sesamoiditis, and gout). Neuralgia and polyneuritis from alcohol ingestion, lead poisoning, or diabetes may produce pain in one or both feet. In addition, these patients frequently complain of burning sensations or paresthesias of the soles of their feet. Decreased tactile and vibratory sensations may be observed on physical examination.

If foot pain is precisely located on the plantar surface between a pair of metatarsal heads, a *Morton's neuroma* should be suspected (Fig. 21–1). This relatively rare condition is more common in females than in males. The usual history is foot pain for 2 or more years that is relieved by shoe removal and unchanged by conservative measures. This pain is often described as "burning," "shooting," "needles," "daggers," or "like walking on a stone." It may radiate to the toes. Patients may complain of numbness and tingling. Physical findings include pain with compression of the toes, a palpable click after the release of pressure in the affected area, occasional swelling, and some sensory changes. The pain is precipitated by walking and is aggravated by compression of the toes and weightbearing.

Patients with Raynaud's disease, in addition to having tingling and numbness, may present with pain in the toes that often is associated with pain in the fingers. These pains may be precipitated by exposure to cold, emotional stress, beta-blockers, or cigarette smoking. Some

DIFFERENTIAL DIAGNOSIS OF FOOT PAIN

CAUSE	NATURE OF PATIENT	NATURE OF SYMPTOMS	PRECIPITATING AND AGGRAVATING FACTORS	PHYSICAL FINDINGS	DIAGNOSTIC STUDIES
Muscular and ligamentous strain	Physically active, especially those unaccustomed to exercise	Pain in region of strained muscles or ligaments	Trauma Unaccustomed or strenuous physical activity	Localized tenderness on palpation	
Foot strain	Older adults Overweight patients	Dull ache in foot, especially forefoot	New shoes Change in heel size Prolonged standing	Forefoot may splay with weightbearing	
Plantar warts and callosities		Pain in plantar surface in metatarsal region	Weightbearing	Plantar callosities	
Jogger's foot	Joggers	Burning in heel Aching in arch		Decreased sensation behind big toe	
Fractures	Patients with history of trauma Joggers		Trauma		May need radiographs to diagnose small fractures of ankle and march fractures of metatarsals

Calcaneal spur or plantar fasciitis		Pain on undersurface of heel Continuous One inch from back of heel	Worse with weightbearing		Radiograph may show calcaneal spur
Achilles tendonitis or bursitis	Joggers	Heel pain over Achilles tendon	Trauma Running	Swelling and tenderness over Achilles tendon	
Apophysitis of calcaneus	Adolescents	Pain in back of heel	Running and jumping	Pain on palpation of Achilles insertion	
Arterial insufficiency	Older adults Diabetics	Rest pain in heel or toes		Coolness Decreased pulses Cornification of heel skin	
Gout	Males, especially over 40 years Postmenopausal females	Acute severe pain in big toe M-P joint, occasionally other toes or ankle	Trauma	Warm, violaceous, tender, swollen joints	Uric Acid Radiographs

patients with rheumatoid arthritis have marked prominence of the metatarsal heads with pain in this region. Foot ulcerations, which are not necessarily associated with significant pain, can occur in patients with diabetes mellitus, tabes dorsalis, leprosy, paraplegia, Raynaud's disease, and thromboangiitis obliterans. These conditions should be suspected whenever there is an ulcer without much pain. They may all cause some degree of neuropathy that interferes with pain perception.

Erythromelalgia is painful dilatation of the superficial vessels of the foot. The pain is burning in quality and may be severe. It may be seen in patients with lead poisoning, polycythemia, or syringomyelia and in some psychologically disturbed patients.

Selected References

Morris, M. A.: Morton's metatarsalgia. Clin. Orthop. Rel. Res. *127*:203–207, 1977.

Rask, M. R.: Medial plantar neuropraxia (jogger's foot): report of three cases. Clin. Orthop. *134*:193–195, 1978.

Scranton, P. E.: Metatarsalgia: diagnoses and treatment. J. Bone Joint Surg. *62*:723–732, 1980.

Swell, J. R., et al.: Quantitative scintigraphs in diagnosis and management of plantar fasciitis (calcaneal periostitis). Con. Comm. J. Nucl. Med. *21*:633–636, 1980.

22
PAIN IN THE LOWER EXTREMITY IN ADULTS

To diagnose pain in the lower extremity accurately, the physician must determine whether the pain is *articular* (hip, knee, or ankle), or whether it is *nonarticular* (muscular, vascular, or neurologic). In addition, it is particularly helpful for the examiner to note whether the pain is present at rest or whether it is primarily associated with exercise. The most likely causes of pain in a child's leg are different from those in an adult. Therefore, lower extremity pain in adults and lower extremity pain and limp in children will be reviewed in separate chapters.

In adults, the most common causes of leg pain include *muscular* and *ligamentous strains, degenerative joint disease* (particularly of the hip and knee), *intermittent claudication* due to arterial insufficiency, *sciatica, night cramps, varicose veins, thrombophlebitis, gout,* and *trauma.* **The major clues to diagnoses are (1) the location of the pain, (2) the age of the patient, and (3) whether the pain is related to exertion.**

NATURE OF PATIENT

The most common cause of leg pain is *muscular* or *ligamentous strain,* seen frequently in "weekend athletes." Questioning usually reveals a history of unusual or strenuous exercise. The usual causes of leg

235

pain in joggers and runners are *shin splints, stress fractures,* and *compartment syndromes.* The most common is shin splints, a musculo-tendinous inflammation of the anterior tibia that occasionally involves the periosteum. The pain is usually on the anterior aspect of the tibia, particularly the distal third along the medial crest, but it can occur on the lateral aspect of the tibia as well. Shin splints are most common in less well conditioned athletes and are most frequently reported early in the running season.

Degenerative joint disease (DJD) is uncommon in patients under 40 years of age unless it has been facilitated by unequal leg length (causing DJD of the hip) or prior trauma such as athletic injuries of the knee. After age 40, pain in the hip or knee is commonly due to DJD.

In patients 50 years or older, calf pain precipitated by walking or exercise that abates with rest is most likely due to *peripheral arterial insufficiency.* **Intermittent claudication pain in the hip is seen in patients with aortoiliac disease.** When exercise-induced calf pain occurs in younger adults—frequently with a history of phlebitis—*venous claudication* is probable. *Gout* is most common in older males but can occur in females, particularly those who have had an early menopause (natural or surgically induced). Patients with gout may or may not have a family history of the condition. Often a history of a prior attack can be elicited. Classic gouty pain occurs in the big toe, but it may occur in other toes, ankles, or knees; it is rare in the hip.

NATURE OF SYMPTOMS

Degenerative Joint Disease. When the knee or hip joints are painful and stiff in the morning, improve during the day, and worsen toward the end of the day, degenerative joint disease is probable. These pains may be exacerbated by certain activities (e.g., descending stairs). Patients with osteoarthritis of the hip may present with pain in the groin or the knee. Therefore, the diagnosis of degenerative joint disease of the hip must be considered in patients who present with knee or groin pain when no pathology is noted in these areas. With degenerative joint disease of the hip, hip motion is usually restricted, and radiographs are generally abnormal. Involvement of the *obturator nerve* also can cause pain in the groin and medial aspect of the thigh and knee. A hernia may be suspected because of groin pain; if no hernia is found, obturator nerve involvement should be considered.

Osteoarthritis of the hip also may present with pain in the buttock; therefore, causes of buttock pain must be considered in the differential diagnosis. Buttock pain caused by *lumbar disc disease* is worse with extension of the spine and relieved by rest in the fetal position. Buttock pain caused by osteoarthritis of the hip is not usually exacerbated by spinal extension or relieved by rest in the fetal position. Likewise, there is usually no evidence of nerve root compression with osteoarthritis of the hip.

Sciatica. Typical sciatica causes pain in the buttock that radiates down the posterolateral aspect of the leg. It may radiate into the dorsum of the foot and tends to follow standard dermatome patterns. Sciatic pain may be sharp or burning. Frequently, it is made worse by coughing, straining at stool (if sciatica is caused by a herniated disc), or walking down steps; it may be precipitated by sudden strenuous movements. The patient may present with pain initiated by an attempt to lift a heavy object or by vigorous turning or twisting with the back flexed (e.g., pulling the rope on a lawn mower or outboard engine).

Effects of Exercise and Rest on Pain. Leg pain that develops during walking occurs in patients with arterial insufficiency, venous insufficiency, spinal stenosis, and thrombophlebitis.

Arterial Insufficiency. The pain of arterial insufficiency (intermittent claudication) usually is described as soreness, a cramp, or a burning sensation in the calf. The discomfort also may be described as a tightness, heaviness, tiredness, or achiness rather than pain. The discomfort usually is precipitated by walking and relieved by rest. It rarely occurs while the patient is at home. It usually develops after the patient has walked a predictable (by the patient) distance and is relieved by rest in a standing position after a predictable (by the patient) period of time. After resting, the patient can resume walking and walk a similar distance before the pain starts again; relief is achieved again after resting. A common mistake is the diagnosis of osteoarthritis of the hip when gluteal claudication is the actual problem. This error is more likely if buttock pain is not associated with pain in the calf. Some patients with vascular disease of the iliac artery complain only of the symptoms of gluteal claudication, which are usually felt when the patient walks outside.

Rest pain (often nocturnal) in the toes or heel is almost pathognomonic of arterial insufficiency. With arterial insufficiency there may be pallor on elevation, rubor on dependency, and loss of hair on the toes. Some men with aortoiliac disease may present with pain in the upper leg or buttock and an inability to develop or sustain an erection. Intermittent claudication pain is usually unilateral but can be bilateral. When the pain is present bilaterally, it rarely occurs in both legs simultaneously. Not uncommonly, the onset of pain in one leg prevents the patient from walking to the point that symptoms in the other leg develop. Physical examination for evidence of arterial insufficiency must be performed on both legs, not only on the one about which the patient complains.

Venous Insufficiency. Venous claudication is very difficult to distinguish from claudication due to arterial insufficiency. In both conditions, walking causes calf pain that may be severe enough for the patient to stop walking. In cases of venous claudication, there usually are no physical signs of arterial insufficiency.

Spinal Stenosis. Spinal stenosis is another cause of leg pain that is exacerbated by exercise. The pain is similar to that associated with arterial insufficiency; it also occurs more frequently in older men. The first clue that the pain in the leg is not due to arterial insufficiency is the presence of normal pedal pulses. **Although both the pain of spinal stenosis and the pain of arterial insufficiency begin with exercise, the former is less typically relieved by rest (Table 22–1).** The pain of intermittent claudication is relieved within a few minutes, whereas the pain of spinal stenosis requires 10 to 30 minutes to subside. Some patients with calf pain from spinal stenosis state that they must sit or lie down with the thighs flexed to relieve the discomfort. The pain of spinal stenosis is caused by a localized narrowing of the spinal canal due to a structural abnormality that results in cauda equina compression. With spinal stenosis, the patients occasionally complain of backache or buttock pain as well as numbness and tingling in the feet with

Table 22–1. **Comparison of Symptoms and Signs in Vascular and Spinal Claudication**

	Vascular Claudication	**Cauda Equina Claudication**
Backache	Uncommon, occurs in aortoiliac occlusion	Common but need not be present
Leg symptoms	Quantitatively related to effort	May be brought on by effort; directly related to posture of extension of spine
Quality	Cramplike, tight feeling; intense fatigue; discomfort; pain may be absent	Numbness, cramplike, burning, paraesthetic; sensation of cold or swelling; pain may be absent
Relief	Rest of affected muscle group	Rest not enough; postural alteration of spine to allow flexion is necessary in most
Onset	Simultaneous onset in all parts affected	Characteristic march up or down legs
Urinary incontinence	Does not occur	Very rare
Impotence	Common in aortoiliac disease (failure to sustain erection)	Very rare (failure to achieve erection?)
Wasting of legs	Global in aortoiliac disease	Cauda equina distribution in severe cases
Trophic changes	May be present; absent in aortoiliac disease	Absent but may be present in combined disease
Sensory loss	Absent	Not uncommon; common after exercise
Ankle jerks	Often absent in patients over 60 years	Common, particularly after exercise
Straight-leg raising	Full	Often full

(From DeVilliers, J. C.: Combined neurogenic and vascular claudication. S. A. Med. J. 57:650–654, 1980.)

walking. Walking uphill is easier than walking downhill for these patients. They have no problem riding a bicycle, probably because the stooped position that they assume during this activity reduces the amount of cauda equina compression. It must be remembered that vascular claudication and spinal stenosis can coexist.

Thrombophlebitis. Unilateral pain and swelling in the calf is usually due to thrombophlebitis. The pain is usually present at rest and is rarely worsened by exercise. In a patient with thrombophlebitis who experiences calf pain when walking, there is an acute exacerbation of the calf pain immediately after he places his foot on the ground. Although the history and physical examination of thrombophlebitis are well known to most physicians (i.e., pain, swelling, tenderness to palpation, and occasionally a history of prior trauma or of previous bouts of phlebitis), this relatively common cause of leg pain often is misdiagnosed. Several studies have suggested that venography should be used to confirm the clinical diagnosis because thrombophlebitis has often been incorrectly diagnosed in the absence of venographic evidence.

Other Conditions. Other causes of painful swelling of the calf include traumatic *rupture of the plantaris tendon* or the *medial head of the gastrocnemius, muscle trauma, muscle stiffness* after unaccustomed exercise, and popliteal *(Baker's) cyst.* This last condition has been called "the pseudothrombophlebitis syndrome" because it causes painful swelling of the calf, thus mimicking thrombophlebitis. Therefore, all patients with painful calf swelling should be examined for a popliteal cyst. In one large series, the majority of patients with painful popliteal cysts also had inflammatory joint disease of the knee, usually rheumatoid arthritis (Table 22–2).

Diffuse aching in one or both calves with no relation to exercise suggests *varicose veins.* Patients with this condition frequently complain that their legs hurt when they go to bed at night, and they often complain of night cramps. The pain of venous insufficiency is vague, nonspecific, and unrelated to any specific muscle groups. Superficial varicosities may suggest the diagnosis, but deep venous insufficiency may be present without noticeable superficial serpiginous varicosities.

Table 22–2. **Disease Entities Associated with Pseudothrombophlebitis Syndrome**

Rheumatoid arthritis	Traumatic arthritis
Psoriatic arthritis	Meniscal injury
Osteoarthritis	Osteochondritis dissecans
Juvenile rheumatoid arthritis	Villonodular synovitis
Reiter's syndrome	Systemic lupus erythematosus
Gonococcal arthritis	Ankylosing spondylitis
Gouty arthritis	Mixed connective tissue disease

(From Katerndahl, D. A.: Calf pain mimicking thrombophlebitis. Postgrad. Med. *68(6)*:107–115, 1980.)

A first attack of *gouty arthritis* of the knee (or, rarely, of the hip) may be difficult to diagnose unless there is a warm, swollen joint in the big toe (podagra) and a prior history of gout. When the first attack is a warm, swollen, painful knee, however, the diagnosis is less apparent and may be confused with *pyogenic arthritis.* Patients with gout do not usually have as many systemic signs (rash, malaise, and fever) as patients with pyogenic arthritis have. With gouty arthritis, there is often a hot, red, tender, swollen joint. The involved joint is very sensitive to external pressure; some patients cannot even tolerate the weight of a sheet or blanket on the joint.

ASSOCIATED SYMPTOMS

Patients with *degenerative joint disease* often have pain and stiffness in other joints. A limp may be present in cases of degenerative joint disease of the hip. Patients with *sciatica* may have numbness, paresthesia, weakness, and sensory deficits as well as abnormal knee or ankle jerks (hyperactive early; diminished to absent later). Patients with *intermittent claudication* may complain of numbness in the foot, which may erroneously suggest a *peripheral neuropathy.* If they also report *impotence,* an *aortoiliac lesion* is probable.

Night cramps, edema of the legs, and stasis abnormalities suggest *chronic venous insufficiency.*

PRECIPITATING AND AGGRAVATING FACTORS

The pain of *degenerative joint disease* worsens with exercise and prolonged weightbearing. *Sciatic* pain is aggravated by coughing, straining at stools, sneezing, walking, stooping, lifting, and spinal extension. As mentioned before, both the pain of *intermittent claudication* and the pain of *spinal stenosis* are brought on by walking and exercise.

AMELIORATING FACTORS

Patients with *degenerative joint disease* will report that their morning stiffness, aches, and pain often abate during the day as they move the joint. *Sciatic* pain often is alleviated by recumbency in the fetal position. The pain of *intermittent claudication* abates within a few minutes after cessation of walking; the pain of spinal stenosis is relieved more slowly and by spinal flexion. The pain of *varicose veins* usually is alleviated somewhat by elevation of the involved limb; the resting (nocturnal) pain of *arterial insufficiency* often is relieved by lowering of the involved limb. **Relief of symptoms with an adequate dose of colchicine is pathognomonic of gout.**

PHYSICAL FINDINGS AND DIAGNOSTIC STUDIES

A careful history and physical examination are essential in all patients complaining of pain in the extremities. During the history, special attention should be paid to any history of previous joint disease, precipitating events, previous diagnoses, and medications, particularly oral contraceptives, which are associated with a higher incidence of thrombophlebitis. Physical examination should include examination and determination of range of motion of all joints, measurement of both calves and both thighs, and inspection and palpation for arterial insufficiency. Examination of the knee and popliteal space should be performed in both the supine and erect positions: Joint effusions are more readily detected in the supine position, whereas cysts are more prominent when the patient is erect.

Muscular and Ligamentous Strains and Tears. When patients complain of pain in the knee, the joint should be palpated (Fig 22–1). Tenderness at the joint line suggests damage to the medial or collateral ligaments, the capsular ligament, or the meniscus. Radiographs and arthroscopic examination may be needed for an accurate diagnosis. The stability of the knee ligaments should be determined by careful physical examination. Tenderness above or below the joint line suggests a muscular pull or strain. With acute muscle tears, there generally are local tenderness, bruising, and possibly a gap in the muscle. With *acute gouty arthritis*, the joint is usually warm, red, tender, and swollen. Although pain can be as severe as that seen in pyogenic arthritis, patients with gouty arthritis do not have comparable systemic symptoms. The serum uric acid usually is elevated, and uric acid crystals may be seen in the joint aspirate.

Degenerative Joint Disease. The major physical findings that suggest degenerative joint disease include joint crepitus, limitation of joint movement, and elicitation of presenting symptoms at extremes of joint movement. In advanced cases, there may be fixed flexion contractures, joint effusions, and radiographic evidence of arthritis. Patients with degenerative joint disease are often iin the same age group as those with vascular insufficiency, in whom the symptoms are referable to soft tissue. **It is essential that the physician remember that both conditions can coexist. A good axiom to keep in mind is that if a careful examination reveals no swelling of the joint, there probably is no serious problem inside the joint.**

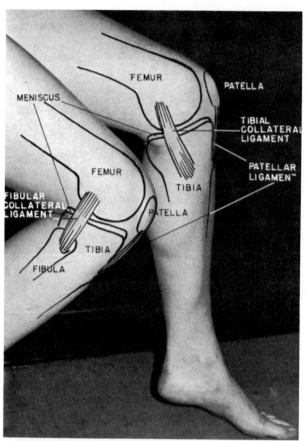

Figure 22–1. Major landmarks in examination of the knee. (From Smith, J. B.: Knee problems in children. Pediatr. Clin. North Am. *24*:4, 1977.)

Sciatica. Some common physical findings in sciatica include restriction of spinal movement (hyperextension often reproduces sciatic pain), limitation of straight-leg raising, and spasm over the sacrospinal muscles (which may be tender to palpation). There may be changes in reflex activity as well as sensory or motor loss over the involved segments. Myelograms and CT scans are rarely necessary for diagnosis. They are used to determine the extent of the spinal cord compression.

Intermittent Claudication. Physical findings in intermittent claudication include pallor on elevation, rubor on dependency (most noticeable in the toes and sole), loss of hair on the toes, and diminished arterial pulsations. The presence of normal pedal pulses at rest and after walking virtually rules out arterial insufficiency.

Patients with *venous claudication* usually have varicose veins. Occasionally, they can identify a tender point in the calf, but examination is nonrevealing. In such cases, the patient should be exercised to the point of discomfort, at which time a group of varices may be noted. Venography may be required for diagnosis.

Thrombophlebitis. The classic findings in patients with thrombophlebitis are swelling and a measurable increase in calf circumference when compared with that of the opposite side. The clinician often can palpate a tender cordlike vein between the heads of the gastrocnemius muscle. There may be dilation of other veins, edema, erythema, and Homan's sign. These findings are variable and not always reliable for the diagnosis of thrombophlebitis. Inflation of a sphygmomanometer around each calf until pain is produced is a sensitive test for the pain of thrombophlebitis. The single most important test is venography. **Because thrombophlebitis may coexist with a popliteal (Baker's) cyst, a venogram should be obtained for all patients with popliteal cysts.**

Other Conditions. The diagnosis of *joint sprain* is made by demonstrating instability of the joint. Tears of joint ligaments often can be demonstrated by the use of stress-view radiographs of the joint involved. With suspected *fractures,* a radiograph including the joints at both ends of the fractured bone always should be performed. Instability of joints suggests ligamentous tears. Angulation in valgus or varus with knee slightly flexed suggests either medial or lateral ligament instability. Abnormal forward or backward shift of the tibia on the femur is indicative of anterior cruciate or posterior cruciate ligament instability, respectively. Occasionally, abnormal rotations may be present; these suggest a complicated combination injury of the knee.

If the diagnosis is still unclear after a complete physical examination is conducted with special attention given to the musculoskeletal, vascular, and nervous systems, noninvasive and invasive studies of the vascular system, electromyography, CT scanning, and myelography may be helpful.

LESS COMMON DIAGNOSTIC CONSIDERATIONS

Sudden onset of pain that sometimes is associated with paralysis, paresthesia, pallor, or absence of arterial pulsation suggests acute arterial embolism. The likelihood of this diagnosis is increased by the presence of atrial fibrillation. Vague arthralgias and muscular aches often are seen with viral and flu-like infections, but no joint abnormality can be detected on physical examination in these cases. Primary bone tumors are rare in adults; pain from metastatic bone disease, however, frequently is seen in patients with breast, lung, and prostatic tumors.

Because cellulitis of the calf can mimic thrombophlebitis, the two conditions must be differentiated. In patients with cellulitis, the pain is described as being on the surface, no palpable cord is present, and Homan's sign is absent. Careful examination will reveal that the pain of cellulitis is induced by light palpation rather than deep palpation over the course of the vein. Likewise, the area of erythema is more clearly demarcated, and there occasionally is an associated open wound. An inflated sphygmomanometer requires high pressure to reproduce the pain, and often there is no difference between the two calves. These findings contrast with those reported in patients with thrombophlebitis.

Chondromalacia patellae, although more common in adolescents than in adults, may be seen in patients in their forties and fifties. These patients characteristically have pain, stiffness, grating, or locking of the knee. The pain is worse when the knee is weightbearing in flexion. Crepitation and pain with manipulation of the patella over the femoral condyle are characteristic. Pain is exacerbated when the patient tenses the quadriceps with the knee in free extension while the examiner depresses the upper pole of the patella.

Meralgia paresthetica, which is slightly more common in male adults, is caused by entrapment of the lateral femoral cutaneous nerve by the tensor fasciae latae. The patient complains of pain, burning, or tingling over the lateral aspect of the thigh that occasionally is worse at night or after exercise. It is alleviated by rest, particularly in the sitting position.

Peripheral neuropathies are more common in diabetic patients but may be seen in nondiabetics. Patients complain of burning, tingling, and numbness, particularly in the feet. They may have a sensation of coldness, but no decrease in vascular pulsations is noted in those with a pure peripheral neuropathy. Diabetics with a peripheral neuropathy often have an associated vascular insufficiency. Physical findings include sensory loss (often symmetric), muscle-wasting, weakness, decreased tendon reflexes, and signs of arterial insufficiency.

Obturator hernias, an uncommon cause of pain, occur more frequently in elderly debilitated women than in other patients. The female-to-male ratio is 6:1. Patients usually present with pain along the anteromedial aspect of the thigh. This pain is increased by adduction of the thigh. Pain also may be felt in the hip or knee. The pain may be associated with intermittent bouts of nausea, vomiting, abdominal pain, and distention—all signs of small bowel obstruction. **Obturator hernia should be given particular consideration in elderly female patients who complain of pain in the hip or knee when there is no objective evidence of degenerative joint disease or other common causes of pain in the hip or knee.**

Pseudothrombophlebitis due to a popliteal (Baker's) cyst has been discussed previously. Fifty per cent of patients with this syndrome have rheumatoid arthritis. It is notable that among patients in whom a popliteal cyst has been confirmed, only 50 per cent had palpable masses, and 12 per cent had masses below the popliteal space. **A Baker's cyst should be suspected in all patients with thrombophlebitis and rheumatoid arthritis and in all patients in whom thrombophlebitis is suspected but for whom no evidence of phlebitis is found on venography.** An arthrogram is essential to the diagnosis of a popliteal cyst. Ultrasonography may help the physician diagnose an intact cyst, but it is not often useful in the diagnosis of a ruptured popliteal cyst.

Rheumatoid arthritis is a relatively uncommon cause of pain in the lower extremity. The joint pain usually lasts for a few weeks, and there is characteristic morning stiffness, joint tenderness, and pain with motion. Frequently, there is joint effusion, soft-tissue swelling, and synovial thickening. As already mentioned, pseudothrombophlebitis should be suspected when calf pain occurs in any patient with rheumatoid arthritis, especially if active inflammation of the knee is present.

Spinal stenosis (neurogenic claudication, cauda equina claudication) is often difficult to differentiate from intermittent claudication due to arterial insufficiency. The patient's history is particularly important because both conditions affect the same age group. Patients with calf pain due to spinal stenosis state that the pain starts insidiously, is exacerbated by walking, and is particularly related to extension of the spine. They may have associated backache or buttock pain, which is relatively uncommon in patients with intermittent claudication. A paresthetic quality to the pain suggests a neurogenic origin. Patients with spinal stenosis do not experience prompt relief of pain with cessation of exercise (as do those with arterial insufficiency); they feel greater relief when they lie or sit down with their thighs flexed. It is noteworthy that patients with spinal stenosis do not have pain when riding a bicycle because the spine is in a flexed position. In any case involving a patient who has signs of intermittent claudication and who rides a bicycle without difficulty, spinal stenosis should be suspected.

Rupture of the gastrocnemius or the plantaris tendon, particularly during athletic activities such as jogging, running, and tennis, is characterized by a sudden onset of pain in the leg ("felt like I got a shot in the leg"). Frequently, the physician can palpate the retracted end of the plantaris muscle.

Trochanteric bursitis, a relatively uncommon cause of leg pain, usually presents with pain over the greater trochanter, in the buttock, and in the lateral thigh along the distribution of the second lumbar dermatone. On physical examination, the patient may limp, and there usually is marked point tenderness over the greater trochanter. The differential diagnosis consists of arthritis of the hip or lumbar spine problems. The major factors in differential diagnosis include pain with palpation over the trochanteric bursa and the absence of sensory loss that would be seen with lumbar disc disease. The pain is not exacerbated by coughing and sneezing but by squatting, climbing stairs, and sitting

DIFFERENTIAL DIAGNOSIS OF LOWER EXTREMITY PAIN IN ADULTS

CAUSE	NATURE OF PATIENT	NATURE OF SYMPTOMS	ASSOCIATED SYMPTOMS	PRECIPITATING AND AGGRAVATING FACTORS	AMELIORATING FACTORS	PHYSICAL FINDINGS	DIAGNOSTIC STUDIES
Muscular or ligamentous strain	Weekend athletes Those with trauma			Unaccustomed or strenuous muscular activity		With ligamentous injury of joint may be tenderness at the joint line and swelling of joint Local tenderness	
Degenerative joint disease	> 40 years (except those with prior trauma)	Knee or hip pain Morning stiffness Gradual onset	Pain and stiffness in other joints Occasional limp	Standing and weightbearing Descending stairs	Movement	Buttock pain not worse with hyperextension No evidence of nerve root compression Crepitation of joint Joint limitation of movement and/or effusion	Radiographs Arthroscopy of knee
Lumbar disc disease (sciatica)	More common in males > 40 years	Pain in buttock and posterolateral aspect of leg Acute onset Lancinating or like toothache Less severe previous episodes	Paresthesias Dysesthesias Weakness	Lifting Turning Twisting Spinal extension Coughing Straining	Fetal position	Spasm of hamstrings Positive straight- or flexed-leg signs Neurologic signs in lower leg Reversal of lordotic curve Pain of sciatic distribution with spinal hyperextension Asymmetric limitation of motion	Myelography and CT scanning to determine extent of pathology Electromyography

Condition	Predisposing factors	Symptoms	Edema and stasis abnormalities	Aggravating factors	Elevation of limb	Physical findings	Diagnostic tests
Varicose veins		Diffuse aching of one or both calves; Worse at night			Elevation of limb	Varicose veins may or may not be apparent	Venography
Thrombophlebitis	History of phlebitis; Use of oral contraceptives	Unilateral; Pain at rest	Swelling	Placing foot on ground		No evidence of arterial insufficiency; Swelling of calf with tenderness and warmth; Palpable cord	Venography
Arterial insufficiency	> 50 years, earlier in diabetics	Pain in calf with walking; Intermittent claudication of hip with aortoiliac disease; Rest pain in calf, toes, or heel suggests severe arterial insufficiency; Usually unilateral	Impotence with aortoiliac disease	Walking	Rest; Dependency of involved limb	Decreased pulses; Pallor on elevation, rubor on dependency; Cool; Loss of hair on toes	Arteriography; Doppler studies
Spinal stenosis	Older men	Calf pain induced by walking and/or leg exercise	Paresthesias; Backache; Buttock pain	Exercise; Not precipitated by exercise with spine flexed (bicycling)	Not quickly relieved by rest; Spinal flexion	Good pedal pulses; Transient neurologic deficit	Electromyography; CT scanning
Gout	More common in men	Acute onset; Toe and knee pain; Rare in hip		Occasionally precipitated by trauma		Joint warm, swollen, exquisitely tender	Serum uric acid test; Uric acid crystals in joint aspirate

with the painful leg crossed over the other one. It is alleviated by infiltration of the trochanteric bursa with local anesthetics or steroids or both.

THE LEG AND SPORTS MEDICINE

The most common causes of chronic leg pain in runners include *shin splints, stress fractures* and *compartment syndromes.* Shin splints represent muscle tenderness, inflammation, and probably subclinical periosteal reaction. With stress fractures there is usually point tenderness over the involved bone, and the diagnosis may be confirmed radiographically. Stress fractures are more common in experienced long-distance runners, particularly in those who attempt to run more than 20 to 30 miles per week. These fractures may occur in the tibia, fibula, or the metatarsus. "Compartment syndromes" occur when the fascial compartment is too small to accommodate the approximately 20 per cent increase in muscle size that occurs with strenuous exercise. This results in a limited venous outflow and tends to produce an ischemic pain of the involved tissue. Patients with compartment syndromes usually present with a gradual onset (over 1 or more years) of pain that is progressive, dull, aching, and particularly worse after long runs. Paresthesias also may be present. The anterior compartment of the leg usually is affected. The next most likely compartment to be affected is the posterior compartment, followed by the posterior superficial compartment. Physical findings include tenderness in the muscle mass itself but not as much in the bone and tendons.

Selected References

Detmer, D. E.: Chronic leg pain. Am. J. Sports Med. *8(2)*:141–144, 1980.
DeVilliers, J. C.: Combined neurogenic and vascular claudication. S. Afr. Med. J. *57*:650–654, 1980.
Goodreau, J. J., et al.: Rational approach to the differentiation of vascular and neurogenic claudication. Surgery *84(6)*:749–757, 1978.
Katerndahl, D. A.: Calf pain mimicking thrombophlebitis. Postgrad. Med. *68(6)*:107–115, 1980.
Noble, J., and Abernathy, P. K.: The painful knee. Br. J. Hosp. Med *22(2)*:169–176, 1979.
Provan, J. L., Moraou, P., and MacNab I.: Pitfalls in the diagnosis of leg pain. Can. Med. Assoc. J. *121*:167–171, 1979.

23

PAIN IN THE LOWER EXTREMITY AND LIMP IN CHILDREN

The physician should approach leg pain or limp in children as in adults—that is, determine whether it originates in joints or in soft tissue. The most common causes of leg pain originating in the soft tissue are unusual or strenuous *exercise* and *trauma*. Other common causes of leg pain include *growing pains, Legg-Calvé-Perthes disease, Osgood-Schlatter disease, chondromalacia patellae,* and *ossification of the Achilles insertion.*

NATURE OF PATIENT

If a limp occurs in a young child when he begins to walk, *congenital dislocation* of one or both hips should be considered. *Legg-Calvé-Perthes disease* (epiphysitis of the hip) usually occurs between 5 and 7 years of age. In adolescents, *slipped femoral epiphyses* and *patellar problems* are more common. In children between the ages of 12 and 14 years, pain in the heel is most often caused by a painful *bursitis* or *irregular ossification of the calcaneal apophysis.*

249

NATURE OF SYMPTOMS

Growing pains is a general diagnosis that is being made less frequently as physicians become more expert in making specific diagnoses. There is no doubt, however, that growing pains do exist, and they are now thought to be a form of *myalgia*. The pain is intermittent and usually located in the leg muscles, particularly in the front of the thigh, the calf, and the back of the knee. The pain is deep and localized to areas outside joints. It is usually bilateral and generally occurs late in the day, although it may awaken the child from a sound sleep. Growing pains may be exacerbated by excessive running during the day, but exercise is not usually a factor. **The findings that the pain is nonarticular, bilateral, and usually unrelated to activity are essential to the accurate diagnosis of growing pains.** There are no abnormal physical findings in children with growing pains.

Most serious diseases that cause leg pain in children (except slipped capital femoral epiphyses) are usually unilateral. Pain in the hip may be due to *Legg-Calvé-Perthes disease*, a disturbance of the epiphyseal ossification of the femoral head in children 4 to 12 years of age (peak age, 5 to 7 years). It often is associated with a limp. Occasionally, the pain is referred to the medial aspect of the knee.

The most common causes of knee pain in children are *acute trauma, Osgood-Schlatter disease,* and *chondromalacia patellae.* Osgood-Schlatter disease is an abnormality of the epiphyseal ossification of the tibial tubercle. It is most common in children 10 to 15 years of age. This condition involves painful swelling of the tibial tubercle at the insertion of the patellar tendon. Pain is worse with contraction of the quadriceps against resistance. It is exacerbated by activity and relieved by rest.

Chondromalacia patellae is an extremely common syndrome in active children and may be a precursor of adult patellofemoral arthritis. In this condition, the patellar cartilage degenerates not because of primary cartilaginous disease but because of abnormal mechanical forces acting on it. These abnormal forces may be due to direct or indirect trauma. Direct injury may occur when a force is applied to the anterior aspect of the patella; this usually results from a fall on the flexed knee. Indirect trauma is more common. This is usually the result of strenuous or repetitive quadriceps activity to which the patient is unaccustomed (e.g., hiking, jogging, calisthenics, or skiing). **The most characteristic symptom of indirect trauma is pain in the lower pole of the patella and adjacent patellar tendon that is precipitated by strenuous activity, especially running, jumping, or squatting.** After resting with the knee flexed, patients with indirect trauma experience a marked increase in pain when they initially extend the knee and begin to move around, but they usually find some relief after standing still or walking a short distance. Patients often describe a grating sensation that may be detected on physical examination when the knee is flexed and extended. The grating is noted particularly when the knee is extended against resistance. Radiographs are usually normal but may show fragmentation of the lower pole of the patella.

Chondromalacia patellae must be differentiated from *patellar osteochondritis, jumper's knee,* and *partial rupture of the patellar tendon.* Children with chondromalacia patella usually have localized tenderness at the lower pole of the patella and the adjacent patellar tendon (see Fig. 22–1). Occasionally, the physician may note separation of the patellar tendon from the lower pole and a palpable defect at that point.

Other conditions that give rise to knee pain include *patellar subluxation, patellar dislocation,* and *meniscal injuries. Rheumatoid arthritis* and *popliteal cysts,* although uncommon, can occur in children.

Limping is a common complaint among children. It is never normal, although its causes are many, ranging from ill-fitting shoes, to a sprained ankle, to the earliest manifestation of a malignant tumor. To determine the exact cause of limping, the physician must approach the problem methodically and thoroughly, obtaining a detailed history and performing a careful examination of the child's gait.

ASSOCIATED SYMPTOMS

Although limping is often due to trauma and the most common cause of leg pain is traumatic injury to the joints or soft tissue, these facts may be misleading in some cases. **In general, when pain or limp is due to mild trauma the symptoms should disappear within 2 to 3 weeks.** If the symptoms do not disappear, despite a report of trauma, the physician must obtain a thorough history and perform a complete physical examination to rule out more serious entities. The physician must determine whether the limp is intermittent or constant, whether it is present at the end of the day or in the morning, whether it is made worse by climbing stairs, and whether it is present only after vigorous exercise (which may be the first clue to an impending stress fracture).

The location of leg pain often provides clues to its etiology, particularly in cases of referred pain. Lower back pathology most commonly refers pain to the buttocks and lateral thigh, whereas hip pathology often refers pain to the groin, medial thigh, or knee. For example, *Legg-Calvé-Perthes disease,* in which unknown factors cause infarction of the femoral head, is a common cause of knee pain and limp in children 4 to 12 years of age.

DIFFERENTIAL DIAGNOSIS OF LOWER EXTREMITY PAIN AND LIMP IN CHILDREN

CAUSE	NATURE OF PATIENT	NATURE OF SYMPTOMS	ASSOCIATED SYMPTOMS	PRECIPITATING AND AGGRAVATING FACTORS	AMELIORATING FACTORS	PHYSICAL FINDINGS	DIAGNOSTIC STUDIES
Epiphysitis of hip (Legg-Calvé-Perthes disease)	4–12 years 5–7 peak incidence	Unilateral hip pain often referred to medial aspect of knee	Limp				Radiograph of hip
Epiphysitis of knee (Osgood-Schlatter disease)	10–15 years	Painful swelling of tibial tubercle		Quadriceps contraction against resistance	Rest		Radiograph of knee
Chondromalacia patellae	Children and adolescents	Pain in lower pole of patella and adjacent patellar tendon		Running Jumping Squatting	Quiet standing or walking	Grating of knee with flexion and extension	Radiograph of knee
Trauma	History of sports participation	Joint or soft tissue			2–3 weeks of rest	Local tenderness	
Growing pains		Intermittent myalgia, especially of thigh, calf, and back of knee Nonarticular and bilateral Not related to activity				No abnormal physical findings	

PHYSICAL FINDINGS

Range of motion of each joint from the hip down should be noted and compared with that of the opposite side, with careful attention given to the patellae. Leg lengths should be measured; a discrepancy of ½ inch or more can cause a *pelvic tilt* and subsequent limp.

When the patient complains of lower leg pain, particularly when there also is a limp, the gait should be examined first. Gait consists of two phases: stance and swing. In the stance phase, the foot is in contact with the floor, and one limb bears all the body weight. In the swing phase, the foot is not touching the floor. This phase begins when the toe comes off the floor and ends with heel strike. A child with a stiff hip would have a short swing phase because of limited hip joint movement. During each phase, the physician should observe one or two of the involved anatomic components: first the feet, and then the knees, the pelvis, and the trunk. The sound of the walk may suggest a steppage gait, with slapping of the foot from foot drop. The shoes should be inspected for abnormal wear: Excessive wear of the toes of the shoes suggests *toe walking,* and excessive wear of the medial aspects of the shoe indicates severe *flat feet.*

If there is joint effusion, the physician must suspect an infectious process, especially if there are systemic signs. Infections may be due to *Gonococcus, Staphylococcus,* or *Hemophilus.*

LESS COMMON DIAGNOSTIC CONSIDERATIONS

Rheumatoid arthritis, popliteal cyst, quadriceps malalignment, supracondylar cortical avulsion, and traumatic epiphyseal injury may cause leg pain or limp or both. Herpes zoster is relatively uncommon in children, but when it does occur, it frequently involves the lower extremity and may cause pain, burning, or itching before the typical herpetic lesion appears. Usually, however, children with herpes zoster of the leg have only a rash and experience no pain.

Selected References

Fixsen, J. A., and Valman, H. B.: Limp in children. Br. Med. J. *283(6294)*:780–781, 1981.
Hensinger, R. N.: Limp. Pediatr. Clin. North Am. *24(4)*:723–730, 1977.
Smith, J. B.: Knee problems in children. Pediatr. Clin. North Am. *24(4)*:841–855, 1977.
Speer, D. P.: Differential diagnosis of knee pain in children. Ariz. Med. *34*:330–332, 1979.

24

PAIN IN THE UPPER EXTREMITY

SHOULDER

After backache, upper extremity pain is the next most common type of musculoskeletal pain. Upper extremity pain usually occurs in the joints (shoulder, elbow, and wrist), with the shoulder being the most common site. Shoulder pain can be referred from the neck, chest, or the diaphragmatic region; usually, however, it is due to a local process. It should be remembered that the "shoulder joint" includes three large bones (the clavicle, scapula, and humerus) and four joints (sternoclavicular, acromioclavicular, glenohumeral, and thoracoscapular). For an excellent description of the anatomy of the shoulder joint and clinical entities that produce shoulder pain, the reader should refer to the 1977 article by Bland and Merrit and the accompanying illustrations (Figs. 24–1 to 24–3).

Several terms are used to describe painful disorders of the shoulder. These terms refer to variations of the same basic process and include *supraspinatus tendonitis, rotator cuff tendonitis, subacromial bursitis, bicipital tendonitis, painful arc syndrome, impingement syndrome, calcific tendonitis, calcific bursitis,* and *calcific bicipital tendonitis.*

Pain may originate in the bursa as well as in the shoulder joint. Many authors suggest that the only signficant bursa in the shoulder is the subacromial bursa and that the subdeltoid, subcoracoid, and supraspinatus bursae are extensions of the subacromial bursa.

255

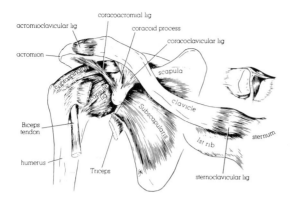

Figure 24–1. Glenohumeral, acromioclavicular, and sterno-clavicular joints. The thoraco-scapular joint is between the anterior scapular surface and the chest wall. (From Bland, J. H., et al.: The painful shoulder. Semin. Arthr. Rheum. 7:21–47, 1977.)

Figure 24–2. Posterior view of shoulder. *A,* Surface muscles, all groups. *B,* Rotator cuff; subscapularis not shown (medial rotator). Note that the rhomboids and levator scapulae displace the scapula medially toward the midline, whereas the scapulohumeral group rotates the humerus laterally. (From Bland, J. H., et al.: The painful shoulder. Semin. Arthr. Rheum. 7:21–47, 1977.)

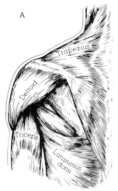
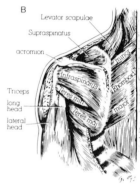

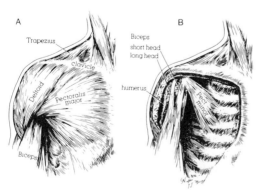

Figure 24–3. Interior view of the shoulder. *A,* Surface muscles. *B,* Deep layer of muscles. (From Bland, J. H., et al.: The painful shoulder. Semin. Arthr. Rheum. 7:21–47, 1977.)

The initial process with shoulder pain is usually a *supraspinatus tendonitis* with extension to other muscles of the rotator cuff. With severe or continuing damage, the inflammatory process spreads first to the subacromial bursa and then to the joint capsule and intra- and extra-articular structures. **The greater the area of pain in the arm and shoulder and the greater the spontaneity of pain (i.e., onset without aggravating events), the greater the likelihood of an extensive lesion.**

Pain in the shoulder (as well as in the elbow and wrist) can be due to *tendonitis, bursitis, trauma, arthritis,* or *referred pain.* Cartilage and bone are not very sensitive to pain. The following are listed in order of decreasing degrees of pain sensitivity: tendons, bursae, ligaments, synovial tissue, capsular reinforcements, and muscles.

Nature of Patient

Acute *subacromial bursitis,* which is painful enough to cause marked limitation of movement, is more common in younger patients. *Calcific tendonitis* is also more common in younger people and rarely is associated with tears; it is more often seen as a sequela to acute bursitis. A *supraspinatus tear,* which permits some movement, is more common in people over 40 to 50 years of age. *Dislocation of the shoulder* is also more common in people over 50 years of age. With first-time dislocations after age 40 to 50 years, there is a much higher incidence of a rotator cuff tear. This is a rare occurrence before 40 years of age.

Nature of Symptoms

Involvement of the Supraspinatus Tendon. Shoulder pain is most commonly located in the lower part of the deltoid region; this is the referral area for pain originating in the supraspinatus tendon. When there is a dull ache in the region of the deltoid insertion that is exacerbated with abduction to 60° or more (painful arc), internal rotation, reaching overhead, or putting on a coat, the physician should suspect a *supraspinatus tendonitis.* Characteristically, patients report that the pain is worse at night or when they lie on the affected shoulder.

Involvement of the Teres Minor, Infraspinatus, and Subscapularis Muscles. If the shoulder is diffusely tender and if moving the humerus posteriorly causes pain, teres minor or infraspinatus muscle involvement should be suspected. If there is pain with resisted medial rotation, there may be subscapularis muscle involvement. In patients with teres minor, infraspinatus, and subscapularis involvement with diffuse shoulder tenderness, pain usually does not radiate into the arm or neck and it commonly is absent or minimal when the arm is dependent.

Tears and Ruptures of the Rotator Cuff. If the patient presents with a sudden onset of shoulder pain in the deltoid area that intensifies within 6 to 12 hours after the initial trauma, a rotator cuff tear should be suspected. With this injury, there may be extreme tenderness over the greater tuberosity as well as pain and restricted motion in one plane of movement at the glenohumeral joint. Patients who present with these findings and recurrent severe pain that awakens them at night may have a rotator cuff tear, even if the arthrogram is normal. In cases of complete rotator cuff rupture, the patient has severe pain and is totally unable to abduct the arm.

Calcific Tendonitis. After a rotator cuff tear, patients may develop calcification and calcific tendonitis of the rotator cuff. Calcification has been reported in the rotator cuff in 8 per cent of the asymptomatic population over 30 years of age. Despite the fact that 8 per cent of the asymptomatic population demonstrate calcific tendonitis, studies have shown that 35 per cent of all patients with calcific tendonitis have had symptoms at some time. If 8 per cent of the population have calcific tendonitis and 35 per cent of these people develop symptoms, approximately 3 per cent of patients over 30 years of age will eventually present with pain referable to a calcific tendonitis. Some studies have related the extent of the symptoms to the size of the calcific area. If the diameter of the calcific mass reaches 1 to 1½ cm, patients invariably develop symptoms. Patients have an abrupt onset of severe, aching pain and find all shoulder movement painful.

Bicipital and Tricipital Tendonitis. When there is generalized tenderness anteriorly in the region of the long head of the biceps (the region of the anterior subacromial bursa), particularly if the pain seems to be worse at night, bicipital tendonitis should be suspected. This pain resembles that of adhesive capsulitis, except that in bicipital tendonitis there is relative freedom of abduction and forward flexion. In patients with bicipital tendonitis, resisted forearm supination causes anterior shoulder pain. This finding is a hallmark of bicipital tendonitis. If there is pain in the triceps region with resisted extension of the elbow, tricipital tendonitis is probable.

Bursitis. When there is point tenderness over the subacromial bursa (often associated with swelling and warmth), subacromial bursitis is probable. Pain in the acromioclavicular joint suggests that this joint is the source of pain. Patients with subacromial bursitis experience particular pain when performing activities such as lifting objects and combing their hair. Virtually all cases of subacromial bursitis are preceded by tendonitis or tenosynovitis in the rotator cuff, biceps, or biceps tendon sheath. When there is an acute onset of excruciating pain in the subdeltoid region of such severity that shoulder movement is totally limited, *calcific bursitis* is probable. Friction of an inflamed bursal surface may be detected with passive motion if the patient is unable to abduct or rotate his upper arm. This acute inflammatory process is probably secondary to calcific deposits in the coracoacromial arch, which ultimately ruptures into the bursal sac and leads to an acute bursitis.

Frozen Shoulder. A frozen shoulder should be suspected when there is a gradual onset of pain with limitation of motion at both the glenohumeral and scapulothoracic joint and when there is limitation of abduction, external rotation, and forward flexion. Although a frozen shoulder is most often due to inflammation of the capsule or rotator cuff, it has many other causes. The hallmark of frozen shoulder is a spontaneous onset of pain that worsens gradually and insidiously. The pain may radiate into the neck and arm, but pain below the elbow is unusual.

Subluxation or Dislocation. When pain in the shoulder follows severe trauma (as opposed to the minor trauma of everyday activity and routine athletic endeavors), it may be due to subluxation or dislocation of the shoulder joint. Patients may state that their shoulder "doesn't feel right," that "something popped," or that "something feels out of place." If this occurs in a child, particularly if there is other evidence of external trauma, child abuse should be considered.

Impingement Syndrome. An impingement syndrome secondary to sports trauma usually occurs in the vulnerable, avascular region of the supraspinatus and biceps tendon. It usually starts as an irritation in the avascular region of the supraspinatus tendon and progresses to an inflammatory response (tendonitis) that involves the biceps tendon and subacromial bursa and then the acromioclavicular joint. This inflammation may finally result in rotator cuff tears and calcification. The most reliable sign of an impingement syndrome is that the pain is reproduced when the arm is flexed forward forcibly against resistance with the elbow extended (Fig. 24–4).

Site of Pain. The location of pain is also useful in differential diagnosis. Pain in the acromioclavicular joint suggests that the source of pain is that joint. Pain occurring in any other part of the arm, shoulder, or neck or in the C5 dermatome may be due to many other shoulder lesions. With supraspinatus tendonitis, the initial symptom frequently is pain in the deltoid insertion area that is precipitated by abduction. As the inflammation spreads to the subacromial bursa, the pain may extend to the distal arm and, occasionally, into the forearm. Pain that involves the forearm as far as the wrist suggests that the inflammatory process has spread to the capsule and has been present for 3 to 6 months. If the entire arm is painful and if there is marked limitation of motion, the inflammation has spread to involve the capsule and synovia. This condition is called frozen shoulder.

Fibrositis Syndrome. Fibrositis syndrome, a form of nonarticular rheumatism, is a common cause of pain in multiple locations, including the upper extremity (Fig. 24–5). Although the existence of this syndrome is doubted by some physicians, others have demonstrated that there is exaggerated, reproducible tenderness at specific anatomic locations in patients with this condition. Even though these sites are normally somewhat tender on palpation, these patients often complain of spontaneous pain over the upper border of the trapezius, the lateral epicondyle of the humerus (the site of tennis elbow pain), and the origin of the supraspinatus muscle near the medial border of the scapula. These patients often complain of insomnia as well. Both the pain and insomnia of fibrositis may respond to tricyclic antidepressants.

Pain Due to Vigorous Physical Activity. Although the traumatic aspects of severe falls and automobile accidents and the recurrent trauma

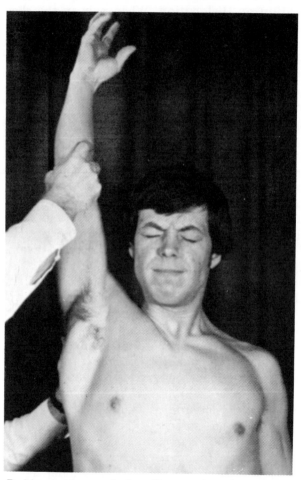

Figure 24–4. Positive impingement sign. The examiner forcibly forward flexes the humerus, jamming the greater tuberosity against the anterior inferior acromial surface. The patient's facial expression on reproduction of the pain confirms the presence of impingement. This may be relieved by the injection of lidocaine directly into the subacromial bursa. (From Hawkins, R. J., and Kennedy, J. C.: Impingement syndrome in athletes. Am. J. Sports Med. 8:151–158, 1980.)

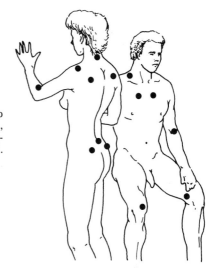

Figure 24–5. Location of 14 typical sites of deep tenderness in "fibrositis." (From Smythe, H. A., and Moldofshy, H.: Two contributions to understanding of the "fibrositis" syndrome. Bull. Rheum. Dis. *28(1)*:928, 1977–1978.)

of competitive sports (e.g., swimming and tennis) are recognized, the fact that trauma to the shoulder can occur as a result of ordinary, vigorous physical activity (e.g., polishing a car for a few hours) is often overlooked. Such physical exertion may cause rotator cuff injuries or subacromial bursitis and severe pain. At rest, pain may be poorly localized; the physician can better determine the source of pain by having the patient repeat the type of activity that apparently induced the pain.

Arthritis. Arthritis of the shoulder is uncommon. When it does occur, it is usually superimposed on a previous injury. With arthritis of the acromioclavicular joint, the pain worsens with adduction of the arm across the chest or circumduction. As with other forms of degenerative arthritis, this pain is often worse in the morning and improves somewhat as the day progresses.

Associated Symptoms

Weakness and atrophy of muscles is uncommon with *supraspinatus tendonitis*. With *rotator cuff tears,* supra- and infraspinatus atrophy may occur in about 3 weeks. With prolonged *frozen shoulder*, there may be atrophy of several shoulder muscles. Patients with *acute bursitis* resist any passive or active shoulder motion.

Arthritis should be suspected if other joints are involved. If paresthesia or hyperesthesia in the region of C8 or T1 is noted, especially with atrophy of the hypothenar eminence, *thoracic outlet syndrome* should be suspected. Patients with this condition also may demonstrate Raynaud's phenomenon.

Precipitating and Aggravating Factors

Prolonged and sustained immobilization with the arm at the side may lead to a *frozen shoulder*. This immobilization may have been recommended by the physician, or the patient may have avoided movement for some other reason for a prolonged period. The *impingement syndrome* often is precipitated by repetitive use of the arm above the horizontal position (as in throwing a baseball or football, swimming, or tennis). Isolated arthritis of the sternoclavicular joint may be due to trauma or weightlifting. *Septic arthritis of the sternoclavicular joint* has been reported in heroin users and in patients with gonococcal arthritis.

Ameliorating Factors

Full trunk and hip flexion allowing the arm to hang limp or supporting the forearm in flexion may help alleviate the pain of rotator cuff tears. This finding may also help the physician establish the diagnosis.

Physical Findings

A careful physical examination with implementation of specific maneuvers is essential to effective diagnosis—and therefore management—of pain in the upper extremity. In most cases, the diagnosis can be made without radiography or arthrography. With *supraspinatus tendonitis,* there is pain on resisted abduction, limitation of joint motion (with or without disruption of the scapulohumeral rhythm), and a normal passive range of motion. Pain is absent or minimal when the arm is dependent. Pain is usually located in the deltoid region, where the supraspinatus tendon inserts.

Patients with *rotator cuff tears* usually have a full range of passive movement and experience pain at extremes of motion. They have pain and restricted movement at the glenohumeral joint and experience pain and weakness with resisted movement. These patients also may demonstrate the "drop arm" sign: weak ability to maintain abduction after passive abduction support is removed. Radiographs may show that the humeral head is high in the glenoid when the arm is in full adduction. Patients with *calcific rotator cuff tendonitis* experience pain with all movements of the shoulder. They usually have associated muscle spasm throughout the shoulder.

Patients with *bicipital tendonitis* experience exacerbation of pain on resisted forearm supination, which causes anterior shoulder pain. Likewise, there is pain with resisted flexion of the shoulder at approximately 80°.

ELBOW

Tennis elbow is a lateral epicondylitis of the humerus that may appear in tennis players of any age or level of expertise, especially those over 40 years of age. It also may occur in people who do not play tennis. Lateral epicondylitis is due to overexertion of the finger and wrist extensors, which originate in the region of the lateral epicodyle. There is pain and acute tenderness at the origin of the extensor muscles of the forearm, which attach just distal to the lateral epicondyle of the humerus. The pain may radiate down the back of the forearm. Patients with epicondylitis also experience pain when performing an activity such as opening a door or lifting a cup or glass.

If pain and swelling is noted in the posterior aspect of the elbow, *bursitis* should be suspected. This may occur after a forced, vigorous extension of the elbow joint. If a child develops pain in the elbow after being swung around by the hand, *radial head dislocation* is probable. *Rheumatoid arthritis* occasionally involves the elbow.

HAND AND WRIST

Pain at the base of the thumb aggravated by movement of the wrist or thumb and reproducible by flexion of the thumb is called *de Quervain's disease*. This is a *tenosynovitis* of the thumb abductors and extensors. Pain in the palm at the base of the third and fourth digits, often associated with a catching or fixation of fingers in flexion, is known as *Dupuytren's contracture*. Examination reveals a painless thickening of the palmar fascia or tendon sheath. If the pain is in the anatomic snuff box, it can be assumed to be due to *navicular bone* fracture unless another cause is determined. Pain or numbness of the fingers is seen in *Raynaud's disease* and associated conditions including *Buerger's disease, disseminated lupus,* and *scleroderma*.

Thoracic outlet syndrome (previously referred to as scalenus anticus syndrome, neurovascular compression syndrome, and hyperabduction syndrome) is most common in middle-aged women and usually occurs on the left side. This syndrome presents with intermittent pain, numbness, or weakness in the hand (occasionally the forearm) after the arm or arms have been in a hyperabducted state for a period of time. Patients often experience this discomfort after working for a long time with the arms over the head or after sleeping with the arms folded behind the neck. Physical examination is normal except when specific maneuvers are employed. For example, forcing the shoulders back and down while in forced inspiration may obliterate the radial pulse on the affected side. Likewise, the radial pulse may be obliterated by the Adson manuever.

Degenerative arthritis usually involves the distal interphalangeal joints, whereas *rheumatoid arthritis* most often involves the proximal interphalangeal and metacarpophalangeal joints. Rheumatoid arthritis also can involve the elbow and the wrist; it rarely involves the shoulder. With active rheumatoid arthritis, there is usually joint stiffness as well as warmth, swelling, and tenderness. The pain is usually polyarticular and migratory rather than monoarticular.

DIAGNOSTIC STUDIES

Precise clinical examination is more useful than radiography in the evaluation of soft-tissue injuries. Arthrography is occasionally helpful. Radiographs should be obtained if fracture is suspected. Electromyograms and nerve conduction studies are helpful tools in the diagnosis of neural entrapment syndromes.

LESS COMMON DIAGNOSTIC CONSIDERATIONS

Less common sources of pain in the upper extremity include some types of local discomfort and referred pain. Apical lung tumors (Pancoast's tumor), cervical disc disease, and cervical spondylosis all can produce shoulder pain. Cervical spondylosis can be due to intervertebral disc protrusion or primary spondylosis. If radiculitis is present, the pain will be sharp and well localized. There may be paresthesias and numbness in the sensory distribution of the compromised nerve root. Fasciculations also may be present, and the pain may be exacerbated by movement of the cervical spine. Despite shoulder pain, a full range of motion may be possible. Cervical spondylosis often can be identified by tenderness over the motor point (where the motor nerve enters the muscle).

Sternoclavicular joint arthritis is rare but occurs in a small number of patients with rheumatic diseases as well as in weightlifters. This pain is usually an anterior chest discomfort that may radiate to the shoulder or arm. When there are significant soft-tissue swelling and warmth in a wide area around the joint, the possibility of a septic arthritis, particularly gonococcal, must be considered.

Shoulder pain can be referred from neck lesions and visceral lesions, including mediastinal disease, subphrenic abscess, and gallbladder disease. Neural entrapment syndromes (e.g., median and ulnar nerve compression) cause pain in the distribution of these nerves. Median nerve compression syndrome is due to compression of the median nerve as it passes beneath the flexor retinaculum, and its symptoms are those of carpal tunnel syndrome. This condition is most common in middle-aged and elderly women. Patients usually complain of pain and pares-

DIFFERENTIAL DIAGNOSIS OF UPPER EXTREMITY PAIN

CAUSE	NATURE OF PATIENT	NATURE OF SYMPTOMS	ASSOCIATED SYMPTOMS	PRECIPITATING AND AGGRAVATING FACTORS	AMELIORATING FACTORS	PHYSICAL FINDINGS
Shoulder Supraspinatus tendonitis	>40 years	Pain in lower part of deltoid region, which is referral area for pain from supraspinatus tendon		Reaching overhead and lying on affected shoulder		Pain worse with resisted abduction Pain worse with abduction to 60° and internal rotation
Subacromial bursitis	<40 years	Severe pain with marked limitation of motion Pain may radiate to distal arm and even forearm		Lifting objects or combing hair		Point tenderness over subacromial bursa, which may be warm and swollen
Bicipital tendonitis		Generalized tenderness anteriorly in the region of long head of biceps (anterior subacromial bursa)				Resisted forearm supination causes anterior shoulder pain Free abduction and forward flexion
Calcific tendonitis	Younger adults	Usually a sequla to acute bursitis				
Rotator cuff tear	Adults	Sudden onset Pain in deltoid area that intensifies 6–12 hours after initial trauma	Recurrent pain		Arm hanging limp	Restricted motion in one plane at glenohumeral joint Weakness and atrophy of supra and infra spinatus Pain over greater tuberosity
Teres minor or infraspinatus tendonitis		Diffuse shoulder pain	No pain radiation into arm or neck		Arm dependent	Pain on moving humerus posteriorly

Table continued on following page

DIFFERENTIAL DIAGNOSIS OF UPPER EXTREMITY PAIN *Continued*

CAUSE	NATURE OF PATIENT	NATURE OF SYMPTOMS	ASSOCIATED SYMPTOMS	PRECIPITATING AND AGGRAVATING FACTORS	AMELIORATING FACTORS	PHYSICAL FINDINGS
Shoulder *Continued* Subscapularis tendonitis		Diffuse shoulder pain	No pain radiation into arm or neck		Arm dependent	Pain with resisted medial rotation
Frozen shoulder		Gradual onset of pain with limitation of motion at the glenohumeral and scapulothoracic joints Limitation of abduction, extension, rotation and forward flexion. Pain may radiate into neck and down arm to elbow	Some atrophy of shoulder muscles	Prolonged immobilization		Marked restriction of motion of shoulder in all directions
Impingement syndrome	Athletes (e.g., participants in baseball, swimming, and tennis)	Tendonitis of the biceps and/or supraspinatus tendon progressing to subacromial bursitis and inflammation of acromio-clavicular joint				Pain on forward flexion of arm with elbow extended
Fibrositis syndrome		Pain at midpoint of upper border of trapezius, origin of supraspinatus near medial border of scapula, 2–3 cm distal to lateral epicondyle of humerus	Sleep disturbance		Tricyclic antidepressants	

Condition				
Lesion of cervical spine and cord		Referred pain to upper extremity, especially back of neck, back of shoulder, and down arm and forearm		Pain and hypesthesia along dermatome distribution
Elbow				
Lateral epicondylitis	Often in tennis players, especially those > 40 years	Pain over lateral epicondyle that may radiate down back of forearm	Resisted extension of wrist and supination of forearm	Tender to palpation over lateral epicondyle
Bursitis		Pain in back of elbow		Swelling, warmth, and tenderness over back of elbow
Radial head dislocation	Child		Swinging child around by hand	Radial head palpable in displaced position
Hand and Wrist				
Tenosynovitis of abductors and extensors of wrist (de Quervain's disease)		Pain at base of thumb	Flexing thumb	
Tenosynovitis of flexors of fingers (Dupuytren's contracture)		Pain in palm at base of third and fourth digits		Catching or fixation of third or fourth digits in flexion Painless thickening of palms, fascia, or tendon sheath
Thoracic outlet syndrome	More common in middle-aged women	Pain, weakness, or numbness in hand (left more often than right) after arms are hyperabducted or on awakening	Prolonged hyperabduction	Decreased radial pulse with Adson's and other maneuvers

thesias in the thumb and in the index and middle fingers. They also may report that they feel clumsy when performing fine movements such as sewing and picking up small objects. Patients may have a sensory loss of median nerve distribution and weakness of the thenar muscles. Both the pain and the paresthesia may be worse at night and on awakening.

Cervical spine and cervical cord lesions often produce referred pain in the upper extremity. Herniation of the disc at C5–C6 or C6–C7 causes pain from the back of the neck, across the back of the shoulder, and down the arm and forearm to the wrist. Patients may have a history of recurrent stiff neck. Their pain is often aggravated by movement, particularly flexion, of the neck. They also may have paresthesias of the thumb and index finger.

Cervical spine spondylosis can cause pain and stiffness in the neck and a radicular distribution of pain in one or both arms. Compression of the cervical cord can cause weakness, wasting, and fibrillations in the upper limbs; paresthesias in the arms or legs; and, occasionally, evidence of pyramidal involvement (e.g., weakness, spasticity, increased deep tendon reflexes, and a positive Babinski sign). The combination of atrophic weakness in the arms and spastic weakness in the legs may suggest amyotrophic lateral sclerosis. Spondylosis can be distinguished from AML by a history of paresthesias and the presence of sensory impairment in the former condition.

Meningeal tumors, Pott's disease, and primary or secondary vertebral body tumors may produce upper extremity pain as a result of root compression. In elderly patients, herpes zoster may cause pain in the arm. These patients often have a history of an eruption and residual pigmented scars.

Angina pectoris is a common cause of pain in the arm and shoulder. This pain is most frequently located in the left upper arm and is usually, but not always, associated with precordial pain. A history of pain in the arm with exertion is the major diagnostic clue for angina pectoris.

Arteritis of the great vessels, Norwegian pulseless disease, is a rare condition that can produce intermittent claudication of one or both arms. It is most common in young women and should be considered in those patients who have diminished blood pressure in one or both arms, especially if they also experience transient episodes of blindness or other cerebral incidents.

Selected References

Bauze, R. J.: Orthopedic pitfalls. Austr. Fam. Phys. 7:1253–1261, 1978.

Bland, J. H., Merrit, J. A., and Boushey, D. D.: The painful shoulder. Semin. Arthr. Rheum. 7:21–47, 1977.

Flechen, P. L.: The painful shoulder. Primary Care 7:271–285, 1980.

Gunn, C. C., and Milbrandt, W. E.: Tenderness at motor points: an aid in the diagnosis of pain in the shoulder referred from the cervical spine. Journal American Osteopathic Association 77:196–212, 1977.

Jenkins, D. G.: Clinical features of arm and neck pain. Psychotherapy 65:102–105, 1979.

Lascelles, R. G., Mohr, P. D., Neary, D., and Bloor, K.: The thoracic outlet syndrome. Braun. 100:601–612, 1977.

Matsen, F. A., and Kirby, R. M.: Office evaluation and management of shoulder pain. Orthop. Clin. North Am. 13:453–475, 1982.

Richardson, A. B., Jobe, F. W., and Collins, H. R.: The shoulder in competitive swimming. Am. J. Sports Med. 8:159–163, 1980.

Smythe, H. A., and Moldofshy, H.: Two contributions to understanding of the "fibrositis" syndrome. Bull. Rheum. Dis. 28:928–931, 1977–1978.

25
PALPITATIONS

Palpitations are defined here as skipped heart beat, irregular heartbeat, rapid or slow heartbeat, or increased awareness of the heartbeat. A patient's awareness of his heartbeat occurs most frequently at rest (e.g., while watching television or while lying in bed). In bed, the mattress serves as a resonator; this facilitates an awareness of the heartbeat, which may be fast, slow, irregular, or normal.

The most common causes of palpitations are *anxiety, stimulants* (e.g., caffeine and alcohol), and *drugs* (e.g., amphetamines, digitalis glycosides, psychotropic agents, and thyroid hormone), and *cardiac disease* (valvular disease, ischemia, myocardiopathy, and mitral valve prolapse). Other common causes include *conduction abnormalities* (e.g., Wolff-Parkinson-White syndrome, sick sinus syndrome, and other conduction disturbances), *hypoglycemia, reactive hypoglycemia, hyperthyroidism, hypoxia,* and *hyperventilation.* If the palpitations occur infrequently or only once, are not associated with other symptoms (e.g., chest pain, syncope, dizzy spells), and develop in an otherwise healthy patient, there is probably little need for concern or extensive work-up. **If palpitations are frequent, are disturbing to the patient, or are associated with syncope, dizzy spells, chest pain, activity, or evidence of heart disease, further investigation is required and should include electrocardiography performed with the patient at rest, exercise electrocardiography, and often 24-hour Holter monitoring.**

NATURE OF PATIENT

In children and adolescents, the complaint of palpitations is most often a sign of *anxiety*. If a rapid arrhythmia is suspected or if the problem is recurrent, the physician should perform electrocardiographic studies and Holter monitoring to determine whether Wolff-Parkinson-White syndrome is present. Children, adolescents, and young adults should be specifically questioned about the use of *stimulants* such as caffeine, alcohol, and nonprescribed illegal drugs.

In adults who have no clinical evidence of heart disease or other systemic disease, the complaint of palpitations is often only an awareness of their normal heartbeat or an occasional atrial or ventricular contraction. The patient should be questioned carefully about the excessive use of stimulants such as caffeine, alcohol, and other agents, including recreational drugs, amphetamines, psychotropic agents, over-the-counter weight-reducing agents, and thyroid-replacement therapy. **With increasing age there is often a decreasing tolerance to agents such as caffeine, alcohol, and drugs.** Although previously tolerated without symptoms, these agents may induce palpitations as the patient gets older. Occasionally, palpitations (often paroxysmal atrial fibrillation) are noted by a patient during the day after unusual but not necessarily excessive alcohol ingestion. This phenomenon has been termed the holiday heart syndrome.

Patients with known cardiac disease who complain of palpitations are more likely to have serious arrhythmias, such as *atrial fibrillation, ventricular tachycardia,* and *sick sinus syndrome.* Those who have poor left ventricular function are particularly prone to ventricular arrhythmias and sudden death. *Mitral valve prolapse* occurs most frequently in young women. One study revealed that the average age of patients with mitral valve prolapse is 38 years and that 70 per cent of patients are women. Palpitations occur in about 44 per cent of patients with documented mitral valve prolapse. Well-conditioned athletes often have a resting bradycardia (sometimes marked). This may be associated with premature ventricular contractions, first A-V block and secondary A-V block; these arrhythmias disappear with exercise.

NATURE OF SYMPTOMS

Patients may complain of a forceful, fast, slow, or irregular heartbeat. It is often useful to have the patient tap out what the rhythm feels like to him. If the patient cannot do this, the physician can tap out a selection of rhythms—slow and regular, slow and irregular, fast and regular, fast and irregular, and the beat of a premature contraction followed by a compensatory pause to assist patients in describing what they mean by "palpitations." Although this procedure is a useful tool, determination of the precise nature of the arrhythmia must be documented by electrocardiography or Holter monitoring.

Various types of arrhythmias are commonly found at different times in the same patient. Arrhythmias that recur in late afternoon and early evening suggest that the arrhythmias are precipitated by *reactive hypoglycemia.* For any patient with unexplained recurrent arrhythmias occurring several hours after eating, the physician should perform a 5-hour glucose tolerance test to rule out reactive hypoglycemia. These arrhythmias are usually supraventricular in origin. Arrhythmias in insulin-dependent diabetics that occur near the time of peak insulin activity are also frequently induced by hypoglycemia. Diabetics often have accelerated coronary artery disease, which is another possible cause of arrhythmias in these patients.

ASSOCIATED SYMPTOMS

Sweating, tremor, and other symptoms of *hypoglycemia* suggest that hypoglycemia is contributing to the arrhythmia. Sticking chest pains that do not usually coincide with the arrhythmia should suggest *mitral valve prolapse,* a condition in which arrhythmias are common. Chest pain, congestive heart failure, syncope, and dizziness all suggest a clinically significant arrhythmia, such as *paroxysmal atrial tachycardia, sick sinus syndrome, complete heart block,* or *ventricular tachycardia.*

PRECIPITATING AND AGGRAVATING FACTORS

Arrhythmias (e.g., premature ventricular contractions) that increase with activity are most likely due to *cardiac disease.* When premature ventricular contractions decrease with exercise (and its associated increase in sinus rate), they are most likely benign. *Digitalis-induced arrhythmias* can be in the form of premature beats, tachyarrhythmias or bradyarrhythmias, supraventricular arrhythmias, supraventricular tachycardia with block, or ventricular tachycardia. Digitalis arrhythmias can be precipitated by increased digitalis dosage, hypokalemia, hypomagnesemia, or decreased renal function. *Antiarrhythmic drugs,* particularly the class I agents (quinidine sulphate, procainamide hydrochloride, lidocaine, disopyramide phosphate, and phenytoin) can both precipitate and suppress arrhythmias. Their prolongation of the Q–T interval makes the patient more vulnerable to the "torsade de pointes" type of ventricular tachycardia, which the patient may perceive as palpitations or dizzy spells.

DIFFERENTIAL DIAGNOSIS OF PALPITATIONS

CAUSE	NATURE OF PATIENT	NATURE OF SYMPTOMS	ASSOCIATED SYMPTOMS	PRECIPITATING AND AGGRAVATING FACTORS	PHYSICAL FINDINGS*	DIAGNOSTIC STUDIES†
Anxiety	Most common cause of palpitations in children and adolescents		Sweaty palms	Hyperventilation	Have patient hyperventilate for 3–4 minutes to see whether arrhythmias can be induced	
Ingestion of stimulants or drugs (caffeine, alcohol, amphetamines)	Patients have decreased tolerance to these agents with increased age		Nervousness Tremor	Caffeine Alcohol Drugs (amphetamines psychotropic agents, thyroid hormone)	PVCs Tachycardia	
Digitalis glycosides			Nausea Anorexia	Increased digitalis dose Hypokalemia Hypomagnesemia Decreased renal function	PVCs Tachyarrhythmias Bradyarrhythmias Second- or third- degree heartblock	Serum digitalis levels Electrocardiography Holter monitoring Serum K Serum Mg Creatinine
β-blockers Antihypertensive Calcium-channel blockers Hydralazine Minoxidil	Patients with angina or hypertension				Bradycardia Sinus tachycardia	
Hypoglycemia	Insulin-dependent diabetics	Arrhythmias occur near the time of peak insulin activity	Sweating Headache Tremor Weakness	Increased insulin Decreased carbohydrate	PVCs Tachycardia	Blood sugar

Reactive hypoglycemia		Recurrent arrhythmias in late afternoon and early evening; Arrhythmias occur several hours after ingestion of carbohydrates	Sweating, Tremor, Headache	Anxiety		5-hour glucose tolerance test
Cardiac Disease						
Mitral valve prolapse	Most common in young women (average age, 38 years)		Sticking chest pain	Exercise	Midsystolic click, Late-systolic murmur, PVCs or premature atrial contractions, Tachycardia	Echocardiography
Wolff-Parkinson-White syndrome	Often detected in children and adolescents	Recurrent palpitations, Frequent paroxysmal tachycardia		Exercise, Digitalis	Paroxysmal tachycardia	Electrocardiography, Holter monitoring
Sick sinus syndrome	Older patients	Bradyarrhythmia, Tachyarrhythmia	Chest pain, Syncope, Congestive heart failure, Dizziness	Exercise	Bradyarrhythmia, Tachyarrhythmia	
Coronary artery disease	Older patients	Palpitations	Angina pectoris, Congestive heart failure		PVCs, Paroxysmal atrial fibrillation	

*Arrhythmias are often absent.
†All arrhythmias should be documented by electrocardiography or Holter monitoring.

Most of the beta blockers, many of the *antihypertensive agents* (e.g., reserpine, methyldopa, clonidine), and the calcium-channel blockers cause bradycardia. Hydralazine and minoxidil can cause sinus tachycardia. Sometimes, discontinuation of drugs (e.g., clonidine, phenytoin, beta-blockers, and antiarrhythmics) is associated with the development of palpitations.

AMELIORATING FACTORS

If the palpitations abate with cessation of stimulants or other drugs, it is most likely that the arrhythmias were caused by the agent or agents that were discontinued. Some patients find that performing a Valsalva maneuver, pressing on their carotid sinus, or gagging themselves to induce vomiting terminates the arrhythmias. In these cases, the arrhythmias are probably supraventricular in origin.

PHYSICAL FINDINGS

Auscultation of a midsystolic click or late-systolic murmur is found in patients with *mitral valve prolapse* (balloon mitral valve, click-murmur syndrome, and Barlow's syndrome). Premature atrial or ventricular contractions occur most commonly in patients with mitral valve prolapse; supraventricular tachycardia or ventricular tachycardia occurs in about 12 per cent of these patients.

There are many different clinical maneuvers (well documented in cardiology texts) that may help the physician determine the nature of arrhythmias. **Precise diagnosis requires electrocardiographic documentation.** In anxious patients complaining of palpitations, the arrhythmias may be precipitated by *hyperventilation*. If this is suspected, the physician can instruct the patient to hyperventilate forcibly for 3 or 4 minutes to determine whether this activity induces an arrhythmia that should be recorded.

DIAGNOSTIC STUDIES

If arrhythmias cannot be documented clinically or electrocardiographically, and if they are frequent or associated with dizziness, syncope, or other cardiac symptomatology, Holter monitoring must be performed. Several studies of 24-hour Holter monitoring have shown that a significant number of patients note palpitations when there is no abnormality detected on their Holter tape and, conversely, that many patients demonstrate arrhythmias on their Holter tape but are unaware of palpitations at that time.

Other studies that may help the physician determine the etiology of palpitations include thyroid function tests, the 5-hour glucose tolerance test, drug screens, determination of serum digitalis levels and blood gases, echocardiography, and, rarely, coronary arteriography.

LESS COMMON DIAGNOSTIC CONSIDERATIONS

Less common causes of palpitations include infiltrative diseases of the myocardium, such as amyloidosis, sarcoidosis, and tumors. Hypothyroidism can cause sinus bradycardia; hyperthyroidism can cause sinus tachycardia, paroxysmal atrial tachycardia, and paroxysmal atrial fibrillation.

Selected References

Chung, E. K.: Wolff-Parkinson-White syndrome—current views. Am. J. Med. 62:252–266, 1977.

Gallagher, J. J., et al.: The Wolff-Parkinson-White syndrome and the preexcitation dysrhythmia—medical and surgical mangagement. Med. Clin. North Am. 60(1):101–122, 1976.

Goldberg, A. D., et al.: Ambulatory electrocardiographic records in patients with transient cerebral attacks or palpitations. Br. Med. J. 4:569–771, 1975.

Kung, G., et al.: What does the symptom "palpitation" mean? Correlation between symptoms and the presence of cardiac arrhythmias in the ambulatory EKG. Z. Kardiol. 66:138–141, 1977.

O'Rourke, R. A., and Crawford, M. H.: The systolic click-murmur syndrome: clinical recognition and management. Curr. Prob. Cardiol. 1(1):1–60, 1976.

Scarpa, W. J.: The sick sinus syndrome. Am. Heart J. 92:648–660, 1976.

Swartz, M. H., et al.: Mitral valve prolapse: a review of associated arrhythmias. Am. J. Med. 62:377–389, 1977.

Zeldis, S. M., et al.: Correlation with cardiac arrhythmias on 24-hour electrocardiographic monitoring. Chest 78:456–461, 1980.

26

SHORTNESS OF BREATH

Dyspnea has been defined as patient awareness of respiratory discomfort, labored breathing, or shortness of breath. Dyspnea can be caused by increased rigidity of lung tissue, increased airway resistance, enhanced ventilation during exercise, or any combination of these factors. Some investigators have suggested that determining the etiology of dyspnea is often facilitated by first classifying it into different types, such as wheezing dyspnea, dyspnea on exertion, paroxysmal nocturnal dyspnea, hyperventilation, and dyspnea of cerebral origin. Perhaps a simple classification is acute, chronic, or recurrent. The common causes of dyspnea incude *chronic obstructive pulmonary disease (COPD), asthma, congestive heart failure, anxiety, obesity,* and *poor physical condition.*

NATURE OF PATIENT

Acute dyspnea in children is most frequently due to *asthma, bronchiolitis, croup,* and *epiglottitis.* Rarely, it may be due to *foreign body aspiration.* An acute onset of dyspnea in a woman who is pregnant or who is taking oral contraceptives suggests *pulmonary embolism.* Pulmonary embolism should also be suspected if dyspnea occurs in patients who are in the postoperative period, in people who have had prolonged recumbency, and in patients who have a history of phlebitis.

The most common cause of chronic and recurrent shortness of breath in children is asthma. In elderly patients, chronic dyspnea is frequently due to chronic obstructive pulmonary disease or heart failure, which are rare conditions in patients under 30 years of age. Chronic dyspnea is more common in people who are heavy smokers because smoking is one of the most important factors in the development of *emphysema, chronic bronchitis,* and *COPD. Obese* and *physically inactive* patients frequently complain of recurrent dyspnea on minimal exertion because of their poor cardiopulmonary reserve.

NATURE OF SYMPTOMS

Acute Dyspnea. In patients with acute dyspnea, the physician should consider the possibility of *pulmonary embolus, asthma, upper airway obstruction, foreign body aspiration, panic disorder, hyperventilation, pneumonia, pneumothorax, pulmonary edema,* and occasionally *respiratory failure.* Asthma is usually episodic and often is precipitated by allergens, exercise, or infections. It is characterized by bilateral wheezing and a decreased respiratory flow rate.

Upper airway obstruction can be caused by *aspiration, vocal cord paralysis, tumors,* and *epiglottic* and *laryngeal edema.* In cases of *foreign body aspiration* (more common in children), the onset of respiratory difficulty is acute. When acute respiratory difficulty occurs during eating, especially in the intoxicated or semiconscious patient, foreign body aspiration is probable. When complete respiratory obstruction occurs, severe respiratory distress, cyanosis, gasping, and loss of consciousness occur quickly. Incomplete respiratory obstruction causes tachypnea, inspiratory stridor, and localized wheezing.

Patients with acute dyspnea due to *hyperventilation* are usually anxious. They often complain of numbness and tingling in the perioral region and the extremities. These patients also often complain of light-headedness, sighing respiration, and an inability to "get enough air in."

A gradual onset of shortness of breath occurs in patients with *congestive heart failure, anemia, lung tumors,* and *parenchymatous lung disease.*

Chronic Dyspnea. Chronic dyspnea in adults is most often due to *chronic pulmonary disease, chronic congestive heart failure,* and *obesity.* It also may be seen with *severe anemia* and *infiltrative pulmonary carcinomatosis.*

ASSOCIATED SYMPTOMS

Dyspnea in Children. When dyspnea occurs in young children, especially when it is associated with coughing and expectoration, *cystic fibrosis* and *bronchiectasis* should be considered.

Acute Dyspnea. *Pulmonary embolism* is a common cause of acute dyspnea in adults. Patients usually appear severely ill and may complain of chest pain, faintness, and occasionally loss of consciousness. Peripheral cyanosis, low blood pressure, and rales may be present. When acute dyspnea is due to severe *anemia* of acute onset, there are usually symptoms of dizziness, weakness, and sweating. There may be signs of hemorrhage (e.g, hypotension, tachycardia, and rapid shallow respirations). When acute dyspnea is a manifestation of *anxiety neurosis* or *panic disorder,* the patient usually also complains of dizziness, lightheadedness, palpitations, and paresthesias. The patients do not appear dyspneic and often complain of "not being able to take in enough air."

Chronic Dyspnea. The most common causes of chronic dyspnea on exertion are *cardiac* and *pulmonary*. **Although paroxysmal nocturnal dyspnea is most frequently due to cardiac pathology, it should be noted that some asthmatics develop symptoms primarily when recumbent, usually at night.** Associated findings are often helpful in differentiating pulmonary from cardiac causes of dyspnea. When dyspnea is primarily due to lung disease, the dyspnea is intensified by effort, the respirations are shallow and rapid, and postural changes generally have little or no effect. When dyspnea is of cardiac etiology, it is intensified by recumbency, and the respirations are shallow but not necessarily rapid.

Other clues also help differentiate pulmonary from cardiac causes of dyspnea on exertion. When the cause is pulmonary, the rate of recovery to normal respiration is fast, and dyspnea abates a few minutes after cessation of exercise. Patients with dyspnea due to cardiac causes, however, remain dyspneic much longer after cessation of exercise. Likewise, in these patients the heart rate also takes longer to return to pre-exercise levels. Patients with pulmonary dyspnea do not usually have dyspnea at rest. Patients with severe cardiac dyspnea demonstrate a volume of respiration that is greater than normal at all levels of exercise; they also experience dyspnea sooner after the onset of exertion.

PRECIPITATING AND AGGRAVATING FACTORS

Smoking is the most frequent precipitating and aggravating factor of chronic pulmonary dyspnea. When *exercise* precipitates wheezing or dyspnea, *bronchial asthma* or *congestive heart failure* may be the diagnosis. *Exposure to cold* often precipitates wheezing and shortness of breath in asthmatics. Bronchial asthma is also probable when *airborn allergens, noxious fumes, or respiratory infections* precipitate dyspnea, cough, or wheezing. *Drugs* (e.g., beta-blockers) may precipitate wheezing or dyspnea in asthmatics. Beta-blockers and calcium-channel blockers may exacerbate dyspnea in cardiac patients. Less common precipitating and aggravating factors include trauma, shock, hemorrhage, and gaseous anesthesia.

AMELIORATING FACTORS OTHER THAN MEDICAL THERAPY

Some patients with severe chronic obstruction lung disease obtain relief by leaning forward while seated or by lying supine with their heads down. These positions increase the efficiency of diaphragmatic movement and facilitate the use of the accessory muscles of respiration. Performance of the Heimlich maneuver may dislodge a foreign body from the upper airway.

PHYSICAL FINDINGS

Patients with *upper airway obstruction* have coarse sonorous rhonchi and impaired inspiration. Stridor as well as suprasternal retraction may be noted with inspiration. Sibilant, whistling expiratory sounds are usually heard in asthmatics. Expiration appears to be prolonged in asthmatics, whereas inspiration seems to be prolonged in patients with upper airway obstruction. The trachea may be shifted to the opposite side in patients with *pneumothorax* or a *large pleural effusion.*

Wheezing dyspnea at rest associated with rhonchi and a productive cough suggests *asthmatic bronchitis.* In contrast, patients with a history of progressive dyspnea that precedes the development of cough or sputum production often have *emphysema.* The physical findings are a hyperinflated lung, decreased breath sounds, decreased diaphragmatic movement, increased AP chest diameter, and hyperresonance to percussion. Classically, emphysematous patients have been described as "pink puffers"; patients with chronic bronchitis are called "blue bloaters."

Bilateral wheezing usually is heard when acute dyspnea is due to *asthma.* Bilateral wheezing also may occur with *pulmonary edema.* Wheezing frequently may be heard prior to the auscultation of rales at the bases and other more classical signs of congestive heart failure. Bilateral wheezing also may be heard in patients with *pulmonary emboli,* but more frequently the wheezing is limited to the side of the pulmonary embolus. Unilateral wheezing may also indicate a *bronchial obstruction* by a foreign body, polyp, or mucous plug. Other causes of dyspneic wheezing include *upper airway obstruction, localized bronchial obstruction,* and *hypersensitivity pneumonitis.*

DIAGNOSTIC STUDIES

Although there are many clinical findings that help the physician differentiate the causes of dyspnea, pulmonary function tests are most helpful and frequently can be performed in an outpatient setting. **Pulmonary function tests should be an integral part of the clinical**

evaluation of all patients with dyspnea. Patients with *simple acute bronchitis* may have a persistent productive cough but demonstrate no signs of airway narrowing on spirometry. In patients with *chronic bronchitis* and a persistent cough, spirometry may indicate widespread narrowing of the airways, but dyspnea may not be present. *Chronic obstructive lung disease* may be diagnosed with simple spirometry. Occasionally, patients with obstructive lung disease demonstrate airway narrowing on spirometry without any other symptoms except cough.

Pulmonary function tests do not provide a specific diagnosis; rather, they demontrate a pattern of the physiologic abnormality. Typical, but not exclusive, patterns of physiologic abnormalities are seen in most patients with chronic pulmonary diseases, in most people with diseases of pulmonary circulation, and in patients with mild cardiac or valvular disease. Pulmonary function tests may help the physician differentiate dyspnea due to hyperventilation or psychologic factors from pulmonary dysfunction.

Pulmonary function tests demonstrate increased obstruction to inspiration when there are extrathoracic (upper airway) obstructive lesions and increased obstruction to expiration when there are intrathoracic obstructive lesions. Expiratory airway obstruction is indicated by decreased airflow rates, decreased forced expiratory volume in one second (FEV_1), decreased peak flow rate (PFR), decreased maximum midexpiratory flow rate (FEF 25–75 per cent), decreased maximum voluntary ventilation (MVV), increased tidal volume, and increased residual volume. These findings are often observed in patients with *asthma, bronchitis, emphysema,* and *bronchial adenoma.* The abnormal findings of bronchospasm can usually be transiently reversed with the inhalation of a bronchodilator drug. Lung volume restriction is indicated by a decreased total lung capacity (TLC), increased respiratory minute volume (VE), and decreased compliance. Decreased compliance is found in patients with *fibrosis, sarcoidosis, pneumoconiosis, pulmonary edema, pneumonia, pleural effusion, kyphoscoliosis, obesity,* and *ascites.* Pulmonary vascular disease is evidenced by increased ventilation (VE) and increased dead space (VD). Ventilation/perfusion scanning and digital subtraction angiography are useful in the diagnosis of pulmonary embolism. An EKG may show P pulmonale and right heart strain.

Chest radiographs may show pulmonary parenchymal disease, pleural effusions, tumors, or signs of congestive heart failure.

LESS COMMON DIAGNOSTIC CONSIDERATIONS

Dyspnea is occasionally the presenting symptom in patients with hyperthyroidism. Pregnant patients may complain of dyspnea. Patients with idiopathic pulmonary hemosiderosis may present with dyspnea on

DIFFERENTIAL DIAGNOSIS OF SHORTNESS OF BREATH

CAUSE	NATURE OF PATIENT	NATURE OF SYMPTOMS	ASSOCIATED SYMPTOMS	PRECIPITATING AND AGGRAVATING FACTORS	AMELIORATING FACTORS	PHYSICAL FINDINGS	DIAGNOSTIC STUDIES
Acute or Recurrent Dyspnea							
Asthma	Most common cause of recurrent dyspnea in children	Acute dyspnea Episodic May rarely be dyspnea only at night	Cough (indicates asthmatic bronchitis)	Allergens Exercise Noxious fumes Respiratory infections Recumbency Exposure to cold B-blockers		Bilateral wheezing Sibilant, whistling sounds Prolonged expiration	Pulmonary function tests: Decreased respiratory flow rates Decreased maximum voluntary ventilation Increased tidal volume Increased residual volume
Pulmonary emboli	Women using birth control pills Patients in postoperative period Long-term recumbent patients Patients with phlebitis Patients in postpartum period	Acute onset of dyspnea	Chest pain Faintness Loss of consciousness	Oral contraceptives Prolonged recumbency		Tachypnea Peripheral cyanosis Low blood pressure Rales Wheezing (usually only on side of emboli) Pleural friction later with pulmonary infarction	Ventilation/perfusion studies Digital subtraction angiography EKG indicates acute right heart strain Pulmonary infarction or effusion on x-ray

Condition	History	Onset/Type	Associated symptoms	Precipitating factors	Treatment	Physical signs	Diagnostic tests
Hyperventilation and anxiety	Usually anxious	Acute dyspnea "Sighing" respirations	Lightheadedness Palpitations Paresthesias (especially in perioral region and extremities)	Stress Panic		Signs of anxiety but no signs of dyspnea	Pulmonary function tests are usually normal
Poor physical conditioning	Obese Physically inactive	Dyspnea on minimal exertion				Obesity After exercise pulse slows very gradually	Pulmonary function tests: Decreased total lung capacity Increased respiratory minute volume Decreased compliance
Foreign body aspiration	Most common in children May occur in intoxicated or semiconscious people during eating	Acute dyspnea			Removal of foreign body Heimlich maneuver	Tachypnea Inspiratory stridor Localized wheezing Suprasternal retraction with respiration May be unilateral wheezing	Chest radiograph may show atelectasis or the foreign body
Chronic Dyspnea							
Chronic obstructive pulmonary disease	Older adults Rarely patients under 30 years Most often smokers	Chronic dyspnea Dyspnea with exertion	Fast rate of recovery to normal respiration after stopping exercise Leaning forward while seated or supine with head down	Smoking Exertion Postural changes have little or no affect	With severe disease patients may obtain some symptomatic relief by leaning forward while sitting	Rapid and shallow respirations	Pulmonary function tests Spirometry

Table continued on following page

DIFFERENTIAL DIAGNOSIS OF SHORTNESS OF BREATH *Continued*

CAUSE	NATURE OF PATIENT	NATURE OF SYMPTOMS	ASSOCIATED SYMPTOMS	PRECIPITATING AND AGGRAVATING FACTORS	AMELIORATING FACTORS	PHYSICAL FINDINGS	DIAGNOSTIC STUDIES
Chronic Dyspnea *Continued* Emphysema		Progressive dyspnea precedes onset of cough Usually no dyspnea at rest				"Pink puffers" Hyperventilated lungs Decreased breath sounds Decreased diaphragmatic movement Increased anterior-posterior chest diameter Hyperresonance	Decreased respiratory flow rate Increased tidal volume Decreased maximum voluntary volume Increased residual volume
Chronic bronchitis		Dyspnea not necessarily presenting symptom Cough precedes dyspnea	Persistent, minimally productive cough			"Blue bloaters" Rhonchi	Same as with emphysema Spirometry shows widespread airway narrowing
Congestive heart failure	Older patients	Chronic dyspnea with gradual onset Paroxysmal nocturnal dyspnea Dyspnea remains long after stopping exercise	Edema	Exercise β-blockers Calcium blockers Recumbency Trauma Shock Hemorrhage Anesthesia	Nocturnal dyspnea may be relieved by sitting	Shallow respirations (not necessarily rapid) Edema Hepatomegaly Jugular venous distention Throat heart sound Basilar rales	Spirometry Respiratory volume is greater than normal at all exercise levels Pulmonary congestion and cardiomegaly on radiograph

exertion, chronic cough, hemoptysis, and recurrent epistaxis. People who work in grain elevators or with hay also may have severe wheezing and dyspnea. Progressive dyspnea and a nonproductive cough may be the presenting symptoms of patients with interstitial pulmonary fibrosis, which may result from drugs (e.g., phenytoin) and from sarcoidosis and other granulomatous diseases. Patients with recurrent pulmonary emboli may present with recurrent episodes of dyspnea. Patients with interstitial pulmonary diseases (e.g., pulmonary fibrosis and pneumoconiosis) as well as those with constrictive cardiomyopathy and constrictive pericarditis may present with dyspnea on exertion, chronic cough, and paroxysmal nocturnal dyspnea.

Selected References

Andrews, J. L.: The clinical roles of pulmonary function testing. Med. Clin. North Am. 63(2):355–377, 1979.

Angelillo, V. A.: Evaluation of dyspnea: Is it really present and, if so, why? Postgrad. Med. 73(2):336–345, 1983.

Campbell, E. J. M., and Howard, J. B. L.: The sensation of breathlessness. Br. Med. Bull. 19:36–40, 1963.

Galish, J. H., Ahmiad, M., and Yarnal, J. R.: Chronic upper airway obstruction; methods of detection and recognition. Cleve. Clin. Q. 47:9–15, 1980.

Gulsvik, A.: Prevalence of and manifestations of obstructive lung disease in the city of Oslo. Scand. J. Respir. Dis. 60:286–296, 1979.

Neff, T. A.: The diagnosis and management of chronic obstructive lung disease. Cleve. Clin. Q. 47:17–24, 1980.

Spiro, G.: Exercise testing in the assessment of respiratory disease. Can. Med. Assoc. J. 122:890–896, 1980.

Williams, M. H.: Expiratory flow rate: their role in asthma therapy. Hosp. Pract. Oct., 1982, pp. 95–105.

27
SKIN PROBLEMS

Skin problems are one of the most common reasons for which patients seek medical attention. The ten most common skin problems for which patients consult dermatologists are *acne, fungal infections, seborrheic dermatitis, atopic* or *eczematous dermatitis, warts,* benign and malignant *skin tumors, psoriasis, hair disorders, vitiligo,* and *herpes simplex.* Other common lesions include infestations such as *scabies* and *pediculosis, contact dermatitis, pityriasis rosea, herpes zoster,* and *seborrheic keratoses.* These are not necessarily the most common skin problems; some of the most prevalent are handled by physicians other than dermatologists. Approximately one third of all patients with a primary dermatologic complaint consult a general physician.

In this chapter, the most common dermatologic problems are presented in tabular form. Because dermatologic diagnosis is generally based on the type of lesion, its configuration, and the distribution of the lesions, the summary table is organized accordingly. Because most of the pediatric exanthems such as measles (rubeola), German measles (rubella), and chicken pox (varicella) are easily diagnosed, they are not discussed in this chapter, and the reader therefore should consult pediatric textbooks for their description.

Skin tumors are most common in later life. The most common malignant lesions are *basal cell epithelioma* and *squamous epithelioma.* **If there is any uncertainty about whether a skin lesion is malignant, it should be biopsied.** For the differential diagnosis of benign and malignant skin tumors, the reader is referred to several excellent texts and articles (see Selected References).

Text continued on page 314

Table 27–1. **Common Areas of Involvement and Causes of Allergic Contact Dermatitis**

Area	Causes
Earlobes	Earrings (nickel)
Postauricular area	Hair dye (paraphenylenediamine) Shampoos (formalin) Hearing aids or glasses (nickel or plastic)
Ear canal	Medications
Face	Hair dye (paraphenylenediamine) Poison ivy Cosmetics Sprays or any airborne contactant
Eyelids	Sprays or any airborne contactant Cosmetics Eyelash curlers (rubber accelerators or nickel) Any contactant on the hands (topical medications, formalin in nail polish)
Perioral area	Lipstick Toothpaste
Neck	Jewelry (nickel) Perfumes Sprays or other airborne contactants
Axilla	Deodorants Clothing (formalin)
Chest	Brassieres (rubber accelerators) Metal objects carried in pockets (nickel)
Back	Metal fasteners (nickel)
Waist	Belt buckles or snaps (nickel) Waist bands or girdles (rubber accelerators)
Extremities	Poison ivy Airborne contacts
Wrists	Jewelry (nickel)
Hands	Rings (nickel) Gloves (rubber accelerators)
Feet	Components of shoes (rubber accelerators, dichromates in leather)
Scrotum	Any contactant on the hands or agent applied in the groin (topical medications)

(From Huff, J. C., and Weston, W. L.: Eczematous dermatitis. Maj. Probl. Clin. Pediatr. *19*:86–122, 1978.)

DIFFERENTIAL DIAGNOSIS OF SKIN PROBLEMS

NATURE OF LESION	DISTRIBUTION OF LESION	ASSOCIATED FINDINGS	NATURE OF PATIENT	LESIONS WITH SIMILAR APPEARANCE	DIAGNOSIS
Papules and pustules	Face, back, and chest (Fig. 27–1)	Comedones	Start at puberty and last several years		Acne
Papules, vesicles and pustules	Face, head, and neck Occasionally diaper area in infants	Oozing, honeycomb-colored crusting	Mostly children		Impetigo (Figs. 27–2 and 27–3)
Scaling and lichenification	Face, extensor surfaces, and exposed areas in children Flexoral folds (antecubital, popliteal), wrists, neck, upper arms, and thighs in adults Symmetric (Fig. 27–4)	Often family history of hayfever or asthma Itching, erythema, often lichenification In blacks, the rash tends to be more papular 10% of general population have atopic dermatitis Erythematous or with plaques Rash in adults is usually localized, dry, excoriated, or lichenfied	Often begin in infancy at 5 months Often clear spontaneously at 5 years Rare in elderly	Seborrheic dermatitis (different location and yellow scales) Psoriasis (typical locations and silvery scales) Contact dermatitis is usually asymmetric	Atopic dermatitis or eczema (Figs. 25–4 and 25–6)
Scaling plaques	Mostly extensor surface of extremities, back, buttocks, and hands, but can occur anywhere	Coin-shaped lesions Itching Oozing	Children and adults	Ringworm (positive KOH) Contact dermatitis (exposed areas) Psoriasis (elbows and knees)	Nummular eczema or nummular dermatitis (Fig. 27–7)
Scaling plaques or patches	Trunk and proximal extremities (Fig. 27–8)	Herald patch (2 × 6 cm), usually on trunk, precedes generalized lesion More common in winter Salmon-colored May itch Oval patches (1 × 2 cm) with long axis along skin lines giving a Christmas tree pattern Collarette scaling	Children Young adults	Fungus, psoriasis, secondary syphilis and drug eruptions	Pityriasis rosea (Figs. 27–9 and 27–10)

Table continued on following page

DIFFERENTIAL DIAGNOSIS OF SKIN PROBLEMS *Continued*

NATURE OF LESION	DISTRIBUTION OF LESION	ASSOCIATED FINDINGS	NATURE OF PATIENT	LESIONS WITH SIMILAR APPEARANCE	DIAGNOSIS
Plaques	Usually on the covered parts of body and face Often multiple	Irregular greasy surface Superficial—on top of skin ("stuck to the skin") Yellow, tan, dark brown or rarely black Sharply defined edges	Adults (mostly elderly)	Actinic keratoses occur in sun-exposed areas and are smaller	Seborrheic keratoses
Erythematous plaques	Extensor surfaces, especially knees and elbows Scalp Coccygeal region Nails Rare on face (Fig. 27–11)	Silvery, loosely adherent scales Occasional itching Arthritis, especially in distal interphalangeal joints Sharp margins Scalp lesions usually stop at hairline	Adults Rare in young children	Seborrheic dermatitis can involve scalp but doesn't stop at hairline Nummular eczema	Psoriasis (Figs. 27–12 to 27–14)
Scaling patches	Scalp Eyebrows Nasolabial fold Midchest Umbilicus (Fig. 27–15)	Yellow, greasy scaling Greasy scaling with poor margain Some erythema Cradle cap in infants	More common in adults	Dandruff with little erythema and no other areas involved Psoriasis involves extensor surfaces Psoriasis of scalp usually stops at hairline with well-defined plaques	Seborrheic dermatitis (Fig. 27–16)
Papules inflamed with excoriation and crusting Linear burrows not always seen	Fingerwebs Wrists Anecubital Elbows Areolar Umbilicus Lower abdomen Genitalia Gluteal cleft	Itching (worse at night) Excoriation Weeping Other in household may have same problem	Adults and children	Pediculosis pubis (nits attached to hair; lice often seen on skin)	Scabies (Fig. 27–17)

Papules inflamed	Usually on trunk Grouped	Itching; flea bites often grouped	Sand flies and fleas in adults on lower legs Flea bites in children can be anywhere	Scabies Drug eruptions Lymphoma	Insect bites (Fig. 27–18)
Depigmentation	Orifices Eyes Extensor surfaces Areas of trauma	Positive Wood's light (bright white) Increased familial incidence	Familial Thyroid disease Addison's disease	Postinflammatory hypopigmentation Tinea versicolor alba Exposure to phenolic compounds	Vitiligo
Depigmentation and pink-red-brown macules	Mainly trunk Upper arms (Fig. 27–19)	Positive Wood's light (pale yellow) Pink-red-brown macules Scaling Positive KOH Mild itching	Young adults	Post-inflammatory hypopigmentation as seen with seborrheic dermatitis and pityriasis rosea, especially in blacks Other fungi	Tinea versicolor (Fig. 27–21)
Depigmentation	Exposed areas, especially hands and arms		Janitors Chemical workers	Vitiligo	Exposure to phenolic compounds
Vesicles	Anywhere (often asymmetric exposed areas)	Itching, oozing May occur hours to a few days after exposure	Adults and children	Allergy to systemic medications Atopic dermatitis	Contact dermatitis (Tab. 27–1)
	Hands				Detergents Chemicals (Fig. 27–21)
	Axilla				Deodorant

Table continued on following page

DIFFERENTIAL DIAGNOSIS OF SKIN PROBLEMS *Continued*

NATURE OF LESION	DISTRIBUTION OF LESION	ASSOCIATED FINDINGS	NATURE OF PATIENT	LESIONS WITH SIMILAR APPEARANCE	DIAGNOSIS
Vesicles on erythematous areas	Exposed areas (especially extremities)	Lesions often in streaks Itching	Adults and children		Plants (ivy, oak, sumac) (Fig. 27–22)
	Near hands, zippers, jewelry (e.g., wrist or earlobe)	Itching			Nickel (Fig. 27–23)
	Where medication is applied (e.g., eye, hair, face, neck)			Eczema	Medication hair preparations Cosmetics
	Hands and other exposed areas Genital region Buttocks				Industrial agents
Vesicles with erythematous base	Genital area	Pain, not itch Positive Tzanck's test	Adults Neonates		Herpes (genitalia) simplex II
	Cold sore (rarely in genital area)	Pain Systemic symptoms Positive Tzanck smear		Acute contact dermatitis Erythema multiforme	Herpes simplex I
Vesicles	Dermatome distribution	Tingling Occasional itch Pain Vesicles	Adults and children	Contact dermatitis (usually itches) Cellulitis	Herpes zoster
	Leg most common site in children	In children, not usually painful Often sciatic distribution			
Patchy alopecia	Scalp	Hairs broken and short Positive KOH *Trichophyton tonsurans* is the most common fungal scalp infection	Preadolescents	Alopecia areata	Fungal infections mostly *Trichophyton tonsurans* (Figs. 27–24 and 27–25)

Presentation	Location	Characteristics	Occurs in	Differential	Diagnosis
Patchy alopecia (possibly scarring)	Scalp	Does not fluoresce; Culture in dermatology test medium (DTM); Microsporum audouini gives apple-green Wood's light	Most common in children	Fungal infection	
	Scalp	Pustular lesion; Boggy scalp; Culture in DTM			Bacterial infection
	Scalp	Pinhead-sized nits on hair shaft; May be superimposed bacterial infection; Itching	More common in children but can occur in adults	Seborrheic dermatitis; Bacterial infection	Pediculosis capitis (Fig. 27–26)
Erythematous; Some scaling; Occasional maceration and oozing	Groin (Figs. 27–28 and 27–29); Under breasts	Border not sharp; pustules at edge; Positive KOH; Moist	Children; Diabetics	May all look similar (KOH required for differentiation) (Fig 27–27)	Candidiasis
	Groin	Border sharp and accentuated; Itch; No pustular edge; Positive KOH	Often complicates simple herpes rash; More common in males; Not seen in children		Tinea cruris (Fig. 27–30)
	Groin; Groin	Moist; Border sharp; Positive Wood's light (coral-red); Reddish-brown macules	Obese adults; Adults		Seborrheic intertrigo; Erythrasma (Corynebacterium)
Scaling, vesicles	Feet (soles)	Scaling; Itch (worse in summer); Positive KOH	Adults and children	May coexist*	Tinea pedis (dyshidrotic form) (Figs. 27–31 and 27–32)
Vesicles	Feet (soles, sides, dorsum)	Negative KOH; Often associated with similar process in hands	Adults	May coexist*	Dyshidrotic eczema

Table continued on following page

*Different forms of tinea pedis may coexist with each other as well as with dyshidrotic eczema.

DIFFERENTIAL DIAGNOSIS OF SKIN PROBLEMS *Continued*

NATURE OF LESION	DISTRIBUTION OF LESION	ASSOCIATED FINDINGS	NATURE OF PATIENT	LESIONS WITH SIMILAR APPEARANCE	DIAGNOSIS
Maceration	Feet (between toes, mainly 4th and 3rd spaces)	Itch (worse in summer) Positive KOH	Adults and children	May coexist*	Tinea pedis (intertriginous form)
Scaling	Feet (soles) Occasionally hands	No itch Positive KOH	Adults and children	May coexist*	Tinea pedis (dry scaly form)
Erythema scaling	Feet (dorsum and toes; toewebs and soles not involved)	Negative KOH	Adults and children	Tinea pedis	Contact dermatitis
Tumor	Most common on face and other sun-exposed areas	Smooth surface Atrophic center Pearly edge Roundish shape Tannish brown Telangiectasia on border	Elderly Those often exposed to sun	Squamous cell cancer Melanoma Sebaceous nevi	Basal cell carcinoma
Tumor	Most common on sun-exposed areas (especially hands, face, and ears)	Smooth or irregular surface Firm Irregular edge May be scaling Tannish brown	Elderly Those often exposed to sun	Basal cell cancer Warts Actinic keratoses	Squamous cell carcinoma
Tumor	Men: mostly on trunk (47%) Women: mostly on legs (39%)	Pigmented, often with different colors in same lesion (blue, purple, white, tan) Irregular border Change in size Satellites	Adults	Mole (melanocytic nevus) Pigmented lesions Seborrheic keratosis Dermatofibroma Angiokeratoma Lentigo	Malignant melanoma

*Different forms of tinea pedis may coexist with each other as well as with dyshidrotic eczema.

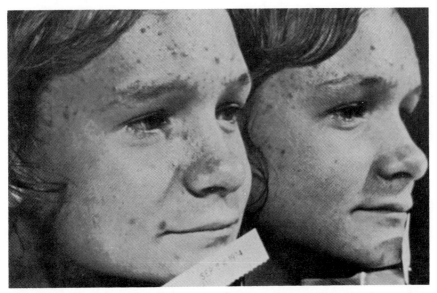

Figure 27–1. Comedones and lesions. Patient posing in front of mirror reveals comedones, papular lesions, and small superficial pustules on both sides of face. (From Chalker, D. K., and Smith, J. G.: Acne vulgaris: causes and preferred regimens. Medical Times, June, 1977, p. 57.)

Figure 27–2. Impetigo. This starts with mild discomfort and is followed in a few hours by serious exudation and crusting. The condition is contagious and can be spread both to other people and to different parts of the body. Culture may grow either *Staphylococcus aureus* or, less commonly, *Streptococcus hemolyticus*. (From Vickers, H. R.: Problems of dermatologic diagnoses. Br. J. Clin. Pract. *32*:159–166, 1978.)

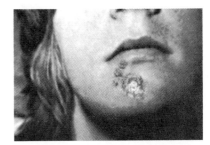

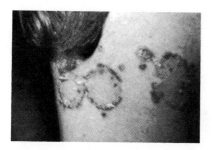

Figure 27–3. Impetigo circinata. Occasionally, the center of an impetigo lesion heals, leaving a ringed, crusted edge culture from which the diagnosis can be established. (From Vickers, H. R.: Problems of dermatologic diagnoses. Br. J. Clin. Pract. *32*:159–166, 1978.)

Figure 27–4. Lichenified pruritic areas in flexual regions and on the face are typical locations for adult atopic dermatitis. (From Lamberg, S. I.: Common problems of the skin. *In* Barker, L. R., Binton, J. R., and Zieve, P. D. [Eds.]: Principles of Ambulatory Medicine. Baltimore, Williams & Wilkins, 1982.)

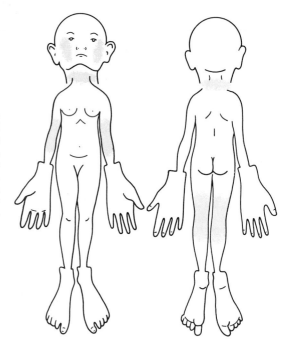

Figure 27–5. Atopic dermatits. Characteristic facial appearance, chronic excoriated dermatitis, and "sad" and "strained" look. (From Huff, J. C., and Weston, W. L. Eczematous dermatitis. Maj. Probl. Clin. Pediatr. *19*:86–122, 1978.)

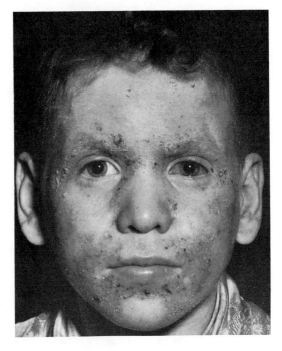

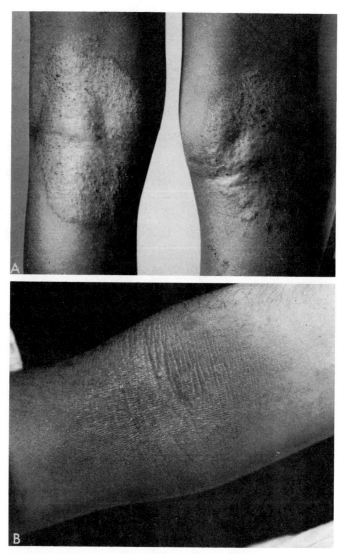

Figure 27–6. Atopic dermatitis—characteristic lesions. *A,* Sharply marginated excoriated lesions of popliteal spaces. *B,* Lichenification and thickening—antecubital fossa. (From Huff, J. C., and Weston, W. L.: Eczematous dermatitis. Maj. Probl. Clin. Pediatr. *19*:86–122, 1978.)

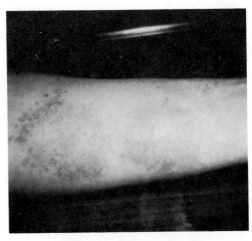

Figure 27–7. Nummular eczema. (From Welton, W.: Dermatology and syphilology. *In* Rakel, R. E., and Conn, H. F. [Eds.]: Family Practice. 2nd ed. Philadelphia, W. B. Saunders Co., 1978.)

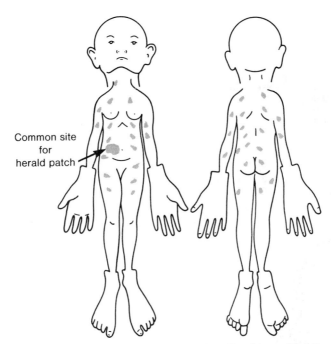

Common site for herald patch

Figure 27–8. Pityriasis rosea typically starts with a "herald patch" followed by oval patches in a fernlike pattern. (From Lansberg, S. I.: Common problems of the skin. *In* Barker, Z. R., Binton, J. R., and Zieve, P. D. [Eds.]: Principles of Ambulatory Medicine. Baltimore, Williams & Wilkins, 1982.)

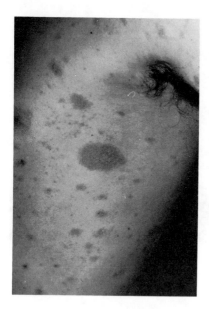

Figure 27–9. Pityriasis rosea. Trunk with central distribution. Discrete papulosquamous lesions. Larger initial plaque ("herald patch"). (From Gilbert, R., and Rosenthal, D.: Dermatology. *In* Rakel, R. C.: Textbook of Family Practice. 3rd ed. Philadelphia, W. B. Saunders Co., 1984.)

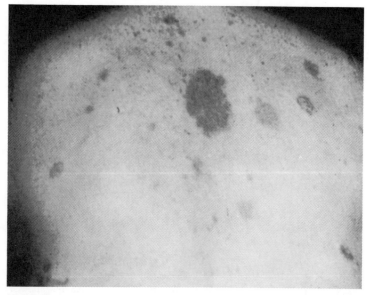

Figure 27–10. Pityriasis rosea with herald patch. (From Welton, W.: Dermatology and syphilology. *In* Rakel, R. E., and Conn, H. F. [Eds.]: Family Practice. 2nd ed. Philadelphia, W. B. Saunders Co., 1978.)

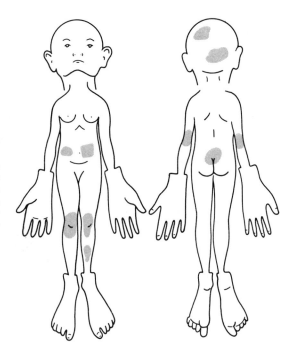

Figure 27–11. Psoriasis tends to be found on extensor surfaces and areas of repeated trauma, such as the waistline. (From Lamberg, S. J.: Common problems of the skin. *In* Barker, L. R., Binton, J. R., and Zieve, P. D. [Eds.]: Principles of Ambulatory Medicine. Baltimore, Williams & Wilkins, 1982.)

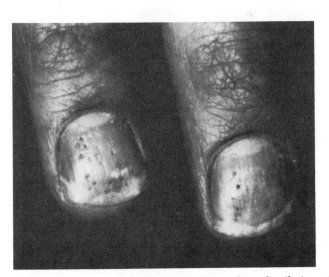

Figure 27–12. Minute pits are commonly seen on the surface of nails in patients with psoriasis. (From Lamberg, S. J.: Common problems of the skin. *In* Barker, L. R., Binton, J. R., and Zieve, P. D. [Eds.]: Principles of Ambulatory Medicine. Baltimore, Williams & Wilkins, 1982.)

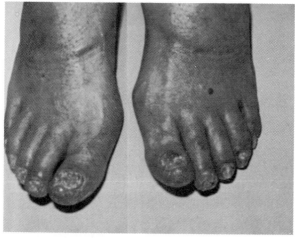

Figure 27–13. Psoriasis of the toes with marked thickening, yellowish discoloration, and crumbling of all toenails. (From Loeffel, E. D. The true heartbreaks of psoriasis. Medical Times, June, 1977, p. 51.)

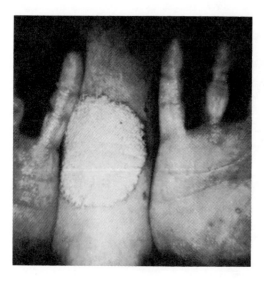

Figure 27–14. Psoriasis. White scale and palm lesions. (From Welton, W.: Dermatology and syphilology. *In* Rakel, R. E., and Conn, H. F. [Eds.]: Family Practice. 2nd ed. Philadelphia, W. B. Saunders Co., 1978.)

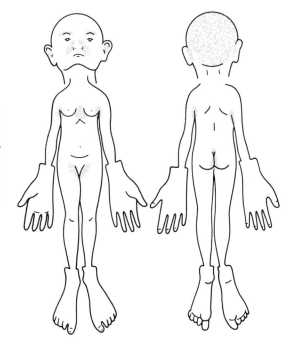

Figure 27–15. Usual location of erythema and scale in seborrheic dermatitis. (From Lamberg, S. I.: Common problems of the skin. *In* Barker, L. R., Binton, J. R., and Zieve, P. D. [Eds.]: Principles of Ambulatory Medicine. Baltimore, Williams & Wilkins, 1982.)

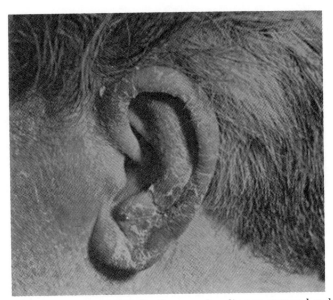

Figure 27–16. Seborrheic dermatitis. Erythema and scaling on ears and scalp is typical of this condition. (From Medical Times. June, 1977, p. 67.)

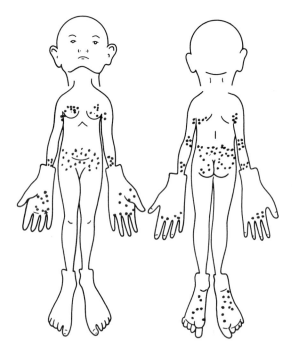

Figure 27–17. Pruritic papules are most prevalent about the waist, pelvis, elbows, hands, and feet in scabies. (From Lamberg, S. I.: Common problems of the skin. *In* Barker, L. R., Binton, J. R., and Zieve, P. D. [Eds.]: Principles of Ambulatory Medicine. Baltimore, Williams & Wilkins, 1982.)

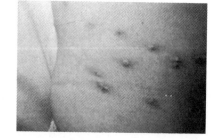

Figure 27–18. Insect bites (clustered itching papules). (From Vickers, H. R.: Problems of dermatological diagnoses. Br. J. Clin. Pract. *32*:159–166, 1978.)

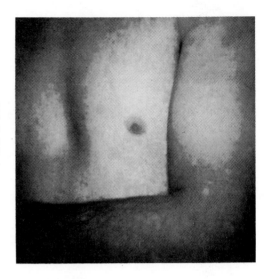

Figure 27–19. Tinea versicolor in varying stages of pigmentation and depigmentation. (From Welton, W.: Dermatology and syphilology. *In* Rakel, R. E., and Conn, H. F. [Eds.]: Family Practice. 2nd ed. Philadelphia, W. B. Saunders Co., 1978.)

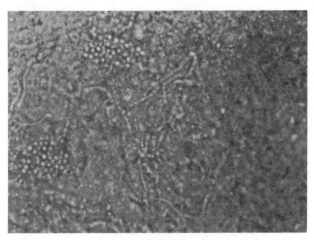

Figure 27–20. Short hyphae and spores of *Malassezia furfur* seen in tinea versicolor (KOH preparation, ×400). (From Lamberg, S. I.: Common problems of the skin. *In* Barker, L. R., Binton, J. R., and Zieve, P. D. [Eds.]: Principles of Ambulatory Medicine. Baltimore, Williams & Wilkins, 1982.)

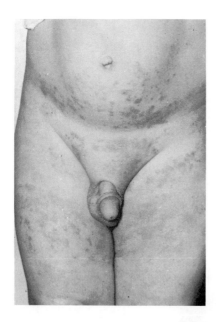

Figure 27–21. Contact dermatitis caused by laundry detergent. Note sparing of the folds. (From Jacob, A. H.: Eruptions in the diaper area. Pediatr. Clin. North Am. *25*:209, 1978.)

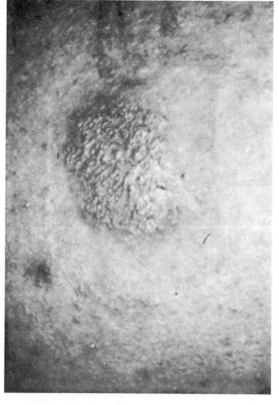

Figure 27–22. Microvesicles and dermal edema in acute contact dermatitis. (From Basler, R. S.: Contact dermatitis. Nebr. Med. J. *65*:296–299, 1980.)

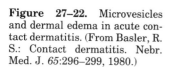

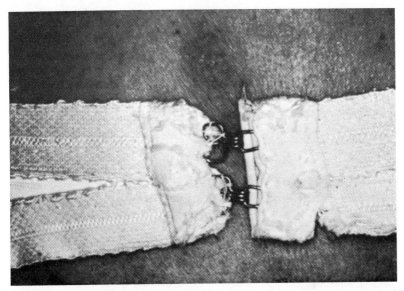

Figure 27–23. Chronic contact dermatitis. (From Basler, R. S.: Contact dermatitis. Nebr. Med. J. *65*:296–299, 1980.)

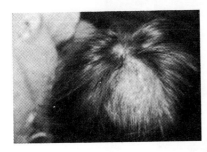

Figure 27–24. Ringworm of scalp *(Trichophyton tonsurans)*. (From Vickers, H. R.: Problems of dermatological diagnosis. Br. J. Clin. Pract. *32*:159–166, 1978.)

Figure 27–25. Tinea capitis Round areas of broken hairs and some scale. (From Welton, W.: Dermatology and syphilology. *In* Rakel, R. E., and Conn, H. F. [Eds.]: Family Practice. 2nd ed. Philadelphia, W. B. Saunders Co., 1978.)

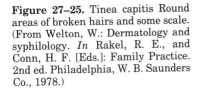

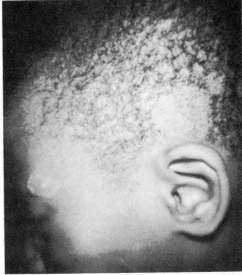

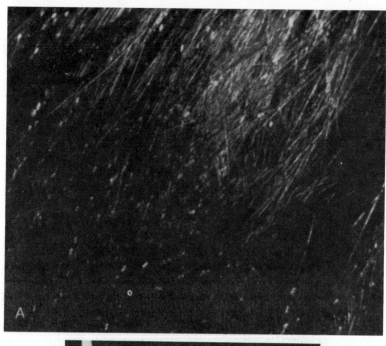

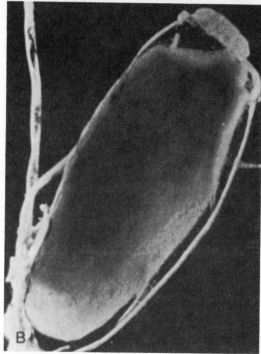

Figure 27–26. Pediculus humanus var. capitis (head louse). *A,* Gross appearance of nits on the hair shaft. *B,* Microscopic appearance (× 100; photograph *B* courtesy of Reed & Carnrick, Kenilworth, N. J.). (From Lamberg, S. I.: Common problems of the skin. *In* Barker, L. R., Binton, J. R., and Zieve, P. D. [Eds.]: Principles of Ambulatory Medicine. Baltimore, Williams & Wilkins, 1982.)

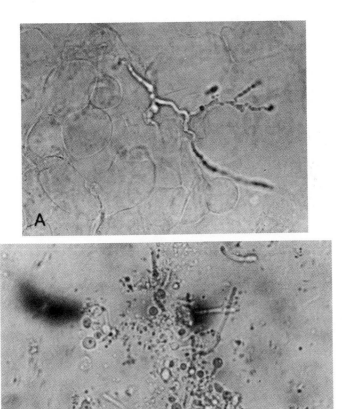

Figure 27–27. *A*, Hyphae of tinea (KOH preparation. × 400). *B*, Pseudohyphae of *Candida* (KOH preparation, × 400; photograph *B* courtesy of William G. Merz, Ph.D.). (From Lamberg, S. I.: Common problems of the skin. *In* Barker, L. R., Binton, J. R., and Zieve, P. D. [Eds.]: Principles of Ambulatory Medicine. Baltimore, Williams & Wilkins, 1982.)

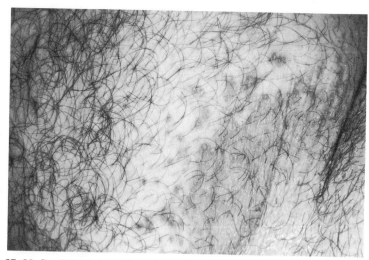

Figure 27–28. Candidiasis (moniliasis). Groin with intense erythema with satellite papules and pustules. Requires blood sugar determination in adult. (From Gilbert, R., and Rosenthal, D.: Dermatology. *In* Rakel, R. E. [Ed.]: Textbook of Family Practice. 3rd ed. Philadelphia, W. B. Saunders Co., 1984.)

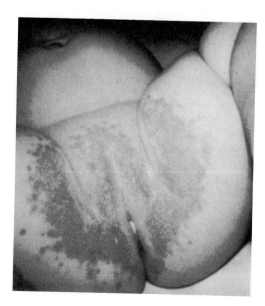

Figure 27–29. Candidiasis. (From Welton, W.: Dermatology and syphilology. *In* Rakel, R. E., and Conn, H. F. [Eds.]: Family Practice. 2nd ed. Philadelphia, W. B. Saunders Co., 1978.)

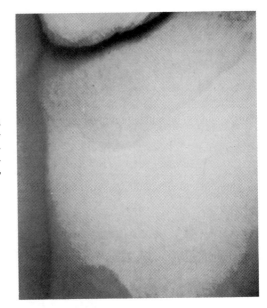

Figure 27–30. Tinea cruris. (From Welton, W.: Dermatology and syphilology. *In* Rakel, R. E., and Conn, H. F. [Eds.]: Family Practice. 2nd ed. Philadelphia, W. B. Saunders Co., 1978.)

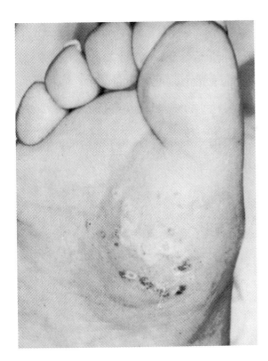

Figure 27–31. Tinea pedis, macerated acute type. (From Welton, W.: Dermatology and syphilology. *In* Rakel, R. E., and Conn, H. F. [Eds.]: Family Practice. 2nd ed. Philadelphia, W. B. Saunders Co., 1978.)

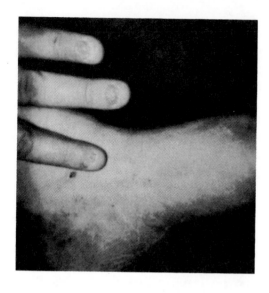

Figure 27–32. Tinea pedis, chronic rubrum type. Nails also are involved. (From Welton, W.: Dermatology and syphilology. *In* Rakel, R. E., and Conn, H. F. [Eds.]: Family Practice. 2nd ed. Philadelphia, W. B. Saunders Co., 1978.)

Selected References

August, P. J.: Iatrogenic skin disease. The Practitioner *224*:471–478, 1980.

Basler, R. S.: Contact dermatitis. Nebr. Med. J. *65*:296–299, 1980.

Cripps, D. J.: Skin care and problems in the aged. Hosp. Pract. *12*:119–127, 1977.

Desk Reference Issue: Skin Disorders. Medical Times *105(6)*:15, 1977.

Epstein, E.: Common skin disorders. Orodell, N.J., Medical Economics Co., 1979.

Feigold, D. S., and Bachta, M.: Common skin diseases seen by the internist. DM *25(8)*:1–39, 1979.

Hanifin, J. M.: Eczematous conditions in the elderly: common and curable. Geriatrics *34*:29–38, 1979.

Huff, J. C., and Weston, W. L.: Eczematous dermatitis. Maj. Probl. Clin. Pediatr. *19*:86–122, 1978.

Lamberg, S. L.: Common problems of the skin. *In* Barker, L. R., Binton, J. R., and Zieve, P. D. (Eds.): Principles of Ambulatory Medicine. Baltimore, Williams & Wilkins, 1982.

McLauria, C. I.: Unusual patterns of common dermatoses in blacks. Cutis, *32(4)*:352–355, 358–360, 1983.

Symposium on Pediatric Dermatology. Pediatr. Clin. North Am. *25(2)*:189–389, May, 1978.

Verou, J. L.: Skin problems in children. The Practitioner *217*:403–415, 1976.

Vickers, H. R.: Problems of dermatological diagnoses. Br. J. Clin. Pract. *32*:159–166, 1978.

White, J. E.: Skin cancer. The Practitioner *224*:501–503, 1980.

28

SORE THROAT

In this chapter, sore throat is defined as pain in the throat at rest that often worsens with swallowing. The most common causes of sore throat without pharyngeal ulcers include *viral pharyngitis, bacterial pharyngitis* and *tonsillitis, allergic pharyngitis, pharyngitis secondary to sinusitis,* and *infectious mononucleosis.* Common causes of sore throat with pharyngeal ulceration include *herpangina, herpes simplex, fuso-spirochetal infection, candidiasis, herpes zoster,* and *chicken pox* (varicella). The less common primary and secondary syphilitic ulcerations are usually not painful.

Pharyngitis is a vexing problem because it is extremely prevalent and it is difficult to establish a precise diagnosis. The annual cost of laboratory tests and medications ordered for patients with sore throats has been estimated to be 300 million dollars. Despite the fact that streptococcal and viral pharyngitis (including infectious mononucleosis) are the most common causes of sore throat, studies have shown that even with careful diagnostic techniques, a precise etiology can be determined only in about 50 per cent of the patients.

Prompt diagnosis and treatment of *streptococccal pharyngitis* are essential to reduction of spread to close contacts; treatment also prevents acute rheumatic fever. For a precise diagnosis of streptococcal pharyngitis, there must be a positive culture for group A streptococci and a fourfold rise in the antistreptolysin (ASO) titer. The carrier state exists when there is a positive culture without antibody response. According to one large study in which these criteria were used, most patients were found to be carriers. Because the ASO titer does not rise until 1 to 6 months after an acute streptococcal infection, the ASO titer in the acute serum is of no value in the diagnosis of a current infection. The foregoing

Table 28–1. **Strategy for Sore Throat Management Displayed in a Decision Table***

	1	2	3	4	5	6	7	8	9	10	11	12
History												
Sore throat duration > 6 days	—	—	—	—	P	—	—	—	—	—	—	—
Age < 25 years	P	—	—	—	—	—	—	—	—	—	—	—
Streptococcus exposure in past week	P	—	—	—	—	—	—	—	—	—	—	—
Anticipated difficulty with follow-up	—	P	—	—	—	—	—	—	—	—	—	—
History of acute rheumatic fever	P	—	P	—	—	—	—	—	—	—	—	—
Diabetic	P	—	P	—	—	—	—	—	—	—	—	—
Known epidemic of Meningococcal meningitis	—	—	—	—	—	—	P	—	—	—	—	—
Diphtheria	—	—	—	—	—	—	P	—	—	—	—	—
Streptococcal pharyngitis	P	—	—	—	—	—	—	—	—	—	—	—
Nephritogenic *Streptococcus*	—	P	—	—	—	—	—	—	—	—	—	—
Mononucleosis symptoms	—	—	—	—	—	X	—	—	—	—	—	—
Physical examination												
Temperature > 37.7 C. by mouth	P	—	—	P	P	—	—	—	—	—	—	—
Epiglottis swollen, red	—	—	—	—	—	—	P	P	—	—	—	—
Unilateral tonsillar swelling	—	—	—	—	—	—	—	—	—	—	P	—
Diphtheritic membrane	—	—	—	—	—	—	P	—	—	—	—	—
Gingivitis	—	—	—	—	—	—	—	—	P	—	—	—
Pharyngeal ulcers	—	—	—	—	—	—	—	—	—	P	—	—
Exudate	P	—	—	P	P	—	—	—	—	—	—	—
Tender anterior cervical nodes	P	—	—	P	P	—	—	—	—	—	—	—

Table continued on opposite page

information does not mean that throat cultures are of no value, but it does reinforce the need for sound clinical judgement in the diagnosis and treatment of patients with sore throats (Table 28–1).

NATURE OF PATIENT

Streptococcal pharyngitis is most prevalent in patients under 25 years of age, particularly those between 6 and 12 years. Likewise, *herpangina, herpes simplex, fusospirochetal infections,* and *candidiasis*

Table 28–1. **Strategy for Sore Throat Management Displayed in a Decision Table** *Continued*

	1	2	3	4	5	6	7	8	9	10	11	12
Posterior cervical nodes	—	—	—	—	—	P	—	—	—	—	—	—
Stiff neck	—	—	—	—	—	—	—	—	—	—	—	P
Scarlatiniform rash	P	P	—	—	—	—	—	—	—	—	—	—
Axillary and inguinal adenopathy	—	—	—	—	—	X	—	—	—	—	—	—
Splenomegaly	—	—	—	—	—	X	—	—	—	—	—	—
Actions												
Culture for group A *Streptococcus*	X	X	—	—	—	—	—	—	—	—	—	—
WBC count/ differential cell counts	—	—	—	—	—	X	—	—	—	—	—	—
Mononucleosis spot test	—	—	—	—	—	X	—	—	—	—	—	—
Culture on appropriate media	—	—	—	—	—	—	X	—	—	—	—	—
Syphilis serology	—	—	—	—	—	—	—	—	—	X	—	—
Evaluate for tuberculosis	—	—	—	—	—	—	—	—	—	X	—	—
Consider lumbar puncture	—	—	—	—	—	—	—	—	—	—	—	X
Treatment: penicillin	—	X	X	X	X	—	—	—	X	—	—	—
Treatment: ampicillin sodium or chloramphenicol	—	—	—	—	—	—	—	X	—	—	—	—
Observe for respiratory obstruction	—	—	—	—	—	—	—	X	—	—	—	—
Incision and drainage	—	—	—	—	—	—	—	—	—	—	X	—

*Each column represents a particular strategy. Any one datum when present (P) leads to an action (X). In the same column, multiple data are required for action in columns 4 and 5. Actions usually involve ordering tests or treatments, but can include the collection of clinical data (column 6). (From Komaroff, A.: A management strategy for sore throat. J.A.M.A. *239*:1429–1432, 1978).

are more common in children. As a cause of pharyngitis, *infectious mononucleosis* is most prevalent in adolescents and young adults. It does occur, although less frequently, in patients over 60 years. It is particularly notable that 70 per cent of elderly patients with infectious mononucleosis do not develop pharyngitis, adenopathy, or splenomegaly.

Neisseria gonorrhoeae presenting with oropharyngeal symptoms is becoming more common as a cause of pharyngitis, yet it is often unrecognized. It has been cultured from the throat in 10 per cent of patients with anogenital gonorrhea. Of those with positive cultures, most do not have pharyngeal symptoms. It is more common in people who engage in orogenital sex. Male homosexuals have a higher incidence of oropharyngeal gonorrheal infections than other groups do.

Common ulcerative and vesicular pharyngeal lesions include *herpes zoster, herpes simplex, fusospirochetal infections*, and *candidiasis* (particularly if the patient is immunosuppressed or taking antibiotics; see Table 28–2). The last three, although common causes of ulcerative pharyngeal lesions in adults, are somewhat more prevalent in children.

Table 28–2. **Common Infections Causing Oropharyngeal Ulceration**

Disease	Location	Vesicu-lation	Pain	Size of Lesion (mm)	Diagnostic Criteria
Local herpangina	Tonsils, pillars, uvula	Yes	Yes	1–2	Characteristic clinical presentation, coxsackievirus in culture of lesion exdudate, positive serological test
Herpes simplex	Lips, gingivae, buccal mucosa, tongue	Yes	Yes	1–2	Multinuclear giant cells with ballooning degeneration in Tzanck smear of ulcer-crater exudate
Fusospirochetal infection	Gingivae, may spread diffusely	No	Yes	2–30	Characteristic lesions, foul breath, anaerobic forms and spirochetes in smear of lesion exudate
Candidiasis	All parts of oropharynx	No	Yes	3–10	*Candida albicans* in Gram-stained smear and culture of scrapings
Primary syphilis	Lips, tonsils, tongue	No	No	5–15	Indurated "heaped-up" lesion, positive serologic test (periodic evaluation necessary)
Herpes zoster	Unilateral involvement of tongue, lip, buccal mucosa	Yes	Yes	2–4	Unilateral involvement, painful prodromes, giant cells in Tzanck smear of lesion exudate
Systemic hand-foot-and-mouth disease	All part of oropharynx	Yes	Yes	1–10	Exanthem on hands and feet, coxsackievirus in culture of lesion exudate, positive serologic test
Varicella	All parts of oropharynx	Yes	No	2–4	Characteristic exanthem
Secondary syphilis	Symmetric involvement of all parts of mouth and orpharynx	No	No	2–10	Other evidence of secondary syphilis, positive serologic test, spirochetes visible on darkfield microscopy

(From Brown, R. B., and Clinton, D.: Vesicular and ulcerative infections of the mouth and oropharynx. Postgrad. Med. *67(2)*:107–116, 1980.)

Although rare, primary and secondary syphilitic lesions occasionally are seen in adults. They should be suspected if the lesion is not painful and if there is an absence of the usual accompanying symptoms of upper respiratory infection.

NATURE OF SYMPTOMS

Marked pain in the throat (frequently associated with dysphagia), an oral temperature exceeding 100° to 101°F, and a rapid onset of symptoms suggest the probability of a *streptococcal* or *viral pharyngitis*. A low-grade temperature, gradual onset of pharyngeal symptoms, and systemic symptoms that are more persistent suggest *infectious mononucleosis*. In reality, it is very difficult for the physician to determine the cause of pharyngitis on the basis of the nature of the chief complaint; predisposing factors and physical examination are frequently more useful indicators.

PREDISPOSING FACTORS

Herpangina, herpes simplex, and *candidiasis* are most common in immunosuppressed patients. *Candidiasis* also is most prevalent in diabetic patients and in those taking broad-spectrum antibiotics. *Herpangina* is most common in children and shows a strong seasonal propensity for summer and autumn, whereas *streptococcal pharyngitis* is most prevalent in fall and winter.

PHYSICAL FINDINGS

Marked erythema and swelling of the throat (often associated with an exudative pharyngitis or tonsillitis), temperature greater than 101°F, tachycardia, and occurrence between September and April all strongly indicate *streptococcal pharyngitis*. Likewise, a history of streptococcal exposure within the family during the past week, prior history of acute rheumatic fever, diabetes, tender anterior cervical nodes, or a scarlatiniform rash increases the likelihood that streptococcal pharyngitis is the correct diagnosis. As mentioned previously, streptococcal pharyngitis is rare after the age of 30 years and is most common between the ages of 6 to 12 years.

Although many authors stress an association between tonsillopharyngeal exudate and *streptococcal pharyngitis*, it is important to note that only 50 per cent of the patients with proven streptococcal pharyngitis have an exudate, and only 50 per cent of all patients with a pharyngeal exudate have streptococcal pharyngitis. Despite this, many physicians presume a streptococcal etiology if an exudate is present and if one or more of the following signs also are demonstrated: temperature greater than 101°F, tender anterior cervical nodes, or duration of sore throat greater than 6 days.

Viral pharyngitis is the most common cause of pharyngitis and, unlike streptococcal pharyngitis, has no particular distribution with regard to age or time of year, although it is slightly more frequent in the winter months. Patients with viral pharyngitis usually have less severe pharyngeal symptoms and more severe systemic symptoms. These patients are less likely to have an exudate or marked erythema of the pharynx. The pharynx is usually slightly injected but also may appear swollen, boggy, or pale. There is usually no exudate or follicular tonsillitis present, but systemic symptoms (malaise, fever, cough, headache, and fatigue) are more prominent than with streptococcal pharyngitis.

Patients with the pharyngitis of *infectious mononucleosis* may present with an exudate, although the majority do not. The enanthem of infectious mononucleosis, palatine petechiae, is almost diagnostic. They resemble small, red, raised grains of sand surrounded by 0.5-mm pale bases. The pharyngitis of infectious mononucleosis is almost invariably (i.e., in 90 per cent of cases) accompanied by posterior cervical adenopathy. Some authors are reluctant to diagnose infectious mononucleosis in the absence of posterior cervical adenopathy.

Epiglottitis, which is not uncommon in children but is rare in adults, is usually caused by a *Hemophilus infection*. When epiglottitis is suspected, appropriate cultures should be performed, and antibiotics should be administered. *Gingivitis* is most often seen in patients with poor oral hygiene. In some cases, it can involve the entire oropharynx. The most common presentation of *ulcerative gingivitis (trench mouth)* is an acute onset of painful bloody gums, foul breath, and a grayish exudate covering the interdental papillae. Ulcerative gingivitis is a *fusospirochetal* infection and responds well to improved oral hygiene and appropriate antibiotics. Pharyngeal involvement with fusospirochetal organisms *(Vincent's angina)* may occur primarily or secondary to a spread of fusospirochetal infection from anterior sites. In patients with this infection, sore throat is the most common complaint, and there may be necrotic, gray, ulcerative lesions about the tonsillar pillars. If the "pseudomembrane" is removed, there is usually bleeding of the undersurface. Although in most cases involvement is initially unilateral, it often spreads and becomes bilateral.

Patients who have frequent sore throats, without evidence of pharyngitis or fever, may have an *allergic pharyngitis*. This is often associated with an intermittent postnasal drip that leads to minor irritation and inflammation of the posterior pharynx. Some patients with recurrent or chronic low-grade *sinusitis* may present with a sore throat induced by a postnasal drip from the affected sinuses. **It is particularly important to note that when a patient complains of a sore throat that becomes worse with swallowing, and when the physical examination of the oropharynx is negative, the physician should suspect thyroiditis and palpate the thyroid for swelling or pain on palpation.** This is a common way by which the uncommon illness of thyroiditis presents.

Retropharyngeal abscess is most common in infants and small children, but it does occur infrequently in adults. There may be an unexplained fever, an upper respiratory infection, loss of appetite, difficulty in swallowing, and stridor. The last sign is particularly common in children. Retropharyngeal abscess is a medical emergency and should be evaluated promptly. Some investigators feel that earlier treatment with antibiotics reduces the incidence of this complication and the need for surgical intervention.

The presence of oropharyngeal ulcerations, with or without vesiculation, is often helpful in differential diagnosis. In patients with *herpangina*, usually children, the painful ulcerations measure 1 to 2 mm and occur on the tonsils, pillars, and the uvula. The pharyngeal ulcers (2 to 30 mm) due to *fusospirochetal infections* are usually present on the gingivae, but they may spread diffusely throughout the oropharynx. These lesions are usually painful, but there is no associated vesiculation. In adults and children with *herpes simplex*, the painful ulcers measure 1 to 2 mm and can occur on the lips, gingivae, buccal mucosa, or rarely on the tongue. The painful ulcerations of *herpes zoster* usually are unilateral and involve the tongue, lip, or buccal mucosa. These lesions are usually 2 to 4 mm and associated with vesiculation. In infants and adults with *candidiasis*, the ulcerations measure 3 to 11 mm and can involve any part of the oropharynx. Vesiculation does not occur with candidiasis.

DIAGNOSTIC STUDIES

Tests that are often helpful in the differential diagnosis of sore throat are a CBC with differential, throat cultures, Gram-staining, Monospot test, and antistreptolysin titers. Komaroff developed a decision table (Table 28–1) that recommends culture if any one of the following is present: age less than 25 years, definite streptococcal exposure during the previous week, history of acute rheumatic fever, diabetes, known epidemic of streptococcal pharyngitis, oral temperature greater than 37.7°C, exudate, tender anterior cervical nodes, or scarlatiniform rash. Difficulty with follow-up, a known epidemic of nephritogenic streptococcal infections, or presence of a scarlatiniform rash is an indication for both throat culture and treatment with penicillin. In addition, if there is a history of rheumatic fever or if diabetes is present, treatment with

DIFFERENTIAL DIAGNOSIS OF SORE THROAT

TYPE OF PHARYNGITIS	NATURE OF PATIENT	NATURE OF SYMPTOMS	PREDISPOSING FACTORS	PHYSICAL FINDINGS	DIAGNOSTIC STUDIES
Without Pharyngeal Ulcers					
Viral	All ages	Pain in the throat Rapid onset Systemic symptoms		Exudate less likely than with streptococcal infections	
Infectious mononucleosis	Adolescents and young adults Uncommon in elderly	Gradual onset		Low-grade temperature Occasional exudate Enanthem, Posterior cervical adenopathy Hepatosplenomegaly	Monospot test
Streptococcal pharyngitis	Patients younger than 25 years, especially those between 6 and 12 years	Pain in throat Rapid onset Few systemic symptoms	Fall and winter Streptococcal infection in family Diabetes	Marked erythema and throat swelling Temperature > 101°F Tachycardia Tender anterior cervical nodes Scarlatiniform rash Exudate more likely than with viral infection	Culture Increased ASO titer
Gonococcal pharyngitis	Most common in male homosexuals and those with anogenital gonorrhea	Often no symptoms	Orogenital sex		Culture

Condition	Patients	Predisposing factors	Symptoms	Signs	Diagnostic tests
Sinusitis with postnasal drip	Adults		Mild throat soreness, Symptoms often worse with recumbency	Evidence of sinusitis, Postnasal drip	Sinus radiographs
Allergic pharyngitis		Seasonal allergies		No fever, Intermittent postnasal drip, Swollen pharynx with minimal injection	Eosinophils in nasal secretions
With Pharyngeal Ulcers					
Herpangina	More common in children	Immunosuppression, Summer and autumn	Painful ulcers on tonsils, pillars, or uvula	Vesicles, 1–2-mm ulcers	Serologic tests
Fusospirochetal infection (Vincent's angina)	Children and those with poor oral hygiene		Painful ulcers, Bleeding gums, Foul breath	No vesicles, Ulcerative gingivits, Gray necrotic ulcers, 2–30-mm ulcers, Pseudomembrane	Spirochetes, Gram stain
Candidiasis	Children and those who are immunosuppressed or taking antibiotics	Immunosuppression, Antibiotics		3–11-mm ulcers, No vesicles	KOH smear shows Candida, Culture
Herpes simplex	Most common in children	Immunosuppression	Not usually a cause of sore throat	1–2-mm painful ulcers, Vesicles present on lips, gingivae, buccal mucosa, or tongue	Tzanck smear shows multinucleated giant cells

penicillin is indicated despite the clinical picture. A patient with a temperature greater than 37.7°C, tonsillar exudate, and tender anterior cervical nodes probably has a *streptococcal pharyngitis*, and immediate treatment is justified. A CBC with a lymphocytosis of greater than 50 per cent or an absolute lymphocytosis of greater than 4500 lymphocytes per mm³ with more than 10 per cent atypical lymphocytes suggests *infectious mononucleosis*. This is confirmed by a positive Monospot test. **There are virtually no false-negative Monospot tests, although some studies have shown 10 per cent false-positive results**. These characteristic hematologic and serologic abnormalities generally occur within 1 week from onset of symptoms in 80 per cent of the patients.

LESS COMMON DIAGNOSTIC CONSIDERATIONS

Patients with thyroiditis may present with a sore throat, dysphagia, or both. In a patient complaining of a sore throat whose throat examination is negative, the thyroid gland should be palpated. If it is tender, thyroiditis should be suspected. Patients with hypothyroidism may complain of a sore throat or hoarseness, regardless of whether a goiter is present. Some patients with seasonal allergy present with a sore throat. In most instances, there is minimal pharyngeal swelling. Occasionally, a postnasal drip is seen, and other allergic symptoms usually can be elicited as well. Patients who have swallowed a coarse foreign body such as a bone, rough vegetable, or piece of meat may complain of a sore throat with or without dysphagia, even if they have successfully swallowed the object. If this complaint persists or is very severe, the possibility that a foreign body is lodged in the posterior pharynx or proximal esophagus should be considered. Patients with leukemia, agranulocytosis, or diphtheria also may present with a sore throat.

Selected References

Komaroff, A. L.: A management strategy for sore throat. J.A.M.A. *239*:1429–1432, 1978.
Brown, R. B., and Clinton, D.: Vesicular and ulcerative infections of the mouth and oropharynx. Postgrad. Med. *67(2)*:107–116, 1980.
Sloan, P. D.: Sore throats. Consultant *22(5)*:110–127, 1972.
Everett, M. T.: The uninflamed sore throat. Practitioner *222*:835–838, 1979.
Gillette, R. D.: Streptococcal throat infections in family practice. J. Fam. Pract. *6*:251–256, 1978.

29

URETHRAL DISCHARGE AND DYSURIA

Dysuria denotes burning or pain associated with urination and can have several causes. Frequency, hesitancy, urgency, and strangury (slow, painful urination) are other symptoms commonly associated with micturition disorders. Urinary urgency occurs as a result of *trigonal* or *posterior urethral irritation* produced by inflammation, stones, or tumor; it most commonly occurs with *cystitis.* Acute inflammatory processes of the bladder cause pain or urgency when only a small quantity of urine is present in the bladder. Frequency of urination, when due to bladder problems, occurs with either a decreased bladder capacity or with pain on bladder distention. Frequency is caused most commonly by lesions of the bladder or urethra, although diseases of the nervous system involving the bladder's nerve supply (either centrally as in tabes and multiple sclerosis or peripherally as in diabetic neuropathy) may produce bladder decompensation with voiding abnormalities. Urinary frequency may also be a manifestation of overflow incontinence; this can occur with either *prostatic hypertrophy* or *neurologic bladder disorders.*

Inflammatory lesions of the prostate, bladder, and urethra are the most common cause of dysuria and frequency and include *prostatitis* in men, *urethrotrigonitis* in women, and *bladder* and *urethral infections* in men and women. Both men and women may have *chronic inflammation of the posterior urethra.* In the United States, women with symptoms of lower urinary tract infections account for more than 5 million office visits per year; only 50 per cent of these women, however, have classic cystitis with urine culture bacteria concentrations greater than 10^5 organisms per milliliter. **Several studies indicate that symptomatic women with urinary bacteria counts less than 10^5 organisms per milliliter (female urethral syndrome) should be considered to have an infectious etiology and be treated accordingly.**

It has been estimated that approximately 2 million cases of urethritis (men and women) occur annually in the United States; about 50 per cent of cases are nongonorrheal. There is increasing evidence that *Chlamydia,* which causes nongonorrheal urethritis, is a major cause of sexually transmitted disease in the United States. Because of the frequency of complaints of dysuria and urethral discharge, the associated public health problem, and the ease of treatment, it is essential that physicians be expert in recognizing the causes of these symptoms.

NATURE OF PATIENT

In children, *meatal stenosis* may cause recurrent lower urinary tract infections. Up to 20 per cent of children with urinary complaints may have some degree of meatal stenosis. Dysuria and urethral discharge are uncommon in children. When these symptoms occur in young girls, they frequently are due to a *chemical vaginitis* or a *mechanical urethritis.* When these findings are seen in young boys, they are often secondary to a mechanical urethritis, which can result from continued jarring of the perineum from bicycle riding, horseback riding, a foreign body, or masturbation.

Bacteriuria is rare in school-age boys and occurs in only 0.1 per cent of male adults. The incidence of bacteriuria increases in men at age 50 years and rises to about 1 per cent at age 60 years and to between 4 and 15 per cent in later years, coinciding with the onset of prostatic disease. Among women under 18 years of age, there is a 5 per cent incidence of asymptomatic bacteriuria. Women between 15 and 34 years of age account for most of the patients who present with symptoms of urinary tract infections. A study in Great Britain showed that 20 per cent of women in this age group developed dysuria and frequency. Dysuria in women is most frequently caused by *cystitis, vaginitis, female urethral syndrome,* and *mechanical irritation of the urethra.* Dysuria in men is most commonly caused by *urethritis, prostatitis, cystitis,* and *mechanical irritation of the urethra.* Urethral discharge, which is essentially limited to men, is usually caused by *gonorrheal* or *nongonorrheal urethritis (Chlamydia* or *Trichomonas).*

NATURE OF SYMPTOMS

Cystitis. In women who complain of frequency and dysuria without clinical evidence of an upper urinary tract infection, *bacterial cystitis* is usually suspected. Several studies, however, have shown that 30 to 50 per cent of women complaining of these symptoms do not have a positive urine culture according to traditional criteria (isolation of a pathogen in concentrations greater than 10^5 bacteria per milliliter of urine in a clean voided specimen). There are several possible reasons for this. First, dysuria often represents a vaginal rather than a urinary tract infection. When carefully questioned, women with dysuria due to cystitis usually describe an internal discomfort, whereas women with dysuria due to vaginitis usually describe a more external discomfort; their burning sensation appears to be in the vagina or the labia and is due to urine flow over an inflamed vaginal mucosa. **All women with dysuria should be questioned about an associated vaginal discharge or irritation.** Second, many women who present with symptoms due to bacterial cystitis (i.e., dysuria and frequency) have colony counts less than 10^5 bacteria per milliliter of urine. Various studies have shown that if pathogens are found in a concentration less than 10^5 per milliliter in symptomatic women, there is probably a significant bacterial infection. Third, *Chlamydia trachomatis* is frequently the causative agent. Patients who are infected with this organism have symptoms and pyuria but a negative routine urine culture. Chlamydial infections of the bladder and urethra in women are somewhat analagous to nongonorrheal urethritis in men; in both, there is pyuria but no growth on routine culture. Although rare, *urinary tract tuberculosis* also may present with pyuria and a negative routine culture.

It is important that the physician inquire about the duration and onset of symptoms. Longer duration and gradual onset of symptoms suggest a chlamydial infection, whereas a history of hematuria and sudden onset of symptoms indicate a bacterial infection. Dysuria that is more severe at the end of the stream, particularly if associated with hematuria, suggests *cystitis;* dysuria that is worse at the beginning of the stream is a sign of *urethritis.* Patients with the *female urethral syndrome* often have dysuria, frequency, suprapubic pain, onset of symptoms over 2 to 7 days, and some pyuria. Besides having dysuria, frequency, and suprapubic pain, patients with *cystitis* demonstrate symptoms that develop quickly—pyuria, bacteriuria, and positive urine cultures (Table 29–1). Fever, nausea, back pain, and leukocytosis are not common findings in either female urethral syndrome or cystitis.

Urethritis. Urethral discharge in male patients is generally accepted as objective evidence of *urethritis,* but patients may have urethritis without a significant urethral discharge. **If the patient has dysuria and more than four polymorphonuclear cells per high-powered field in a urethral smear, urethritis is probable.** Nongonorrheal urethritis is currently defined to include inflammations in men who have negative urethral cultures for *Neisseria gonorrhoeae* and a urethral discharge or more than four polymorphonuclear cells per high-powered field in the urethral smear. *Chlamydia trachomatis* is the most common

Table 29–1. **Clinical Features of Female Urethral Syndrome and Cystitis**

Clinical Features	Female Urethral Syndrome	Cystitis
Dysuria, frequency, suprapubic pain	+	+
Fever, nausea, back pain, other systemic signs	–	–
Duration of symptoms (days)	2–7	1–2
Leukocytosis	–	–
Urinalysis:		
Pyuria	+ or –	+
Bacteriuria	–	+
Hematuria	–	+ or –
WBC casts	–	–
Urine cultures	–	+
Blood cultures	–	–

(From Meadows, J. C. The acute urethral syndrome: diagnosis, management, and prophylaxis. Continuing Education, December, 1983, pp. 112–120.)

isolate from patients with nongonorrheal urethritis (Table 29–2). Other causative organisms may include *Mycoplasma,* group D *Streptococcus, Trichomonas,* and, rarely, *Candida albicans.* Although a significant number of patients with nongonorrheal urethritis are asymptomatic, most have mild dysuria and a minimal or absent urethral discharge. When a discharge does appear, it is usually clear or whitish. In contrast, approximately 80 per cent of patients with gonorrheal urethritis have a moderate to heavy urethral discharge that is usually purulent. Dysuria with a mucoid or mucopurulent urethral discharge generally develops 1 to 3 weeks after coitus with an infected partner.

Urethral discharges are usually observed on awakening, after a long period without urination, or after penile stripping. Other symptoms include urgency, frequency, and meatal or urethral irritation. The usual presentation of nongonorrheal urethritis is a low-grade inflammation; the symptoms of gonorrheal urethritis tend to be more acute and severe and include a urethral discharge that is purulent, spontaneous, and greater in volume. **It is important to recognize that a patient may have gonorrheal as well as nongonorrheal urethritis at the same time.** Both may be contracted simultaneously from the same contact.

ASSOCIATED SYMPTOMS

When hematuria accompanies dysuria, *cystitis* is most probable, although the possibility of a *tumor* or *stone* also should be considered. If dysuria and frequency are associated with a high fever or chills, an upper urinary tract infection such as *pyelonephritis* may be present. When frequency and dysuria are associated with backache or costovertebral angle tenderness, *pyelonephritis* or *prostatitis* should be suspected.

Table 29–2. **Comparison Between** *Chlamydia trachomatis* **and** *Neisseria gonorrhoeae* **as Venereal Disease Agents**

Subject	*C. trachomatis*	*N. gonorrhoeae*
Organism	Obligate intracellular parasite	Gram-negative diplococcus often found within cells (as leukocytes on Gram stain)
Transmission	Venereal	Venereal
Incubation period	8–21 days	2–6 days (can be longer, up to 10–16 days in rare cases)
Major infection	Urethritis (men); cervicitis (women)	Urethritis (men); cervicitis (women)
Local complications	Yes: epididymitis, bartholinitis, urethral syndrome, salpingitis, others	Yes: same, and others, including prostatitis
Systemic complications	Possibly: arthritis, perihepatitis, peritonitis, and endocarditis reported	Well known: gonococcal septicemia, with resultant arthritis, dermatitis, endocarditis, and meningitis; perihepatitis and peritonitis also reported
Pharyngitis	Yes	Yes
Conjunctivitis	Yes	Yes
Proctitis	Cultured from the rectum; infection not yet documented	Yes: common venereal infection in homosexuals
Maternal infection with effect on newborn or infant	Well known: inclusion conjunctivitis and pneumonia	Less well established
Carrier state	Recognized, especially in women; can last for months	Recognized, especially in women; can last for months
Reservoir	Cervix (male urethra a minor role)	Cervix (male urethra a minor role)
Treatment	Tetracycline (antibiotic of choice) Erythromycin, sulfonamides, streptomycin, and tri-methoprimsulfamethoxazole also effective Regimen of 14 days often used	Current CDC recommendation involves procaine penicillin, ampicillin, amoxicillin, tetracycline, or spectinomycin; probenecid used; shorter treatment regimen
Treatment of sexual contacts	Yes	Yes

(From Greydanus, D. E., and McAnarney, E. R.: *Chlamydia trachomatis:* an important sexually transmitted disease in adolescents and young adults. J. Fam. Pract., *10*:611–615, 1980.)

Patients who have prostatitis often present with an unexplained back-ache, with or without fever. The physician should perform a gentle rectal examination of any man who complains of frequency, dysuria, and fever to determine whether the prostate is tender to palpation. Pyelonephritis should be suspected if nausea and vomiting accompany dysuria. Patients who demonstrate prostatic enlargement or experience severe pain on micturition that causes them to resist voiding have outflow obstruction. This causes bladder distention, which may also induce nausea, vomiting, or mild ileus, resulting in abdominal distention.

Frequency of urination without discomfort on voiding may be due to a *diminished bladder capacity, overflow incontinence,* or *habit* in patients with a normal bladder. It also is observed in patients who pass a large volume of urine owing to diabetes, hypercalcemia, hypokalemia, congestive heart failure, loss of renal concentrating capacity, or the use of diuretics. The absence of nocturia in a patient with urinary frequency suggests that the increased frequency of urination may be of psychogenic origin. Rarely, this may be due to a polyp or irritative lesion in the posterior urethra that is relieved by recumbency.

PRECIPITATING AND AGGRAVATING FACTORS

Patients who have multiple sexual contacts are more likely to develop a sexually transmitted disease such as *gonorrheal* or *nongonorrheal urethritis* or *cervicitis.* An abrupt alteration in the frequency of ejaculation may result in symptoms of *prostatitis.* This often occurs upon the patient's return from a vacation during which the frequency of intercourse and subsequent ejaculation were increased. The use of vaginal sprays, douches, and bubble baths (particularly in children) may induce a *chemical vaginitis* that may present with dysuria. It is important for the physician to ask women who complain of dysuria whether a vaginal discharge is present because, in the absence of a recognizable discharge, *vaginitis* is an unlikely cause of dysuria.

AMELIORATING FACTORS

Some patients with *cystitis* feel that they can alleviate their pain by avoiding urination; they actually mean that the pain is made worse with micturition, particularly at the end of urination, when the inflamed bladder walls become apposed. Some symptoms of cystitis are ameliorated by warm tub baths. Patients who complain of persistent frequency, nocturia, terminal hematuria, and suprapubic pain relieved by voiding may have *chronic interstitial cystitis,* a condition that is most common in middle-aged women.

If *Neisseria gonorrhoeae* is the offending organism, the symptoms of urethritis occasionally abate without treatment after a few months. In contrast, the symptoms of nongonorrheal urethritis, although low-grade, usually persist if not treated appropriately.

PHYSICAL FINDINGS

The physical findings of gonorrheal urethritis in men include a spontaneous urethral discharge or one that can be elicited by penile stripping. The most common physical finding in patients with dysuria due to cystitis is suprapubic tenderness to palpation or percussion. When dysuria is due to vaginitis, a vaginal discharge is apparent on pelvic examination.

DIAGNOSTIC STUDIES

In men, *urethritis* is present if a urethral smear shows more than four polymorphonuclear cells per high-power field. All urethral discharges should be examined by Gram stain and culture. A culture should be obtained for *Neisseria gonorrhoeae* and, when indicated, for *Chlamydia*. Urine cultures should be obtained for all patients with symptoms of cystitis. When sterile pyuria is demonstrated on routine culture, the urine should be cultured for *Chlamydia* and for tuberculosis-causing species of *Mycobacterium*.

Laboratory tests are required to distinguish gonorrheal from nongonorrheal urethritis. Because it is frequently difficult to culture *Chlamydia,* physicians often diagnose nongonorrheal urethritis by establishing the presence of urethritis and then excluding gonorrheal infection by smear and culture. *Trichomonas vaginalis* and *Candida albicans* are uncommon causes of urethritis and need not be considered at the initial visit. A Gram smear or a KOH preparation may help identify patients with candidal urethritis, and a saline wet mount should be examined if trichomonal urethritis is suspected.

The following are considered indications for urologic evaluation: an initial urinary infection in a child, initial urinary tract infection in men, urinary infections in pregnant women, recurrent urinary tract infections (three per year) in women, severe acute urinary tract infections suggesting upper tract involvement, and painless hematuria.

LESS COMMON DIAGNOSTIC CONSIDERATIONS

Less common causes of dysuria and urinary frequency include genital herpes simplex virus, *Trichomonas,* and *Candida* urethritis.

DIFFERENTIAL DIAGNOSIS OF URETHRAL DISCHARGE AND DYSURIA

CAUSE	NATURE OF PATIENT	NATURE OF SYMPTOMS	ASSOCIATED SYMPTOMS	AMELIORATING FACTORS	PRECIPITATING AND AGGRAVATING FACTORS	PHYSICAL FINDINGS	DIAGNOSTIC STUDIES
Cystitis	Most common in women aged 15–34 years	Dysuria (worse at end of flow) Urgency Frequency "Internal" discomfort Acute onset of symptoms with bacterial infection	Hematuria Nocturia Fever	Avoidance of urinating Warm baths	Meatal stenosis may cause recurrent UTI in children	Suprapubic tenderness to palpation or percussion Fever	Urine culture positive Cystoscopy Special test for *Chlamydia* Pyuria
Female Urethral Syndrome		Dysuria Frequency Gradual onset of symptoms over 2–7 days	Suprapubic pain			Suprapubic pain No fever	Minimal pyuria Urine culture usually negative
Vaginitis (see Chapter 30)	Candidiasis more common in diabetics	Dysuria "External burning"	Vaginal itching			Vaginal discharge on pelvic exam	KOH and saline wet mounts for *Candida* and *Trichomonas* Gram stain and culture for gonococci
Chemical vaginitis	Common cause of dysuria and urethral discharge in young girls	Dysuria "External burning" Urethral discharge (minimal)			Bubble baths Vaginal sprays and douches	Vaginitis	
Prostatitis	Men over 50 years of age	Dysuria Frequency	Backache Fever Decreased or intermittent stream		Abrupt change in frequency of ejaculation (e.g., after a vacation)	May be CVA tenderness Prostate tender to palpation on rectal examination	Examination and culture of prostatic secretions

Meatal Stenosis	Children	Dysuria Recurrent urinary tract infection symptoms			
Urethritis Gonorrheal	Most common in men	Sexually transmitted Urethral discharge is moderate to large, purulent, mucoid, or mucopurulent and develops 1–3 weeks after coitus with infected partner Dysuria (worse at beginning of urine flow)	Sexual contact	Urethral discharge is spontaneous or elicited by penile stripping	Gram stain and culture of urethral smear
Nongonorrheal (chlamydial or trichomonal)	Most common in men	Sexually transmitted Symptoms usually minimal or absent Discharge (if present) is observed on awakening and is thin and clear or whitish Dysuria (ranges in severity) Urgency Frequency	Meatal or urethral irritation Multiple sexual partners	Thin, scanty, and whitish Urethral discharge appears on penile stripping	Gram stain and culture of urethral smear Special test for *Chlamydia* Saline wet mount for *Trichomonas*
Mechanical	Most common in young boys and girls	Dysuria Minimal urethral discharge	Horseback or bike riding Masturbation Foreign body		

Rarely, frequency is an early symptom of a bladder tumor or of carcinoma in situ of the bladder.

Relatively uncommon causes of urethritis include infections with *Mycoplasma hominis*. Urethritis secondary to *Mycoplasma* is most common in lower socioeconomic groups and in men and women who have multiple sexual partners. T mycoplasma have been associated with nongonorrheal urethritis. Another uncommon cause of urethritis is Reiter's syndrome, which frequently begins with a urethritis after sexual contact and is followed in a few days by conjunctivitis, mucocutaneous lesions (including balanitis), and arthritis. Generally, this type of urethritis is characterized by mucopurulent discharge and dysuria, but it may be asymptomatic. Reiter's syndrome sometimes may be initiated by a gonorrheal urethritis. In such cases, the urethritis responds to penicillin so that the purulent discharge disappears and is replaced by the less purulent, mucoid discharge of nonspecific urethritis.

Selected References

Felman, V. M., and Nikitas, J. A.: Nongonococcal urethritis—a clinical review. J.A.M.A. *245*:381–386, 1981.
Graham, J. B.: The female urethral syndrome? Urol. Clin. North Am. *(7)1*:59–62, 1980.
Greydanus, D. E., and McAnarney, E. R.: *Chlamydia trachomatis:* an important sexually transmitted disease in adolescents and young adults. J. Fam. Pract. *10*:611–615, 1980.
Komaroff, A. L., and Friedland, G.: The dysuria–pyuria syndrome. N. Engl. J. Med. *303*:452–453, 1980.
Komaroff, A. L.: Acute dysuria in women. N. Engl. J. Med. *310(6)*:368–374, 1984.
Martin, D. H., Pollock, S., Kuo, C. C., et al.: *Chlamydia trachomatis* infections in men with Reiter's syndrome. Ann. Int. Med. *100*:207–213, 1984.
Meadows, J. C.: The acute urethral syndrome: diagnosis, management, and prophylaxis. Continuing Education, December, 1983, pp. 1112–1129.
Stamm, W. E., et al.: Causes of the acute urethral syndrome in women. N. Engl. J. Med. *303*:409–415, 1980.

30
VAGINAL DISCHARGE AND ITCHING

Vaginal discharge, which may be accompanied by vulvar itching or burning, is one of the commonest problems seen in the physician's office. Usually, these symptoms indicate *moniliasis (Candida albicans), trichomoniasis (Trichomonas),* or *Gardnerella vaginalis (Hemophilus vaginalis).* Other common causes of vaginal discharge include *acute cervicitis, gonorrhea,* and *herpes genitalis.* Many discussions of vaginitis emphasize a "typical" appearance of the discharge: cheesy, frothy, or mucoid. Appearances, however, may be quite misleading. **In addition, 15 to 20 per cent of patients in one series had two coexistent infections.** Other studies of patients with vaginitis have shown that 35 per cent had a *Gardnerella vaginalis,* 25 per cent had moniliasis, and 20 per cent had trichomoniasis. The remaining 20 per cent had less common types of vaginitis.

Vaginitis, in contrast to cervicitis, is an inflammatory change of the vaginal mucosa in the absence of profuse discharge from the cervix. A vaginal discharge can be produced by cervicitis without a significant vaginal infection, as can be the case with *gonorrhea. Chlamydia* also causes a mucopurulent cervicitis.

NATURE OF PATIENT

Prepubertal Patients. Prepubertal girls may develop a vaginal discharge in association with *vulvovaginitis* or an *exocervicitis.* These

335

young girls are particularly susceptible to vulvovaginitis because of the anterior location of the vagina, the proximity of the vagina to the anus, the lack of labial fat pads, a neutral to alkaline vaginal pH, a thin, atrophic vaginal wall, and, occasionally, poor hygiene. *Trichomonas vaginitis* is rare in children and in women over 60 years of age but does occur in newborns of infected mothers. Conversely, *monilial vaginitis* can occur at any age. It is a common cause of vulvovaginitis in children. In prepubertal girls, vulvovaginitis is more common than vaginitis. Vulvovaginitis can be caused by *bubble baths, other chemical irritants, tight nylon panties, mixed bacterial infections,* and *foreign bodies. Gardnerella infections* are rare in premenarchal girls. **Gonorrheal infections in premenarchal children are rare but do occur. In such cases, sexual abuse must be suspected.** Although a girl may be asymptomatic when a gonococcal infection is present, vulvovaginitis and exocervicitis are usually present.

Adolescents. After puberty, a vaginal discharge may be due to physiologic factors, to cervicitis, or to vaginitis. Although *trichomonas vaginitis* and *monilial vaginitis* may occur in adolescents, the commonest cause of vaginitis with discharge in adolescent girls is *Gardnerella.* Adolescents are especially susceptible to *Gardnerella* because the changes in vaginal secretions at menarche provide a favorable environment for the *Gardnerella vaginalis* bacillus to grow. *Monilia* is the second most common cause of specific leukorrhea in adolescents. There is a high and increasing incidence of *gonorrhea* among postpubertal women. Among young mothers, the growing prevalence of gonorrhea may increase the incidence of this infection among neonates and some children. It is important to question the patient about genital or urinary infections in other family members (male or female) or sexual partners (male or female).

It must be remembered that a *physiologic leukorrhea* may occur in menarchal girls. This is not usually profuse or associated with itching. Although these girls may be concerned about a vaginal discharge, they may not present with it as a chief complaint. Therefore, the physician should provide reassurance concerning this and other normal changes that may occur with menarche. The discharge that occurs just before and after menarche is often thick, grayish-white, and odorless, and it has a pH of 4.5 to 6.0. There are no signs of inflammation because this discharge is a physiologic reaction to the initial phase of cyclic estrogen production.

Adults. In adult women of reproductive age, the common causes of vaginitis are *Candida, Gardnerella,* and *Trichomonas,* in decreasing order of frequency. The three most common causes of cervicitis are *Chlamydia trachomatis, Neisseria gonorrhoeae,* and *herpes simplex virus.* In elderly, postmenopausal women, *senile atrophic vaginitis* often causes a discharge, as do other specific forms of vaginitis.

NATURE OF SYMPTOMS

Vulvovaginitis in premenarchal girls usually causes only minor discomfort, which may include perineal pruritis, burning, and a discharge that may be profuse or scanty.

The duration and type of symptoms do not consistently distinguish the common infectious causes of vaginitis. Certain symptoms and findings, however, strongly suggest the diagnosis. For instance, although an acute onset of vaginal discharge or vulvar irritation indicates that a yeast infection is the probable cause, these symptoms are often unreliable. Likewise, a curdlike discharge (resembling cottage cheese) strongly suggests a yeast vaginitis; **however, the gross appearance is less sensitive and less specific in establishing the diagnosis than is a microscopic examination of the vaginal discharge.** A curdlike apearance virtually eliminates the possibility of a trichomonas vaginitis, which usually produces a profuse, frothy, white or grayish-green, malodorous discharge. The discharge in *trichomonas vaginitis* is typically described as frothy, whereas the discharge in *Gardnerella vaginalis (Hemophilus)* may also be frothy in 15 per cent of the cases.

Because itching and burning may occur with virtually all forms of vaginitis, these symptoms are not particularly helpful in the differentiation of the cause. Itching is most prominent in *monilial vaginitis* and least prominent in *Gardnerella*. Itching and burning are uncommon with *gonococcal* infections, but a significant percentage of patients with a gonococcal infection have a combined infection. They may have gonorrhea with their itching caused by *Trichomonas* or *monilia.*

If a vaginal discharge is sticky, brown, or yellowish and occurs in an elderly woman, an *atrophic vaginitis* should be suspected.

ASSOCIATED SYMPTOMS

Dysuria may be a symptom of both a vaginal infection and a urinary tract infection. **Therefore, all women complaining of dysuria should be asked about the presence of a vaginal discharge or irritation or both.** Approximately 30 per cent of patients who have vaginitis but no evidence of urinary tract infection complain of dysuria. Usually, these patients complain of "external" dysuria (pain felt in the inflamed vaginal labia as the urinary stream passes) rather than "internal" dysuria (felt inside the body). Internal dysuria seems to correlate with urinary tract infections, whereas external dysuria usually corresponds to vaginal infections.

Dyspareunia in association with a purulent discharge suggests *acute cervicitis. Trichomonas vaginitis* is often associated with gonococcal or *Bacteroides* cervicitis. *Trichomonas* and *Chlamydia* may produce a vaginitis as well as a coexisting urethritis that causes dysuria and frequency. If dysuria, rectal infections, or pain on walking or climbing stairs is present, *gonorrhea* should be suspected.

If there are symptoms of diabetes or ingestion of birth control pills or antibiotics, a *monilial vaginitis* is probable. Refractory fungal vulvovaginitis may be secondary to undiagnosed diabetes.

PRECIPITATING AND AGGRAVATING FACTORS

Oral contraceptives, antibiotics, and pregnancy predispose the patient to a *Candida vaginitis*. Uncontrolled diabetes and long-term use of tetracycline for acne increase the intestinal reservoir of *Candida,* which predisposes the patient to recurrent monilial vaginitis. *Gardnerella* vaginitis is common and increasing in incidence. It is most frequently spread through venereal contacts. *Trichomonas vaginitis* is usually transmitted by sexual intercourse; in children, however, it may be spread by direct nonsexual contact. The increasing incidence of venereal diseases such as gonorrhea, *Gardnerella,* and trichomoniasis is due to earlier sexual activity, multiple partners, and failure to use protective barrier contraceptives (e.g., diaphragms and condoms).

In young children and in some adults, inappropriate genital hygiene (i.e., wiping the perineal region from back to front) may increase the incidence of recurrent vaginal infections. *Chemical vaginitis* is precipitated by douches, bubble baths, and vaginal sprays. It may be aggravated by powders and panties made of synthetic fibers.

PHYSICAL FINDINGS

Physical examination should include thorough evaluation of the genital and pelvic areas. The appearance of the labia, vulva, entire vagina, and cervix should be noted, and the vaginal discharge should be inspected. Nonspecific vaginitis, which occurs particularly in premenarchal girls, usually does not extend above the lower one third of the vagina. Atrophic vaginitis can occur in premenarchal girls, as can infections due to insertion of foreign bodies into the vagina. When atrophic vaginitis occurs in postmenopausal women, there is often a sticky, brownish vaginal discharge, and the vaginal mucosa is usually thick, pale, and smooth, demonstrating loss of normal rugosal folds. The pelvic examination should include adnexal palpation and cervical manipulation so that the physician can determine whether there are any masses or points of tenderness. Adnexal tenderness and pain on motion of the cervix ("chandelier sign") suggest *pelvic inflammatory disease*—not

Table 30–1. **Classification of Vaginitis**

Type of Vaginitis	Symptom	pH	Wet Smear Findings
Candidiasis (moniliasis)	Pruritis	4.2–4.9	Hyphae or spores
Gardnerella vaginitis	Odor	5.6–6.3	"Clue" cells
Trichomoniasis	Profuse discharge	4.9–5.6	Protozoa and white blood cells
Atrophic vaginitis	Discharge	7	Parabasal cells

merely cervicitis. When these findings occur in conjunction with a vaginal discharge, a *gonococcal* infection is probable. In such cases, if smear and culture are negative for gonorrhea, *Chlamydia* should be suspected and appropriately treated.

DIAGNOSTIC STUDIES

Ninety per cent of patients with vaginitis can be classified into one of four major clinical categories on the basis of symptomatology, vaginal pH, and wet smear findings; the importance of vaginal pH and wet smear findings, therefore, is readily apparent.

In patients whose only symptom of vaginitis is vaginal discharge, a Gram stain is not indicated because it is not specific. However, if a patient has a purulent discharge from the cervical os, a Gram stain that reveals more that three polymorphonuclear leukocytes per high-power field (with typical intracellular gram-negative diplococci) is highly specific for a gonococcal infection. False-positive results are rare. A Gram stain is recommended whenever there is a purulent discharge from the cervical or urethral os. If this discharge is not accompanied by pelvic pain or fever, a gonococcal infection is unlikely.

In some populations in which there is a high prevalence of asymptomatic gonococcal carriers, a cervical culture for *Neisseria gonorrhoeae* on Thayer-Martin medium is considered appropriate whenever a patient has a pelvic examination. It certainly should be performed in any woman with a purulent discharge from the cervical os or urethra.

In all patients with a vaginal discharge, saline and KOH wet mounts should be examined. The saline mount should be inspected for "clue cells" (epithelial cells with bacilli adherent to their surface), which are virtually pathognomonic of *Gardnerella vaginalis*. *Gardnerella vaginalis* may also be diagnosed on the basis of a positive culture in Casman's broth or blood agar. These cultures must be done promptly because the organisms are susceptible to drying and alkaline pH. The pH range of secretions in patients with *Gardnerella* infection is usually 5.6 to 6.3.

DIFFERENTIAL DIAGNOSIS OF VAGINAL DISCHARGE AND ITCHING

CAUSE	NATURE OF PATIENT	NATURE OF SYMPTOMS	ASSOCIATED SYMPTOMS	PRECIPITATING OR AGGRAVATING FACTORS	PHYSICAL FINDINGS	DIAGNOSTIC STUDIES
Vulvovaginitis due to: Candida Chemical irritants Douches Vaginal sprays Bubble baths Bacteria Foreign bodies	Most common cause of vaginal discharge in prepubertal girls	Variable discharge (scanty to profuse) Perineal pruritus Burning	May be "internal" dysuria		Vulvovaginitis does not usually extend above lower third of vagina Thin atrophic vaginal wall	pH of discharge is 4.5–6.0
Physiologic discharge	Menarchal girls	Discharge is thick, grayish-white, odorless, but not profuse No pruritus		Beginning estrogen effect occurs just before or after menarche	No signs of inflammation	
Moniliasis (candidiasis)	Any age Common cause of vulvovaginitis in children Common during reproductive years	Acute onset of discharge or vulvar irritation Discharge is often curdlike (resembles cottage cheese) Pruritus is prominent	May be "external" dysuria	Diabetes Antibiotics Birth control pills Pregnancy	Vaginitis	Saline or KOH wet mount shows hyphae or spores Vaginal pH is 4.2–4.9

Trichomoniasis	Common cause of vaginal discharge in women of childbearing age Rare in children Rare in women over 60 years old May occur in newborns of infected mothers	Discharge is usually profuse, frothy, gray-greenish and malodorous Varying degrees of pruritus	May be associated with gonococcal or *Bacteroides* infection Urethritis may cause dysuria and frequency	Often sexually transmitted Multiple sex partners	Vaginitis Vaginal petechiae Mucosal inflammation	Vaginal pH is 4.9–5.6 Saline wet mount shows WBCs and motile protozoa
Gardnerella vaginalis (*Hemophilus vaginalis*)	Most common cause of vaginitis in adolescents Common during reproductive years Rare in premenarchal girls	Discharge is malodorous but not usually frothy Pruritus not prominent	Urethritis may cause dysuria and frequency	Change in vaginal secretions at menarche Sexually transmitted Multiple sex partners	Vaginitis	Saline wet mount shows "clue" cells Vaginal pH is 5.6–6.3
Gonorrhea	Increased incidence in newborns of infected mothers Rare in premenarchal girls (if present, sexual abuse must be suspected)	Itching/burning uncommon Purulent cervical discharge Pelvic pain Fever	Dysuria Rectal infection (often asymptomatic) Pain on walking or climbing stairs	Symptoms often worse near time of menstrual period Sexually transmitted	Cervicitis and cervical discharge Pain with cervical manipulation Adnexal tenderness	Gram stain of discharge reveals intracellular gram-negative diplococci Positive culture on Thayer-Martin medium
Chlamydia			Dysuria	Sexually transmitted	Cervicitis and cervical discharge Pain with cervical manipulation	Culture for *Neisseria gonorrhoeae* is negative

Table continued on following page

DIFFERENTIAL DIAGNOSIS OF VAGINAL DISCHARGE AND ITCHING *Continued*

CAUSE	NATURE OF PATIENT	NATURE OF SYMPTOMS	ASSOCIATED SYMPTOMS	PRECIPITATING OR AGGRAVATING FACTORS	PHYSICAL FINDINGS	DIAGNOSTIC STUDIES
Herpes genitalis	Most commonly sexually active adolescents Less frequently patients over 35 years	Pain can be excruciating Vulvar pruritus uncommon Burning Vulvar tenderness	Dyspareunia Dysuria	Secondary *Streptococcus* or *Candida* infection	Cervicitis Widespread clusters of vesicles over vulvar and perineal areas, vagina, and cervix Herpetic lesions: Affect vulva and adjacent areas Begin as vesicles Progress in 5–10 days to shallow, painful ulcers Ulcers last 3–10 days Recurrent Does not usually produce vaginitis	Tzanck smear
Senile atrophic vaginitis	Elderly women	Discharge is sticky, brown, or yellowish		Loss of estrogen effect	Vaginal mucosa is thin, pale, and smooth (owing to loss of rugosal folds)	Vaginal pH is 7.0 Parabasal cells

The saline wet mount is the most reliable laboratory test for confirmation of the motile protozoan *Trichomonas*. It should be done as soon as possible after the specimen is obtained. The pH of the vaginal secretions in patients with *Trichomonas* infection ranges from 4.9 to 5.6.

The most accurate test for detection of *monilial* vaginitis is microscopic examination of the discharge in a KOH preparation; this will show the *Candida* mycelia. The pH in patients with monilial vaginitis ranges from 4.2 to 4.9.

LESS COMMON DIAGNOSTIC CONSIDERATIONS

Dermatoses (e.g., psoriasis and seborrheic dermatitis) and infestations with parasites (e.g., pinworms and lice) can cause vaginal discharge in rare cases. Vaginal and cervical neoplasms can cause a serosanguinous discharge. Poor anal and vulvar hygiene also may produce vaginal discharge and itching. Tuberculosis is a rare cause of vulvovaginitis. In premenarchal girls, particularly young children, coliform bacterial infections may produce vaginitis. This is usually a low-grade, somewhat chronic infection and may be associated with pinworm infestation or insertion of foreign body into the vagina.

Herpes simplex type II, herpes genitalis, is a relatively uncommon cause of vaginal discharge (although a common cause of cervicitis), but it is increasing in frequency. It is certainly receiving much attention from the media and the public. It is most common in adolescents and appears less frequently in patients over the age of 35 years. Herpetic lesions, which can be excruciating, affect not only the vulva but also adjacent areas (thighs, buttocks, vagina, and cervix). The lesions begin as vesicles that progress in 5 to 10 days to shallow, exquisitely painful ulcerations with a clear watery discharge. The ulcers last 3 to 10 days and are prone to secondary infections, especially with *Streptococcus* and *Candida*. Unfortunately, genital herpes is often recurrent; some patients experience repeated flare-ups for many years. The presenting symptoms may include pain, vulvar pruritus, burning, and frequently extreme vulvar tenderness that makes intercourse unbearable. Micturition also may be excrutiating. Examination reveals widespread clusters of vesicles that may involve the vulvar and perineal areas as well as the vagina and cervix. It is important for the physician to remember that herpes does not usually produce vaginitis, although it may infect the vagina and cervix. A Tzanck smear of the base of the vesicle is a simple, definitive diagnostic test.

Selected References

Adler, M. W.: ABC of sexually transmitted diseases. Vaginal discharge: diagnosis. Br. Med. J. *287*(6404):1529–1531, 1983.

Friedrich, E. G.: Vaginitis. Am. Fam. Phys. *28*:238–242, 1983.

Hard, J. K.: Vaginitis. Med. Clin. North Am. *63*:423–432, 1979.

McCue, J. D., et al.: Strategies for diagnosing vaginitis. J. Fam. Pract. *9*:395–402, 1979.

Schneider, G. T.: Vaginal infections. How to identify and treat them. Postgrad. Med. *73*:255–262, 1983.

Singleton, A. E.: Vaginal discharge in children and adolescents—evolution and management: a review. Clin. Pediatr. *19*:799–804, 1980.

Woodruff, J. D.: Vulvar disease. A spectrum of clinical pictures. Postgrad. Med. *73*:232–245, 1983.

31
WEIGHT GAIN

Without doubt, the commonest cause of weight gain is *increased caloric intake*, regardless of what the patient states. Weight gain due to *fluid retention* occurs in patients with the nephrotic syndrome, congestive heart failure, or cirrhosis with ascites; in these patients, there are clear signs of edema. *Hypothyroidism* can lead to decreased metabolic needs and to weight gain, but, for significant weight gain to occur, hypothyroidism must be pronounced, and it is usually clinically apparent. *Physiologic weight gain* occurs as a result of pregnancy and premenstrual fluid retention. Commonly prescribed *drugs* (e.g., steroids and antidepressants) can cause weight gain by promoting salt and water retention or by stimulating appetite.

NATURE OF PATIENT

Although the most common type of obesity in children is *exogenous*, this diagnosis requires that endocrine and genetic causes of obesity be considered. Children with exogenous obesity often show accelerated or at least normal linear growth and may reach puberty early. **Most children with endogenous obesity are short for their age and generally have other associated abnormalities. All obese children with short stature should be evaluated promptly and carefully.**

There are no particularly distinguishing characteristics of patients who are obese other than excessive weight. Although it is said that fat people are "jolly," they may experience *depression*, which can be either the result of their being overweight or the cause of their overeating. There are rare instances of *familial obesity;* in most instances, however,

345

this probably represents an acquired propensity to overeat. In cases of familial obesity, various members of the family are short and obese. Their obesity tends to be proximal but can have a generalized distribution.

Weight increase in patients with *edema syndromes* (cirrhosis, nephrosis, and congestive heart failure) usually is accompanied by symptoms that suggest a deteriorating clinical status.

NATURE OF SYMPTOMS

Patients may present complaining of weight gain, uncontrollable appetite, inability to diet, or too-tight garments. The weight gain associated with fluid retention in the *premenstrual period* usually is described as "bloating" and often is accompanied by breast tenderness, breast-swelling, or finger-swelling. Some patients with *hypothyroidism* comment that their skin seems puffy or that they are unable to lose weight on diets that previously had resulted in weight loss.

ASSOCIATED SYMPTOMS AND AMELIORATING FACTORS

Sudden, marked changes in weight that occur over 1 to 2 days usually are related to changes in fluid balance. Changes may range from a few pounds gained because of *premenstrual edema* or *salt-retaining drugs* to many pounds added as the result of *cyclic edema*. The weight gain of premenstrual edema usually dissipates after menstruation. Patients usually can alleviate fluid retention that occurs with *cyclic edema* by maintaining a recumbent posture for 48 to 72 hours. The weight gain caused by salt-retaining *drugs* is not continuously progressive; it levels off after a weight increase of several pounds. When weight gain is progressive and the patient appears to be obese without evidence of edema, it is reasonably certain that the patient's weight gain is due to *overeating*.

PRECIPITATING AND AGGRAVATING FACTORS

Weight gain results from ingestion of more calories than are metabolized. Thus, although weight gain usually is related to increased caloric intake, it also can be produced by reduction of either physical activity or metabolic rate. These weight changes occur gradually.

Although most people eat less when they are tense or upset, 15 to 25 per cent respond to stress with increased caloric intake, or *reactive hyperphagia*. These patients are often overweight. They eat excessively when they are depressed or anxious and likewise celebrate good times with elaborate meals.

Drug ingestion is an important factor in weight gain. Steroids, nonsteroidal anti-inflammatory agents, phenylbutazone, and lithium all may cause fluid retention and produce a weight gain of several pounds. Birth control pills increase weight by causing fluid retention, increasing appetite, and creating an anabolic effect. Psychotropic agents (e.g., tricyclic antidepressants, some phenothiazines, and some other antipsychotics) may produce a "carbohydrate craving" in patients taking these drugs. In addition, when antidepressant drugs alleviate the anorexia of depression, a pronounced weight gain may occur. Propranolol may cause weight gain through its induction of hypoglycemia.

PHYSICAL FINDINGS

In obese patients adipose tissue is usually generally distributed, but it occasionally is proximally concentrated in the extremities. Proximal obesity associated with a "buffalo hump," hirsutism, hypertension, or diabetes suggests *Cushing's disease*. Marked weight gain due to *edema* usually is associated with pitting edema of the legs, ascites, gallop rhythm or, in the nephrotic syndrome, swelling of the eyelids and facial edema. The physical findings of *hypothyroidism* may include somewhat coarse, dry skin; coarse hair; loss of the outer third of the eyebrows; a low, hoarse voice; an enlarged thyroid; and "hung-up" ankle jerks (delayed contraction and relaxation phase of deep tendon reflexes). The "hung-up" ankle jerk is often more readily detected when the patient kneels on a bed, chair, or examining table with his feet extended over the edge. Tapping the Achilles tendon with a reflex hammer may show a prompt contraction phase but a more readily perceived slowed relaxation phase.

DIAGNOSTIC STUDIES

Although hypothyroidism is an uncommon cause of obesity, it is readily diagnosed by thyroid function tests.

LESS COMMON DIAGNOSTIC CONSIDERATIONS

Endogenous causes of obesity are rare but usually can be diagnosed by other associated findings. Several causes are associated with short stature. Pseudohypoparathyroidism is characterized by short stature,

DIFFERENTIAL DIAGNOSIS OF WEIGHT GAIN

CAUSE	NATURE OF PATIENT	NATURE OF SYMPTOMS	ASSOCIATED SYMPTOMS	PRECIPITAT-ING FACTORS	AMELIORAT-ING FACTORS	PHYSICAL FINDINGS
Physiologic Factors Pregnancy	Females of reproductive age					
Premenstrual fluid retention	Menstruating females	Premenstrual weight gain	Breast tenderness and breast-swelling Finger-swelling	End of menstrual cycle	End of menstruation	
Excessive Ca-loric Intake (most common cause of weight gain)	Patients who over-eat	Gradual, pro-gressive weight in-crease	Children Show normal linear growth May reach pu-berty early Adults Show depression or psychologic dependency on food	Increased stress ("reactive hy-perphagia")	Decreased caloric intake and/or in-creased caloric needs	No evidence of edema Obesity is gener-ally distributed (may have proxi-mal concentra-tion)
Drugs	Users of: Steroids Nonsteroidal anti-inflam-matory agents				Cessation of drug	

Phenylbutazone Lithium Antipsychotics Antidepressants Propanolol Birth control pills			
Edema Syndromes Nephrotic syndrome Congestive heart failure Cirrhosis (with ascites)	Weight increase may be sudden and rapid (over 24–48 hours)	Edema Signs of deteriorating clinical status Signs of primary condition	Depends on primary disease Edema (may be pitting in legs) Periorbital edema Gallop rhythm Ascites
Metabolic Causes Hypothyroidism	Patient unable to lose weight on previously successful plan	Constipation Intolerance of cold weather Skin is puffy, coarse, and dry	Enlarged thyroid "Hung-up" ankle jerk Coarse hair Loss of outer one third of eyebrows Low, hoarse voice
Cushing's disease	Proximal obesity	Diabetes Proximal obesity	"Buffalo hump" Hirsutism Hypertension

short metacarpals, hypocalcemia, and occasionally mental retardation. The Prader-Willi syndrome is characterized by short stature, mental retardation, and hypogenitalism. The Laurence-Moon-Biedl syndrome is characterized by short stature, mental retardation, hypogonadism, and retinal pigmentation.

Other rare causes of obesity that are not particularly associated with short stature include Cushing's syndrome and insulinomas. Patients with insulinomas invariably have symptoms of hypoglycemia. Patients with hypothalamic tumors may present with obesity, but there usually are other findings suggestive of an intracranial tumor. Cyclic edema is more common in women than in men. Postencephalitic obesity, tumors of the third ventricle, obesity that develops after cerebral trauma, and certain brain tumors (e.g., chromophobe adenomas and craniopharyngiomas) are other rare causes of hyperphagia.

Selected References

Acherman, S.: The management of obesity. Hospital Practice, March, 1983, pp. 117–139.

Hart, F. D. (Ed.): French's Index of Differential Diagnosis. 11th ed. Chicago: Distributed by Year Book Medical Publishers, 1979, pp. 579–586.

Kalucy, R. S.: Drug induced weight gain. Drugs 19:278–288, 1980.

Richmond, D. A., Blyer, E. M., and Linscheid, T. R.: The obese child. Am. Fam. Phys. 28:129–134, 1983.

INDEX

Note: Page numbers in *italics* indicate illustrations; those followed by (t) indicate tables.

Diarrhea *(Continued)*
  diagnostic studies in, 100, 102(t)–105(t)
  differential diagnosis of, 102(t)–105(t)
  drug-induced, 99, 103(t)
  functional, 96, 97, 99, 105(t)
  in children, 95–96, 101–106
    and abdominal pain, 22
    chronic, 101–106
  in colorectal carcinoma, 101
  in diabetes mellitus, 96, 100, 105(t)
  in fecal impaction, 101
  in gastroenteritis, 95–98, 100, 102(t)
  in giardiasis, 96, 97, 98, 100, 105(t)
  in inflammatory bowel disease, 101, 104(t)
  in irritable colon, 96, 97, 105(t)
  in lactose intolerance, 96, 98, 99, 100,
    105(t)
  in malabsorption, 101
  in obstipation, 101
  in pseudomembranous enterocolitis, 99,
    103(t)
  in ulcerative colitis, 98
  less common causes of, 100–102
  patient type in, 95–96, 102(t)–105(t)
  physical findings in, 99, 102(t)–105(t)
  precipitating and aggravating factors in,
    99, 102(t)–105(t)
  rotavirus, 96, 102(t)
  Salmonella, 96, 98, 100, 102(t)
  Shigella, 96, 98, 100, 102(t)
  small bowel, 97–98, 104(t)
  staphylococcal, 98, 104(t)
  symptoms in, 97, 102(t)–105(t)
  traveler's, 99
Diethylstilbestrol (DES) daughters, 200
Digitalis, and arrhythmias, 273, 274(t)
  and vomiting, 219, 223(t)
Disc disease, 30, 31(t), 42(t)
  as surgical emergency, 33, 38
  backache in, amelioration of, 34
    associated symptoms in, 33
    nature of pain in, 32
    physical findings in, 36
  lumbar, leg pain in, 237, 240, 242, 246(t)
Dislocation, of radial head, 263, 267(t)
  of shoulder, 257, 259
Diverticular disease, abdominal pain in,
    14(t)
  location of, 6, 7, 8
  patient types in, 4
  physical findings in, 12
  bloating and flatulence in, 49, 50
Dizziness, 107, 110–116, 114(t)–115(t). See
  also *Vertigo.*
Duodenal ulcer, pain in, location of, 5, *6*
Dupuytren's contracture, 263, 267(t)
Dysentery syndrome, 97–98, 104(t)
Dysfunctional uterine bleeding, 197–198,
    206(t)
  and estrogen preparations, 198
  and foreign bodies, 193, 203(t)

Dysfunctional uterine bleeding *(Continued)*
  and intrauterine devices, 206(t)
  and uterine fibroids, 196, 197, 206(t)
  anovulatory, 198–199
    vs. dysfunctional ovulatory bleeding,
      192(t)
  associated symptoms in, 198, 204(t)–207(t)
  diagnostic studies in, 199–200,
    204(t)–207(t)
  differential diagnosis of, 204(t)–207(t)
  during menstrual life, 196–198, 199(t)
  estrogen-breakthrough, 190–191, 195,
    204(t)
  estrogen-withdrawal, 190, 193–195, 204(t)
  in bleeding disorders, 200
  in cancer, 196, 198, 200, 206(t)
  in ectopic pregnancy, 195–196, 199–200,
    205(t)
  in endocrinopathies, 199
  in endometriosis, 106, 200, 206(t)
  in neonate, 198
  in pregnancy, 195, 198, 205(t)
  in salpingitis, 196, 206(t)
  in spontaneous abortion, 198, 205(t)
  less common causes of, 200
  ovulatory, 191, 192(t), 198, 205(t)
  patterns of, 191, 192(t)
  physical findings in, 199, 204(t)–207(t)
  post-menopausal, 198
  precipitating factors in, 198–199,
    204(t)–207(t)
  prepubertal, 198
  progesterone-breakthrough, 191, 204(t)
  progesterone-withdrawal, 191, 204(t)
  symptoms of, 195–196, 204(t)–207(t)
Dysmenorrhea, 209–215
  ameliorating factors in, 212(t)–213(t), 214
  and cervical stenosis or occlusion, 210
  and emotional stress, 214
  and intrauterine devices, 210, 214
  and intrauterine synechiae, 210
  and uterine fibroids, 211, 213(t)
  and uterine retroversion, 214
  associated symptoms in, 211, 212(t)–213(t)
  diagnostic studies in, 212(t)–213(t), 215
  differential diagnosis of, 212(t)–213(t)
  in adenomyosis, 211
  in pelvic inflammatory disease, 211, 213(t)
  nature of pain in, 210–211, 212(t)–213(t)
  patient type in, 210, 212(t)
  physical findings in, 212(t)–213(t), 214
  precipitating and aggravating factors in,
    212(t)–213(t), 214
  primary, causes of, 210, 212(t)
    defined, 209
    with superimposed secondary
      dysmenorrhea, 211
  secondary, causes of, 210, 213(t)
    defined, 209–210
  symptoms of, 210–211, 212(t)–213(t)